DRUG COMPARISON HANDBOOK

Third Edition

Robert Reilly, Pharm. D.

Skidmore-Roth Publishing, Inc.

SR
PUBLISHING

Developmental Editor: Molly Sullivan, B.A.
Copy Editor: Kathryn Head, B.A.
Cover Design: Martha A. Romero
Typesetting: Jeannine Parker, Affiliated Executive Systems

Notice: The author and the publisher of this volume have taken care to make certain that all information is correct and compatible with the standards generally accepted at the time of publication. Because technology is constantly changing and expanding, new techniques and concepts are continually implemented. Therefore, the reader is encouraged to stay abreast of new drug developments and to be aware that policies vary according to the guidelines of each school or institution.

Reilly, Robert
The Drug Comparison Handbook/Reilly, Robert
Third Edition

ISBN 1-56930-075-5
1. Nursing — nurses' instruction.
2. Nursing — patient care planning.

SKIDMORE-ROTH PUBLISHING, INC.
400 Inverness Drive South, Suite 260
Englewood, Colorado 80112
1-800-825-3150
Fax 303-662-8079
web site: www.skidmore-roth.com

PREFACE

The third edition of *The Drug Comparison Handbook* has been updated to provide a quick reference for the generic or brand name of a drug.

Often, physicians order medications by the generic name, or pharmacists fill orders by the generic name. Because generic names are generally long chemical names, they are more difficult to memorize than brand names. Therefore, this uncomplicated, quick reference will give the reader either the generic or brand name as quickly as he or she can look it up alphabetically.

In the first section, generic names are listed alphabetically along with a complete list of the brand names. Then, in the second section, the brand names are listed alphabetically with the corresponding generic names. New to this edition are pertinent investigational drugs and orphan drugs.

It is hoped that this will be an important reference for the nurse who wishes to find the names of drugs without having to wade through a great deal of other information. The third edition of *The Drug Comparison Handbook* will provide the nurse with information essential to preventing medication errors in an easy-to-use format.

CONTENTS

Section I — Generic to Brand

Section II — Brand to Generic

Section I — Generic to Brand

GENERIC NAME	BRAND NAME

2-chlorodeoxyadenosine
Classification:
Antineoplastic (Orphan)

2-Chlorodeoxyadenosine

2-O-desulfated heparin
Classification:
Anticoagulant (Orphan)

Aeropin

3,4-diaminopyridine
Classification:
Anti-myasthenia agent (Orphan)

3,4-diaminopyridine

4-aminosalicylic acid
Classification:
Anti-inflammatory (Orphan)

Pamisyl
Rezipas

5,6-dihydro-5-azacytidine
Classification:
Antineoplastic (Orphan)

5,6-dihydro-5-azacytidine

5-aza-2 deoxycitidine
Classification:
Antineoplastic (Orphan)

5-aza-2 deoxycitidine

9-[3-pyridylmethyl]-9-deazaguanine
Classification:
Antineoplastic (Orphan)

9-[3-pyridylmethyl]-9-deazaguanine

9-cis retinoic acid
Classification:
Antineoplastic (Orphan)

9-cis retinoic acid

24,25-diphydroxycholecalciferol
Classification:
Vitamin, fat soluble (Orphan)

24,25-dihydroxydcholecalciferol

A

ABCIXIMAB
Classification:
Antiplatelet

ReoPro

absorbable gelatin
Classification:
Hemostatic

Gelfilm
Gelfilm Ophthalmic
Gelfoam

GENERIC NAME	BRAND NAME

acarbose
Classification:
Antidiabetic

Precose
Prandase*

acebutolol HCl
Classification:
Beta-adrenergic blocker

Acebutolol HCl
Monitan*
Sectral

acemannan
Classification:
Antiviral (Investigational)

Carrisyn

acetaminophen
Classification:
Analgesic, antipyretic

Abenol 120 mg*
Abenol 325 mg*
Abenol 650 mg*
Acephen
Acetaminophen
Acetaminophen Uniserts
Aceta
Apacet
Arthritis Foundation Pain Reliever
    Aspirin Free
Aspirin Free Anacin Maximum Strength
Aspirin Free Pain Relief
Atasol*
Campain*
Children's Dynafed Jr.
Children's Feverall
Dapacin
Extra Strength Dynafed E.X.
Fem-Etts
Feverall, Infants
Genapap
Genapap Children's
Genapap Extra Strength
Genapap Infant's Drops
Genebs
Genebs Extra Strength
Halenol Children's
Junior Strength Feverall
Liquiprin Drops for Children
Maranox
Mapap Children's
Mapap Extra Strength
Mapap Infant Drops
Mapap Regular Strength
Meda Cap

GENERIC NAME	BRAND NAME

acetaminophen
(cont'd)

Meda Tab
Neopap
Oraphen-PD
Panadol
Panadol Children's
Panadol Infant's Drops
Panadol Junior Strength
Redutemp
Ridenol
Robigesic*
Rounax*
Silipap Children's
Silipap Infants
Tapanol Extra Strength
Tapanol Regular Strength
Tempra
Tempra 2 Syrup
Tempra 3
Tempral
Tylenol
Tylenol Caplets
Tylenol Chewable
Tylenol Children's
Tylenol Children's Suspension*
Tylenol Extended Relief
Tylenol Extra Strength
Tylenol Infant's Drops
Tylenol Infant's Suspension*
Tylenol Junior Strength
Uni-Ace

acetaminophen, buffered
Classification:
Analgesic; antipyretic

Bromo Seltzer

acetazolamide
Classification:
Diuretic, carbonic anhydrase inhibitor

Acetazolamide
Dazamide
Diamox
Diamox Sequel

acetazolamide sodium
Classification:
Diuretic, carbonic anhydrase inhibitor

Diamox Parenteral

acetohexamide
Classification:
Antidiabetic; sulfonylurea

Acetohexamide
Dimelor*
Dymelor

*Available in Canada Only

GENERIC NAME	BRAND NAME
acetohydroxamic acid (AHA) Classification: Urinary urease inhibitor	Lithostat
acetorphan Classification: Antidiarrheal (Investigational)	Acetorphan
acetylcarbromal Classification: Sedative-hypnotic, non-barbiturate	Paxarel
acetylcholine chloride, intraocular Classification: Miotic	Miochol-E
acetylcysteine Classification: Mucolytic	Acetylcysteine Airbron* Mucomyst Mucosil-10 Mucosil-20
acetylcysteine Classification: Biologic response modifier (Investigational)	Fluimucil
acetylcysteine, intravenous Classification: Mucolytic (Orphan)	Mucomyst 10 IV
acitretin Classification: Antipsoriatic	Soriatane
aconiazide Classification: Antitubercular (Orphan)	Aconiazide
acyclovir Classification: Antiviral	Acyclovir Zovirax
acyclovir sodium Classification: Antiviral	Acyclovir Sodium Zovirax

GENERIC NAME	BRAND NAME

AD-439
Classification:
Antiviral (Investigational)

AD-439

AD-519
Classification:
Antiviral (Investigational)

AD-519

ADCI
Classification:
Anticonvulsant (Investigational)

ADCI

adapalene
Classification:
Anti-acne product

Differin

adefovir dipivoxil
Classification:
Antiviral (Investigational)

Adefovir Dipivoxil

adenosine
Classification:
Antiarrhythmic

Adenocard

adenosine
Classification:
In vivo diagnostic aid

Adenoscan

adenosine phosphate (A_5MP)
Classification:
Nucleoside

Adenosine Phosphate

aerosol talc (sterile)
Classification:
Sclerosing agent (Orpahn)

Aerosol Talc

AIDS vaccine
Classification:
Vaccine (Investigational)

VaxSyn HIV-1

AL-721
Classification:
Antiviral (Investigational)

AL-721

alatrofloxacin mesylate
Classification:
Antibiotic, fluoroquinolone

Trovan I.V.

GENERIC NAME	BRAND NAME
albendazole Classification: Anthelmintics	Albenza
albumin human 5% Classification: Blood derivative	Albuminar-5 Albunex Albutein 5% Buminate 5% Plasbumin-5
albumin human 25% Classification: Blood derivative	Albuminar-25 Albutein-25% Buminate 25% Plasbumin-25
albuterol sulfate Classification: Bronchodilator; beta-adrenergic agonist	Albuterol Airet Proventil Proventil HFA Proventil Repetabs Salbutamol* Ventolin Ventolin Nebules Ventolin Rotacaps Volmax
alclometasone dipropionate Classification: Glucocorticoid	Aclovate
aldesleukin (interleukin-2, IL-2) Classification: Antineoplastic; biologic response modifier	Proleukin
alendronate sodium Classification: Bone resorption inhibitor	Fosamax
alfentanil HCl Classification: Opioid analgesic	Alfenta
alglucerase Classification: Enzyme	Ceredase
allopurinol Classification: Uricosuric	Allopurinol Apoallopurinol* Lopurin

*Available in Canada only

GENERIC NAME	BRAND NAME

**allopurinol
(cont'd.)**

Novapurol*
Purimol*
Zyloprim

alpha-1-antitrypsin (human)
Classification:
Enzyme replacement (Orphan)

Alpha-1-antitrypsin

**alpha-1-proteinase inhibitor
(human)**
Classification:
Enzyme replacement

Prolastin

alpha-d-galactosidase enzyme
Classification:
Food modifier

Beano

alpha-galactosidase A
Classification:
Enzyme replacement (Orphan)

Fabrase

alprazolam
Classification:
Antianxiety; benzodiazepine

Alprazolam
Alprozolam Intensol
Xanax

alprostadil (PGE$_1$)
Classification:
Prostaglandin

Caverject
Edex
Muse
Prostin VR Pediatric

alteplase, recombinant
Classification:
Antithrombotic

Activase

**altretamine
(hexamethylmelamine)**
Classification:
Antineoplastic, miscellaneous

Hexalen

aluminum acetate solution
Classification:
Astringent

Bluboro Powder
Boropak Powder
Burow's Solution
Domeboro
Modified Burow's Solution
Pedi-boro Soak Paks

aluminum carbonate gel
Classification:
Antacid

Basaljel

GENERIC NAME	BRAND NAME

aluminum chloride hexahydrate
Classification:
Antihyperhydrosis agent

Drysol

aluminum hydroxide gel
Classification:
Antacid

Alternagel
Alu-Cap
Aluminum Hydroxide
Aluminum Hydroxide Gel
Alu-Tab
Amphojel
Basaljel*
Concentrated Aluminum Hydroxide
Dialume

alvircept sudotox
Classification:
Antiviral (Investigational)

Alvircept Sudotox

amantadine HCl
Classification:
Antiviral; antiparkinson agent

Amantadine HCl
Symmetrel

ambenonium chloride
Classification:
Anticholinesterase

Mytelase

amcinonide
Classification:
Glucocorticoid

Cyclocort

amifostine
Classification:
Antineoplastic adjuvant; cytoprotective

Ethyol

amikacin sulfate
Classification:
Aminoglycoside

Amikacin
Amikin

amiloride HCl
Classification:
Potassium-sparing diuretic

Midamor

amino acid solution
Classification:
Nitrogen product

Aminosyn
Aminosyn II
Aminosyn-PF
FreAmine III
Novamine
ProcalAmine
Travasol
TrophAmine

*Available in Canada only

GENERIC NAME	BRAND NAME

amino acid solution, hepatic
Classification:
Nitrogen product

HepatAmine

amino acid solution, renal
Classification:
Nitrogen product

Aminess
Aminosyn-RF
NephrAmine
RenAmin

amino acid solution, stress
Classification:
Nitrogen product

Aminosyn-HBC
BranchAmin
FreAmine HBC

aminocaproic acid
Classification:
Hemostatic

Amicar
Aminocaproic Acid

aminoglutethimide
Classification:
Adrenal steroid inhibitor

Cytadren

aminohippurate sodium (PAH)
Classification:
In vivo diagnostic

Aminohippurate Sodium

aminophylline (theophylline ethylenediamine)
Classification:
Bronchodilator; xanthine

Aminophylline
Corophyllin*
Phyllocontin
Truphylline

aminosalicylate sodium
Classification:
Anti-inflammatory (Orphan)

Aminosalicylate Sodium

aminosalicylic acid
Classification:
Antitubercular

Paser

aminosidine
Classification:
Antitubercular (Orphan)

Gabbromicina
Paromomycin

amiodarone HCl
Classification:
Antiarrhythmic

Cordarone

amitriptyline HCl
Classification:
Antidepressant, tricyclic

Amitriptyline HCl
Apo-Amitriptyline*
Elavil

*Available in Canada Only

GENERIC NAME	BRAND NAME

amitriptyline HCl (cont'd.)

Enovil
Levate*
Meravil*
Novotriptyn*
Rolavil*

amlexanox
Classification:
Anti-inflammatory

Aphthasol

amlodipine
Classification:
Calcium channel blocker

Norvasc

ammonium chloride
Classification:
Acidifier

Ammonia Chloride

ammoniated mercury
Classification:
Antipsoriatic

Emersal

amobarbital/amobarbital sodium
Classification:
Sedative-hypnotic; barbiturate

Amytal Sodium

amoxapine
Classification:
Antidepressant, tricyclic

Amoxapine
Asendin

amoxicillin and potassium clavulanate
Classification:
Antibiotic; aminopenicillin

Augmentin
Clavulin*

amoxicillin trihydrate
Classification:
antibiotic; aminopenicillin

Amoxican*
Amoxicillin
Amoxil
Amoxil Pediatric Drops
Apo-Amoxi*
Biomox
Novamoxin*
Polymox
Polymox Drops
Trimox 125
Trimox 250
Trimox 500
Wymox

GENERIC NAME	BRAND NAME
amphetamine sulfate Classification: Cerebral stimulant	Amphetamine Sulfate
amphotericin B Classification: Antifungal	Amphotericin B Fungizone* Fungizone Intravenous Fungizone Oral
amphotericin B, cholesteryl Classification: Antifungal	Amphotec
amphotericin B, liposomal Classification: Antifungal	Abelcet AmBisome
amphotericin B, topical Classification: Antifungal	Fungizone
ampicillin, oral Classification: Antibiotic; aminopenicillin	Ampicillin Marcillin Omnipen Polycillin Polycillin Pediatric Drops Principen Totacillin
ampicillin sodium, parenteral Classification: Antibiotic; aminopenicillin	Ampicillin Sodium Omnipen-N Polycillin-N Totacillin-N
ampicillin sodium and sulbactam sodium Classification: Antibiotic; aminopenicillin	Unasyn
ampicillin with probenecid Classification: Antibiotic; aminopenicillin	Polycillin-PRB Probampacin
ampligen Classification: Biologic response modifier (Investigational)	Ampligen

GENERIC NAME	BRAND NAME

amrinone lactate
Classification:
Cardiac inotropic agent

Inocor

amsacrine
Classification:
Antineoplastic (Investigational)

Amsacrine

amyl nitrite
Classification:
Antianginal

Amyl Nitrite
Amyl Nitrite Aspirols
Amyl Nitrite Vaporole

anagrelide HCl
Classification:
Antiplatelet

Agrylin

ananain
Classification:
Enzyme (Orphan)

Vianain

anaritide acetate
Classification:
Renal allograft function (Orphan)

Auriculin

anastrazole
Classification:
Antineoplastic; hormone

Arimidex

ancrod
Classification:
Antithrombotic (Orphan)

Arvin

anisindione
Classification:
Anticoagulant

Miradon

anisotropine methylbromide
Classification:
Anticholinergic

Anisotropine Methylbromide

anistreplase (APSAC)
Classification:
Thrombolytic enzyme

Eminase

anthralin (dithranol)
Classification:
Antipsoriatic

Anthra-Derm
Drithocreme
Drithocreme HP 1%
Dritho-Scalp
Micanol

GENERIC NAME	BRAND NAME

antiepilepsirine
Classification:
Anticonvulsant (Orphan)

Antiepilepsirine

antihemophilic factor (AHF, factor VIII)
Classification:
Hemostatic

Antihemophilic Factor (Porcine)
   Hyate:C
Bioclate
Hemofil M
Helixate
Humate-P
Koāte HP
Kogenate
Kryobulin VH*
Monoclate-P
Recombinate

anti-inhibitor coagulant complex
Classification:
Hemostatic

Autoplex T
Feiba VH Immuno

antithrombin III, human
Classification:
Antithrombin

ATnativ
Thrombate III

antithrombin III concentrate, intravenous
Classification:
Anithrombin (Orphan)

Kybernin

anti-thymocyte serum
Classification:
Immunosuppressive (Orphan)

Anti-thymocyte Serum

antivenin (crotalidae) polyvalent
Classification:
Antivenin

Antivenin (Crotalidae) Polyvalent

antivenin (crotalidae) purified (avian)
Classification:
Antivenin (Orphan)

Antivenin (crotalidae) Purified (avian)

antivenin (micrurus fulvius)
Classification:
Antivenin

Antivenin (Micrurus Fulvius)

*Available in Canada Only

GENERIC NAME	BRAND NAME

antivenin, polyvalent crotalid
Classification:
Antivenin (Orphan)

CroTab

APL 400-200
Classification:
Antineoplastic (Orphan)

APL 400-200

apomorphine HCl
Classification:
Antiparkinson agent (Orphan)

Apomorphine HCl

apraclonidine HCl
Classification:
Adrenergic agonist

Iopidine

aprobarbital
Classification:
Sedative-hypnotic; barbiturate

Alurate

aprotinin
Classification:
Hemostatic

Trasylol

AR-121
Classification:
Antifungal (Investigational)

Nystatin-LF I.V.

AR177
Classification:
Antiviral (Investigational)

AR177

arbutamine
Classification:
In vivo diagnostic

GenESA

arcitumomab
Classification:
In vivo diagnostic (Orphan)

Arcitumomab

arcitumomab-Tc99m sodium pertechnetatein
Classification:
In vivo diagnostic

CEA-Scan

ardeparin sodium
Classification:
Anticoagulant

Normiflo

GENERIC NAME	BRAND NAME

arginine butyrate
Classification:
Blood modifier (Orphan)

Argine Butyrate

arginine HCl
Classification:
Pituitary function test

R-Gene 10

arnica
Classification:
Irritant

Arnica Tincture

aromatic ammonia spirit
Classification:
Ammonia inhalant

Aromatic Ammonia
Aromatic Ammonia Aspirols
Aromatic Ammonia Spirit
Aromatic Ammonia Vaporole

artificial tear insert
Classification:
Ophthalmic lubricant

Lacrisert

artificial tears solution
Classification:
Ophthalmic lubricant

Adsorbotear
Akwa Tears
AquaSite
Artificial Tears Plus
Artificial Tears Solution
Bion Tears
Cellufresh
Celluvisc
Comfort Tears
Dakrina
Dry Eyes
Dry Eye Therapy
Dwelle
Eye-Lube-A
HypoTears
HypoTears PF
Isopto Alkaline
Isopto Plain
Isopto Tears
Just Tears
Lacril
Liquifilm Forte
Liquifilm Tears
LubriTears
Moisture Drops
Murine
Murocel

GENERIC NAME	BRAND NAME
artificial tears solution (cont'd.)	Nature's Tears Nu-Tears Nu-Tears II OcuCoat OcuCoat PF Puralube Tears Refresh Tear Drop TearGard Teargen Tearisol Tears Naturale Tears Naturale II Tears Naturale Free Tears Plus Tears Renewed Ultra Tears Viva-Drops
AS-101 Classification: Biologic response modifier (Investigational)	AS-101
ascorbic acid (vitamin C) Classification: Vitamin, water soluble	Ascorbic Acid Ascorbicap Cecon Cenolate Cetane Cevalin Cevi-Bid Ce-Vi-Sol Cebid Timecelles Dull-C Flavorcee N'ice Vitamin C Drops Redoxon* Sunkist Vitamin C Vita-C
asparaginase Classification: Antineoplastic, miscellaneous	Elspar
aspirin Classification: Salicylate analgesic; antipyretic	Alka-Seltzer Ancasal* Arthritis Foundation Pain Reliever Arthritis Pain Formula

*Available in Canada only

GENERIC NAME	BRAND NAME

aspirin
(cont'd)
	A.S.A
	Ascriptin
	Ascriptin A/D
	Ascriptin Extra Strength
	Aspergum
	Aspirin
	Asprimox
	Bayer
	Bayer Children's Aspirin
	Bayer Extra Strength Enteric 500
	    Aspirin
	Bayer Low Adult Strength
	Bayer Regular Strength Enteric Coated
	    Caplets
	Bufferin
	Buffex
	Cama Arthritis Pain Reliever
	Easprin
	Ecotrin
	Ecotrin Adult Low Strength
	Ecotrin Maximum Strength
	8-Hour Bayer Timed Release
	Empirin
	Enteric Coated Caplets
	Enteric 500 Aspirin
	Entrophen*
	Genprin
	½ Halfprin
	Halfprin 81
	Heartline
	Magnaprin
	Magnaprin Arthritis Strength Aspirin
	Maximum Bayer
	Norwich Extra-Strength
	Novasen*
	Sal-Adult*
	Sal-Infant*
	St. Joseph Adult Chewable Aspirin
	Supasa*
	Tri-Buffered Bufferin
	ZORprin

astemizole Classification: Antihistamine	Hismanal

GENERIC NAME	BRAND NAME
atenolol Classification: Antihypertensive; beta-adrenergic blocker	Apo-Atenol* Atenolol Tenormin
ateviridine mesylate Classification: Antiviral (Investigational)	Ateviridine Mesylate
atorvastatin calcium Classification: Antilipemic	Lipitor
atovaquone Classification: Antiprotozoal	Mepron
atracurium besylate Classification: Nondepolarizing neuromuscular blocker	Tracrium
atropine sulfate Classification: Anticholinergic	Atropine Sulfate Sal-Tropine
atropine sulfate, ophthalmic Classification: Mydriatic	Atropine-1 Atropine Care Ophthalmic Atropine Sulfate Atropine Sulfate Ophthalmic Atropisol Isopto Atropine
attapulgite Classification: Antidiarrheal	Kaopectate Advanced Formula
auranofin Classification: Gold compound	Ridaura
aurothioglucose Classification: Gold compound	Solganal
azacitidine Classification: Antineoplastic (Investigational)	Azactidine
azatadine maleate Classification: Antihistamine	Optimine

*Available in Canada only

GENERIC NAME	BRAND NAME
azathioprine Classification: Immunosuppressive	Azathioprine Sodium Imuran
azelastine Classification: Antihistimine	Astelin
azelic acid Classification: Anti-acne product	Azelex
azidouridine Classification: Antiviral (Investigational)	AzdU
azithromycin Classification: Antibiotic; macrolide	Zithromax
AZT-P-ddl Classification: Antiviral (Investigational)	Scriptene
aztreonam Classification: Antibiotic; monobactam	Azactam

B

bacampicillin HCl Classification: Antibiotic; aminopenicillin	Penglobe* Spectrobid
bacitracin Classification: Antibacterial (Orphan)	Altracin
bacitracin, intramuscular Classification: Antibacterial	Baci-IM Bacitracin U.S.P.
bacitracin, ophthalmic Classification: Antibacterial	AK-Tracin Bacitracin

GENERIC NAME	BRAND NAME

bacitracin, topical
Classification:
Antibacterial

Baciguent
Bacitin*
Bacitracin

baclofen
Classification:
Skeletal muscle relaxant, direct acting

Baclofen
Lioresal
Lioresal Intrathecal

barium sulfate
Classification:
Radiopaque agent

Anatrast
Barium Sulfate U.S.P.
Baro-Cat
Baroflave
Barosperse Powder for Suspension
Barosperse 110 Powder for Suspension
Enecat
Entrobar
Epi-C
Flo-Coat
HD 85
HD 200 Plus
Liquid Barosperse
Liquipake
Prepcat
Tomocat
Tonopaque

BCG, intravesical
Classification:
Antineoplastic, miscellaneous

ImmuCyst*
Oncoticce*
Pacis*
TheraCys
TICE BCG

BCG vaccine, percutaneous
Classification:
Vaccine

TICE BCG

becaplemin
Classification:
Growth factor

Regranex

beclomethasone dipropionate
Classification:
Glucocorticoid

Becloforte Inhaler*
Beclovent
Vanceril
Vanceril Double Strength

beclomethasone dipropionate, nasal
Classification:
Glucocorticoid

Beconase AQ Nasal
Beconase Inhalation
Vancenase AQ Nasal
Vancenase Nasal Inhaler
Vancenase Pockethaler

*Available in Canada only

GENERIC NAME	BRAND NAME
belladonna Classification: Anticholinergic	Belladonna Tincture
belladonna alkaloids Classification: Anticholinergic	Bellafoline
benazepril HCl Classification: Antihypertensive, angiotensin converting enzyme inhibitor	Lotensin
bendroflumethiazide Classification: Thiazide diuretic	Naturetin
bentiromide Classification: Gastrointestinal function test	Chymex
benzalkonium chloride Classification: Germicidal	Benza Benzachlor-50* Benzalkonium Chloride Ionax Scrub* Mycocile NS Sabol Shampoo* Zephiran Zephiran Chloride*
benzocaine Classification: Local anesthetic	Detane Diet Ayds Slim-Mint
benzocaine, oral Classification: Local anesthetic	Baby Anbesol Baby Orajel Baby Orajel Nighttime Formula Benzodent Maximum Strength Anbesol Mycinettes Orabase-B Orabase Baby Orabase Gel Orajel SensoGARD Spec-T Toothache Gel Trocaine

GENERIC NAME	BRAND NAME

benzocaine, oral (cont'd.)

Tyrobenz
Vicks Children's Chloraseptic
Zilactin-B Medicated
ZilaDent

benzocaine, topical
Classification:
Local anesthetic

Americaine
Americaine Anesthetic
Americaine Anesthetic Lubricant
Benzocaine
Bicozene
Boil-Ease
Chigger-Tox
Dermoplast
Foille
Foille Medicated First Aid
Foille Plus
Hurricaine
Lanacane
Medicane
Solarcaine

benzoin
Classification:
Protectant

AeroZoin
Benzoin Compound
Benzoin Tincture
TinBen
TinCoBen

benzonatate
Classification:
Non-narcotic antitussive

Benzonatate Softgels
Tessalon Perles

benzoyl peroxide
Classification:
Anti-acne product

Acne 5
Acne 10
Ambi 10
Ben-Aqua 10
Benoxyl 5
Benoxyl 10
Benzac AC 2½
Benzac AC 5
Benzac AC 10
Benzac AC Wash 2½
Benzac AC Wash 5
Benzac AC Wash 10
Benzan W Wash 2½
Benzac W Wash 5
Benzac W Wash 10
Benzac W 5
Benzac 5

GENERIC NAME	BRAND NAME
benzoyl peroxide (cont'd.)	Benzac 10
	Benzac W 10
	5-Benzagel
	10-Benzagel
	Benzashave
	Benzoyl Peroxide
	BlemErase
	Brevoxyl
	Clear by Design
	Clearasil Maximum Strength
	Del Aqua-5
	Del Aqua-10
	Desquam-E
	Desquam-E 5
	Desquam-E 10
	Desquam-X5
	Desquam-X10
	Desquam-X5 Wash
	Desquam-X10 Wash
	Dryox 2.5
	Dryox 5
	Dryox 10
	Dryox 20
	Dryox Wash 5
	Dryox Wash 10
	Exact
	Fostex
	Fostex 10% BPO
	Loroxide
	Oxy 5
	Oxy 10
	Oxy 10 Wash
	PanOxyl 5
	PanOxyl 10
	PanOxyl AQ 2½
	PanOxyl AQ 5
	PanOxyl AQ 10
	Peroxin A5
	Peroxin A10
	Persa-Gel
	Persa Gel W 5%
	Persa Gel W 10%
	Triaz
	Vanoxide

*Available in Canada Only

GENERIC NAME	BRAND NAME
benzphetamine HCl Classification: CNS stimulant; anorexiant	Didrex
benzthiazide Classification: Thiazide diuretic	Exna
benztropine mesylate Classification: Anticholinergic	Benztropine Mesylate Cogentin
benzylpenicilloyl-polylysine Classification: Skin-test antigen	Pre-Pen
bepridil HCl Classification: Calcium channel blocker	Vascor
beractant Classification: Lung surfactant	Survanta
beta-carotene Classification: Vitamin, fat soluble	Max-Caro
betaine anhydrous Classification: Antihomocystinuria agent	Cystadane
betamethasone Classification: Glucocorticoid	Celestone
betamethasone dipropionate Classification: Glucocorticoid	Alphatrex Betamethasone Dipropionate Diprosone Maxivate Teladar
betamethasone dipropionate, augmented Classification: Glucocorticoid	Diprolene Diprolene AF

GENERIC NAME	BRAND NAME

betamethasone sodium phosphate
Classification:
Glucocorticoid

Betamethasone Sodium Phosphate
Celestone Phosphate
Cel-U-Jec

betamethasone sodium phosphate and betamethasone acetate
Classification:
Glucocorticoid

Celestone Soluspan
Betamethasone Sodium Phosphate and
   Betamethasone Acetate

betamethasone valerate
Classification:
Glucocorticoid

Beta Cort*
Betaderm*
Betamethasone Valerate
Betatrex
Beta-Val
Valisone
Valisone Reduced Strength

betaxolol HCl
Classification:
Beta-adrenergic blocker

Betoptic
Betoptic S
Kerlone

bethanechol chloride
Classification:
Cholinergic stimulant

Bethanechol Chloride
Duvoid
Myotonachol
PMS-Bethanechol Chloride*
Urecholine

bicalutamide
Classification:
Antineoplastic; hormone

Casodex

biperiden HCl/biperiden lactate
Classification:
Anticholinergic

Akineton

bisacodyl
Classification:
Laxative, irritant

Apo-Bisacodyl*
Bisacodyl
Bisacodyl Uniserts
Bisco-Lax
Dulcagen
Dulcolax
Fleet Laxative
Fleet Bisacodyl

GENERIC NAME	BRAND NAME

bisacodyl tannex
Classification:1
Laxative, irritant

Clysodrast

bismuth subgallate
Classification:
Systemic deodorizer

Devrom

bismuth subsalicylate
Classification:
Antidiarrheal

Bismatrol
Bismatrol Extra Strength
Pepto-Bismol
Pepto-Bismol Maximum Strength
Pink Bismuth

bisoprolol fumarate
Classification:
Antihypertensive; beta-adrenergic blocker

Zebeta

bithionol
Classification:
CDC anti-infective

Lorothidol
Bitin

bitolterol mesylate
Classification:
Bronchodilator; beta-adrenergic blocker

Tornalate

black widow spider species antivenin
Classification:
Antivenin

Antivenin (Latrodectus mactans)

bleomycin sulfate
Classification:
Antineoplastic; antibiotic

Blenoxane

boric acid ointment
Classification:
Protectant

Boric Acid
Borofax

botulinum toxin, type A
Classification:
Ophthalmic paralytic (Orphan)

Botox
Dysport

botulinum toxin type B
Classification:
Paralytic (Orphan)

Botulinum Toxin Type B

---

*Available in Canada only

GENERIC NAME	BRAND NAME

botulinum toxin type F
Classification:
Paralytic (Orphan)

Botulinum Toxin Type F

botulinum toxoid, pentavalent (ABCDE)
Classification:
Toxoid

Botulinum Toxoid, Pentavalent
(ABCDE)

botulism equine trivalent antitoxin (ABE)
Classification:
Antitoxin

Botulism Equine Trivalent Antitoxin
(ABE)

botulism immune globulin
Classification:
Immune serum (Orphan)

Botulism Immune Globulin

bovine colostrum
Classification:
Antidiarrheal (Orphan)

Bovine Colostrum

bretylium tosylate
Classification:
Antiarrhythmic (Class III)

Bretylate*
Bretylium Tosylate
Bretylol

brimonidine tartrate
Classification:
Adrenergic agonist

Alphagan

bromfenac sodium
Classification:
Nonsteroidal anti-inflammatory

Duract

bromhexine
Classification:
Mucolytic (Orphan)

Bromhexine

bromocriptine mesylate
Classification:
Dopamine receptor agonist; ovulation
stimulant

Parlodel

bromodeoxyuridine
Classification:
Antineoplastic adjuvant (Orphan)

Bromodeoxyuridine

GENERIC NAME	BRAND NAME

brompheniramine maleate
Classification:
Antihistamine

Brompheniramine
Cophene-B
Diamine T.D.
Dimetane Extentabs
ND Stat
Nasahist-B
Veltane

buclizine HCl
Classification:
Antiemetic; anticholinergic

Bucladin-S Softabs

budesonide
Classification:
Glucocorticoid

Pulmicort Turbuhaler

budesonide, nasal
Classification:
Glucocorticoid

Rhinocort
Rhinocort Turbuhaler*

bumetanide
Classification:
Loop diuretic

Bumetanide
Bumex

bupivacaine HCl
Classification:
Local anesthetic

Bupivacaine HCl
Marcaine HCl
Marcaine Spinal
Marcaine with Epinephrine
Sensorcaine
Sensorcaine with Epinephrine
Sensorcaine MPF

buprenorphine HCl
Classification:
Opioid agonist-antagonist analgesic

Buprenex

bupropion HCl
Classification:
Antidepressant

Wellbutrin
Wellbutrin SR

bupropion HCl
Classification:
Smoking deterrent

Zyban

buspirone HCl
Classification:
Antianxiety

BuSpar

GENERIC NAME	BRAND NAME

busulfan
Classification:
Antineoplastic; alkylating agent

Myleran

butabarbital sodium
Classification:
Sedative-hypnotic; barbiturate

Butabarbital Sodium
Butisol Sodium

butamben picrate
Classification:
Local anesthetic

Butesin Picrate

butenafine HCl
Classification:
Antifungal

Mentax

butoconazole nitrate, vaginal
Classification:
Antifungal

Femstat 3

butorphanol, nasal
Classification:
Opioid agonist-antagonist analgesic

Stadol NS

butorphanol tartate
Classification:
Opioid agonist-antagonist analgesic

Stadol

butyrylcholinesterase
Classification:
Antidote (Orphan)

Butyrylcholinesterase

C

C1 inhibitor
Classification:
Immunosuppressive (Orphan)

C1 inhibitor

C1-esterase-inhibitor
Classification:
Immunosuppressive (Orphan)

C1-esterase-inhibitor

cA2
Classification:
Antitumor necrosing factor
(Investigational)

CenTNF

GENERIC NAME	BRAND NAME

cabergoline
Classification:
Dopamine receptor agonist

Dostinex

caffeine
Classification:
Analeptic

Caffedrine
Caffeine
Caffeine and Sodium Benzoate
Nō-Dōz
Quick Prep
Tirend
Vivarin

calanolide A
Classification:
Antiviral (Investigational)

Calanolide A

calcifediol
Classification:
Vitamin, fat soluble

Calderol

calcipotriene
Classification:
Antipsoriatic

Dovonex

calcitonin (human)
Classification:
Parathyroid agent

Cibacalcin

calcitonin (salmon)
Classification:
Parathyroid agent

Calcimar
Miacalcin
Osteocalcin
Salmonine

calcitriol (1,25-dihydroxycholecalciferol)
Classification:
Vitamin, fat soluble

Calcijex
Rocaltrol

calcium acetate
Classification:
Electrolyte replacement; calcium

Phos-Lo
Caphron

calcium ascorbate
Classification:
Vitamin, water soluble

Calcium Ascorbate

calcium carbonate
Classification:
Antacid; calcium supplement

Alka-Mints
Amitone
Cal Carb-HD
Calci-Chew

*Available in Canada only

GENERIC NAME	BRAND NAME

calcium carbonate (cont'd.)

Calci-Mix
Calciday 667
Calcium 600
Calcium Carbonate
Cal-Plus
Caltrate 600
Caltrate Jr.
Chooz
Dicarbosil
Equilet
Extra Strength Alkets Antacid
Gencalc 600
Maalox
Mallamint
Nephro-Calci
Os-Cal 500
Oystercal 500
Oysco 500
Oyst-Cal 500
Oyster Shell Calcium 500
Rolaids Calcium Rich
Tums
Tums 500
Tums E-X Extra Strength
Tums Ultra

calcium caseinate
Classification:
Food modifier

Casec

calcium chloride
Classification:
Electrolyte replacement; calcium

Calcium Chloride

calcium citrate
Classification:
Electrolyte replacement; calcium

Citracal
Citracal Liquitab

calcium glubionate
Classification:
Electrolyte replacement; calcium

Neo-Calglucon

calcium gluceptate
Classification:
Electrolyte replacement; calcium

Calcium Gluceptate

GENERIC NAME	BRAND NAME
calcium gluconate Classification: Electrolyte replacement; calcium	Calcium Gluconate
calcium gluconate gel 2.5% Classification: Antidote (Orphan)	H-F Gel
calcium lactate Classification: Electrolyte replacement; calcium	Calcium Lactate
calcium pantothenate (B_5, pantothenic acid) Classification: Vitamin, water soluble	Calcium Pantothenate
calcium salts of sennosides A&B Classification: Laxative, irritant	Ex-Lax Gentle Nature
capreomycin sulfate Classification: Antitubercular	Capastat Sulfate
capsaicin Classification: Analgesic	Capsin Capzasin●P Dolorac No Pain-HP Zostrix Zostrix-HP
captopril Classification: Antihypertensive; angiotensin converting enzyme inhibitor	Capoten Captopril
carbachol, intraocular Classification: Miotic	Miostat
carbachol, topical Classification: Miotic	Isopto Carbachol Carboptic
carbamazepine Classification: Anticonvulsant	Apo-Carbamazepine* Carbamazepine Epitol Mazepine* Tegretol

*Available in Canada only

GENERIC NAME	BRAND NAME
carbamazepine, extended release Classification: Anticonvulsant	Carbatrol Tegretol-XR
carbamide peroxide, otic Classification: Emulsifier	Auro Ear Drops Debrox E•R•O Ear Mollifene Murine Ear
carbamide peroxide (urea peroxide) Classification: Antiseptic	Gly-Oxide Liquid Orajel Perioseptic Proxigel
carbenicillin indanyl sodium Classification: Antibiotic; extended spectrum penicillin	Geocillin
carbidopa Classification: Antiparkinson agent	Lodosyn
carboplatin Classification: Antineoplastic; alkylating agent	Paraplatin
carboprost tromethamine Classifications: Oxytocic, prostaglandin	Hemabate
carbovir Classification: Antiviral; protease inhibitor (Orphan)	Carbovir
cardioplegic solution Classification: Cardioplegic solution	Plegisol
carisoprodol Classification: Skeletal muscle relaxant, centrally acting	Carisoprodol Soma
carmustine (BCNU) Classification: Antineoplastic; alkylating agent	BiCNU Gliadel

GENERIC NAME	BRAND NAME
carteolol HCl Classification: Beta-adrenergic blocker	Cartrol Ocupress
carvedilol Classification: Antihypertensive	Coreg
cascara sagrada Classification: Laxative, irritant	Cascara Sagrada Cascara Sagrada Aromatic Fluid Extract
castor oil Classification: Laxative, irritant	Castor Oil Emulsoil Fleet Flavored Castor Oil Neoloid Purge
CD4, recombinant soluble human (rCD4) Classification: Immune serum (Orphan)	Receptin
CD4-IgG Classification: Immune serum (Investigational)	CD4-IgG
cefaclor Classification: Antibiotic; cephalosporin	Ceclor Ceclor CD
cefadroxil Classification: Antibiotic; cephalosporin	Cefadroxil Duricef
cefamandole nafate Classification: Antibiotic; cephalosporin	Mandol
cefazolin sodium Classification: Antibiotic; cephalosporin	Ancef Cefazolin Sodium Kefzol Zolicef
cefdinir Classification: Antibiotic; cephalosporin	Omnicef

GENERIC NAME	BRAND NAME
cefepime HCl Classification: Antibiotic; cephalosporin	Maxipime
cefixime Classification: Antibiotic; cephalosporin	Suprax
cefmetazole sodium Classification: Antibiotic; cephalosporin	Zefazone
cefonicid sodium Classification: Antibiotic; cephalosporin	Monocid
cefoperazone sodium Classification: Antibiotic; cephalosporin	Cefobid
cefotaxime sodium Classification: Antibiotic; cephalosporin	Claforan
cefotetan disodium Classification: Antibiotic; cephalosporin	Cefotan
cefoxitin sodium Classification: Antibiotic; cephalosporin	Mefoxin
cefpodoxime proxetil Classification: Antibiotic; cephalosporin	Vantin
cefprozil Classification: Antibiotic; cephalosporin	Cefzil
ceftazidime Classification: Antibiotic; cephalosporin	Ceptaz Fortaz Tazicef Tazidime
ceftibutin Classification: Antibiotic; cephalosporin	Cedax

*Available in Canada Only

GENERIC NAME	BRAND NAME
ceftizoxime sodium Classification: Antibiotic; cephalosporin	Cefizox
ceftriaxone sodium Classification: Antibiotic; cephalosporin	Rocephin
cefuroxime axetil Classification: Antibiotic; cephalosporin	Ceftin
cefuroxime sodium Classification: Antibiotic; cephalosporin	Cefuroxime Sodium Kefurox Zinacef
cellulose sodium phosphate Classification: Antihypercalciuria agent	Calcibind Calcisorb*
cephalexin HCl monohydrate Classification: Antibiotic; cephalosporin	Keftab
cephalexin monohydrate Classification: Antibiotic; cephalosporin	Biocef Cefanex Cephalexin Ceporex* Keflex Novolexin*
cephalothin sodium Classification: Antibiotic; cephalosporin	Cephalothin Sodium Ceporacin*
cephapirin sodium Classification: Antibiotic; cephalosporin	Cephapirin Sodium
cephradine Classification: Antibiotic; cephalosporin	Cephradine Velosef
cervistatin sodium Classification: Antilipemic	Baycol
cetirizine HCl Classification: Antihistamine	Zyrtec

*Available in Canada only

GENERIC NAME	BRAND NAME

charcoal
Classification:
Antiflatulent

Charcoal
CharcoCaps

charcoal, activated
Classification:
Adsorbent

Actidose-Aqua
Actidose, with Sorbitol
CharcoAid
CharcoAid 2000
Charcoal, Activated
Liqui-Char

chenodiol
Classification:
Antilithic (Orphan)

Chenix

chimeric Mab (C2B8) to CD20
Classification:
Biologic response modifier (Orphan)

Chimeric Mab (C2B8) to CD20

chloral hydrate
Classification:
Sedative-hypnotic; non-barbiturate

Aquachloral Supprettes
Chloral Hydrate
Novochlorhydrate*

chlorambucil
Classification:
Antineoplastic; alkylating agent

Leukeran

chloramphenicol, ophthalmic
Classification:
Antibacterial

AK-Chlor
Chloramphenicol
Chloromycetin
Chloroptic
Chloroptic S.O.P.
Fenicol*
Isopto Fenical*
Pentamycin*

chloramphenicol, otic
Classification:
Antibacterial

Chloromycetin Otic
Sopamycetin*

chloramphenicol sodium succinate
Classification:
Antibacterial; antirickettsial

Chloramphenicol
Chloramphenicol Sodium Succinate
Novochlorocap*

chlordiazepoxide HCl
Classification:
Antianxiety; benzadiazepine

Chlordiazepoxide HCl
Libritabs
Librium
Medilium*

*Available in Canada Only

GENERIC NAME	BRAND NAME
chlordiazepoxide HCl (cont'd.)	Mitran Novopoxide* Reposans-10 Solium*
chlorhexidine gluconate, oral Classification: Antibacterial	Peridex PerioGard
chlorhexidine gluconate, topical Classification: Germicidal	BactoShield Dyna-Hex Skin Cleanser Dyna-Hex 2 Skin Cleanser Exidine Skin Cleanser Exidine-2 Scrub Exidine-4 Scrub Hibiclens Hibiclens Antiseptic/Antimicrobial Skin Cleanser Rinse Hibistat Germicidal Hand
chlormezanone Classification: Antianxiety	Trancopal Caplets
chlorophyll derivatives Classification: Systemic deodorizer	Chloresium Chlorophyllin Derifil PALS
chloroprocaine HCl Classification: Local anesthetic	Nesacaine Nesacaine-MPF
chloroquine HCl Classification: Antimalarial	Aralen HCl
chloroquine phosphate Classification: Antimalarial	Aralen Phosphate Chloroquine Phosphate Novochloroquine*
chlorothiazide Classification: Thiazide diuretic	Chlorothiazide Diurigen Diuril Sodium Diuril
chlorotrianisene Classification: Estrogen	Tace

*Available in Canada only

GENERIC NAME	BRAND NAME

chloroxine
Classification:
Antiseborrheic

Capitrol

chlorphenesin carbamate
Classification:
Skeletal muscle relaxant, centrally acting

Macil*
Maolate

chlorpheniramine maleate
Classification:
Antihistamine

Aller-chlor
Chlo-Amine
Chlor-100
Chlor-Pro
Chlorate
Chlorpheniramine Maleate
Chlor-Pro 10
Chlorspan-12
Chlor-Trimeton
Chlor-Trimeton Allergy
Chlor-Trimeton Allergy 8 Hour
Chlor-Trimeton 12 Hour Allergy
Efidac 24 Chlorpheniramine
Pedia Care Allergy Formula
Pfeiffer's Allergy

chlorpromazine HCl
Classification:
Antipsychotic

Chlorpromanyl*
Chlorpromazine HCl
Ormazine
Thorazine
Thorazine Spansules

chlorpropamide
Classification:
Antidiabetic; sulfonylurea

Chloronase*
Chlorpropamide
Diabinese
Novopropamide*

chlorthalidone
Classification:
Thiazide-like diuretic

Chlorthalidone
Hygroton
Novothalidone*
Thalitone

chlorzoxazone
Classification:
Skeletal muscle relaxant, centrally acting

Chlorzoxazone
Paraflex
Parafon Forte DSC
Remular-S

cholecalciferol (D$_3$)
Classification:
Vitamin, fat soluble

Delta-D
Vitamin D$_3$

*Available in Canada Only

GENERIC NAME	BRAND NAME
cholera vaccine Classification: Vaccine	Cholera Vaccine
cholestyramine Classification: Antilipemic	Cholestyramine Prevalite Questran Questran Light
choline Classification: Amino acid	Choline Choline Bitartrate Choline Chloride Choline Dihydrogen Citrate
choline chloride Classification: Amino acid (Orphan)	Choline Chloride
choline magnesium trisalicylate Classification: Salicylate analgesic	Trilisate
choline salicylate Classification: Salicylate analgesic	Arthropan Teejel*
chondroitinase Classification: Enzyme (Orphan)	Chondroitinase
chorionic gonadotropin human (HCG) Classification: Chorionic gonadotropin	A.P.L. Chorex-5 Chorex-10 Chorionic Gonadotropin (Chorionic Gonadotropine) Choron 10 Gonic Pregnyl Profasi
chromic phosphate P32 Classification: Antineoplastic; radiopharmaceutical	Phosphocol P32
chromium Classification: Trace element	Chroma-Pak Chromic Chloride Chromium Chromium Chloride

*Available in Canada only

GENERIC NAME	BRAND NAME

chymopapain
Classification:
Enzyme

Chymodiactin

chymotrypsin
Classification:
Enzymes

Catarase 1:5000

CI-1020
Classification:
Antiviral (Investigational)

CI-1020

ciclopirox olamine
Classification:
Antifungal

Loprox

cidofovir
Classification:
Antiviral; nucleotide

Vistide

ciliary neurotrophic factor
Classification:
Anti-amyotrophic lateral sclerosis agent
(Orphan)

Ciliary Neurotrophic Factor

**ciliary neurotrophic factor
recombinant human**
Classification:
Anti-amyotrophic lateral sclerosis agent
(Orphan)

Ciliary Neurotrophic Factor
Recombinant Human

cimetidine
Classification:
Histamine H_2 receptor antagonist

Cimetidine
Tagamet
Tagamet HB

cinoxacin
Classification:
Urinary anti-infective

Cinobac
Cinoxacin

ciproflaxacin HCl
Classification:
Antibiotic; fluroquinolone

Cipro
Cipro I.V.

ciprofloxacin, ophthalmic
Classification:
Antibiotic; fluoroquinolone

Ciloxan

GENERIC NAME	BRAND NAME
cisapride Classification: Gastrointestinal stimulant	Propulsid
cistracurium besylate Classification: Nondepolarizing neuromuscular blocker	Nimbex
cisplastin (CDDP) Classification: Antineoplastic; alkylating agent	Platinol-AQ
citrate and citric acid Classification: Systemic alkalinizer	Bicitra Citrolith Oracit Polycitra Polycitra-LC Polycitra-K
cladribine Classification: Antineoplastic, miscellaneous	Leustatin
clarithromycin Classification: Antibiotic; macrolide	Biaxin
clemastine fumarate Classification: Antihistamine	Antihist-1 Clemastine Fumarate Tavist
clidinium bromide Classification: Anticholinergic	Quarzan
clinafloxacin (CI-960) Classification: Antibiotic; fluroquinolone (Investigational)	Clinafloxacin
clindamycin HCl Classification: Antibiotic; lincosamide	Cleocin Clindamycin HCl Dalacin C*
clindamycin palmitate HCl Classification: Antibiotic; lincosamide	Cleocin Pediatric

*Available in Canada only

GENERIC NAME	BRAND NAME

clindamycin phosphate
Classification:
Antibiotic; lincosamide

Cleocin Cream
Cleocin Phosphate
Clindamycin Phosphate

clindamycin, topical
Classification:
Anti-acne product

C/T/S
Cleocin T
Clinda-Derm
Clindamycin Phosphate
Clindets

clioquinol
(iodochlorhydroxyquin)
Classification:
Antifungal

Vioform

clobetasol propionate
Classification:
Glucocorticoid

Cormax
Temovate
Temovate Emollient

clocortolone pivalate
Classification:
Glucocorticoid

Cloderm

clofazimine
Classification:
Leprostatic

Lamprene

clofibrate
Classification:
Antilipemic

Atromid-S
Claripen*
Claripex*

clomiphene citrate
Classification:
Ovulation stimulant

Clomid
Clomiphene Citrate
Serophene

clomipramine HCl
Classification:
Antidepressant, tricyclic

Anafranil
Clomipramine HCl

clonazepam
Classification:
Anticonvulsant; benzodiazepine

Klonopin

clonidine HCl
Classification:
Antihypertensive, centrally acting

Catapres
Clonidine HCl
Dixarit*

*Available in Canada Only

GENERIC NAME	BRAND NAME

clonidine HCl
Classification:
Analgesic

Duraclon

clonidine HCl-transdermal
Classification:
Antihypertensive, centrally acting

Catapres-TTS-1
Catapres-TTS-2
Catapres-TTS-3

clopidogrel
Classification:
Antiplatelet

Plavix

clorazepate dipotassium
Classification:
Antianxiety; benzodiazepine

Gen-Xene
Tranxene
Tranxene-SD
Clorazepate dipotassium
Tranxene-SD half strength

clostridial collagenase
Classification:
Enzyme (Orphan)

Clostridial Collagenase

clotrimazole, oral
Classification:
Antifungal

Mycelex Troches

clotrimazole, topical
Classification:
Antifungal

Fungoid Solution
Lotrimin
Lotrimin AF Lotion
Mycelex
Mycelex OTC

clotrimazole, vaginal
Classification:
Antifungal

Canesten*
Clotrimazole
Gyne-Lotrimin
Gyne-Lotrimin Combination Pack
Mycelex-G
Mycelex-7
Mycelex-7 Combination Pack
Mycelex Twin Pack

clotrimidazole
Classification:
Anti-sickle cell disease agent (Orphan)

Clotrimidazole

cloxacillin sodium
Classification:
Antibiotic, penicillinase-resistant
penicillin

APO Cloxi*
Bactopen*
Cloxacillin Sodium
Cloxapen
Novocloxin*

GENERIC NAME	BRAND NAME

cloxacillin sodium (cont'd.)

Orbenin*
Tegopen

clozapine
Classification:
Antipsychotic

Clozaril

coal tar
Classification:
Keratolytic

Advanced Formula Tegrin
Balnetar
Creamy Tar
Cūtar Bath Oil
Denorex
DHS Tar
Doctar
Duplex T
Extra Strength Denorex
High Potency Tar
Iocon
Ionil T Plus
MG 217 Medicated
Neutrogena T/Gel
Packer's Pine Tar
Pentrax
Pentrax Gold
Polytar
Polytar Bath
Protar Protein
PsoriNail
Tegrin Medicated
Theraplex T
Zetar
Zetar Emulsion

cocaine
Classification:
Local anesthetic

Cocaine HCl
Cocaine Viscous

coccidioidin
Classification:
In vivo diagnostic

BioCox
Spherulin

codeine
Classification:
Opioid analgesic; antitussive

Codeine Phosphate
Codeine Sulfate

GENERIC NAME	BRAND NAME
colchicine Classification: Antigout	Colchicine
colestipol HCl Classification: Antilipemic	Colestid
colistimethate sodium Classification: Antibiotic; polymyxin	Coly-Mycin M
collagen (purified Type II) Classification: Antirheumatic (Orphan)	Colloral
collagenase Classification: Enzyme (Orphan)	Plaquase
collagenase Classification: Topical enzyme	Santyl
copper Classification: Trace element	Copper Cupric Sulfate
corn oil Classification: Modular supplement	Lipomul
corticorelin ovine trifultate Classification: In vivo diagnostic	Acthrel
corticotropin injection Classification: Anterior pituitary hormone	ACTH Acthar Corticotropin
corticotropin injection, repository Classification: Anterior pituitary hormone	ACTH-80 Duracton* H.P. Acthar Gel
cortisone Classification: Glucocorticoid	Cortisone Acetate Cortone Acetate

*Available in Canada only

GENERIC NAME	BRAND NAME

cosyntropin
Classification:
Anterior pituitary hormone

Cortrosyn

co-trimoxazole (trimethoprim and sulfamethoxazole) see trimethoprim and sulfamethoxazole
Classification:
Sulfonamide

APO-Sulfatrim*

cromolyn sodium (disodium cromoglycate)
Classification:
Antiasthmatic

Cromolyn Sodium
Gastrocrom
Intal
Intal P*
Nasalcrom
Rynacrom*

cromolyn sodium, ophthalmic
Classification:
Anti-inflammatory

Crolom
Opticrom 4%

crotamiton
Classification:
Scabicide; pediculicide

Eurax

cryptosporidium hyperimmune IgG concentrate
Classification:
Immune serum (Orphan)

Cryptosporidium Hyperimmune IgG Concentrate

cryptosporidium parvum bovine immune globulin
Classification:
Immune serum (Orphan)

Cryptosporidium Parvum Bovine Immune Globulin

curdian sulfate
Classification:
Antiviral (Investigational)

Curdian Sulfate

cyanocobalamin (vitamin B_{12})
Classification:
Vitamin, water soluble

Bedoz*
Crystamine
Crysti 12
Crysti 1000
Cyanabin*
Cyanoject
Cyomin

*Available in Canada Only

GENERIC NAME	BRAND NAME
cyanocobalamin (vitamin B$_{12}$) (cont'd.)	Ener-B Nascobal Rubion* Vitamin B$_{12}$
cyclandelate Classification: Peripheral vasodilator	Cyclospasmol
cyclizine Classification: Antiemetic; anticholinergic	Marezine
cyclobenzaprine HCl Classification: Skeletal muscle relaxant, centrally acting	Cyclobenzaprine HCl Flexeril
cyclopentolate HCl Classification: Mydratic	AK-Pentolate Cyclogyl Cyclopentolate HCl Pentolair
cyclophosphamide Classification: Antineoplastic; alkylating agent	Cytoxan Neosar Procytox*
cycloserine Classification: Antitubercular	Seromycin Pulvules
cyclosporine (cyclosporin A) Classification: Immunosuppressive	Neoral Sandimmune
cyclosporine, opthalmic Classification: Immunosuppressive (Orphan)	Optimmune
cyproheptadine HCl Classification: Antihistamine	Cyproheptadine HCl Periactin Vimicon*
cysteamine bitartrate Classification: Anticystine agent	Cystagen
cysteine HCl Classification: Nitrogen product	Cysteine HCl

*Available in Canada only

GENERIC NAME	BRAND NAME
cytarabine (ARA-C; cytosine arabinoside) Classification: Antineoplastic; antimetabolite	Cytarabine Cytosar-U
cytolin Classification: Immune serum (Investigational)	Cytolin
cytomegalovirus immune globulin intravenous (human) (CMV-IGIV) Classification: Immune serum	CytoGam

D

GENERIC NAME	BRAND NAME
dacarbazine (DTIC, imidazole carboxamide) Classification: Antineoplastic, miscellaneous	DTIC-Dome
daclizumab Classification: Immunosuppressive	Zenapax
dactinomycin (actinomycin D; ACT) Classification: Antineoplastic; antibiotic	Cosmegen
dalteparin sodium Classification: Anticoagulant	Fragmin
danaproid Classification: Anticoagulant	Orgaran
danazol Classification: Androgen	Cyclomen* Danazol Danocrine
dantrolene sodium Classification: Skeletal muscle relaxant, direct acting	Dantrium Dantrium Intravenous

*Available in Canada Only

GENERIC NAME	BRAND NAME

dapiprazole HCl
Classification:
Alpha-adrenergic blocker

Rēv-Eyes

dapsone (DDS)
Classification:
Leprostatic

Avlosulfon*
Dapsone

daunorubicin citrate liposomal
Classification:
Antineoplastic; antibiotic

DaunoXome

deferoxamine mesylate
Classification:
Chelating agent

Desferal

defibrotide
Classification:
Blood modifier (Orphan)

Defibrotide

dehydrex
Classification:
Ophthalmic (Orphan)

Dehydrex

dehydrocholic acid
Classification:
Hydrocholeretics

Dehydrocholic acid
Decholin
Cholan-HMB

dehydroemetine
Classification:
CDC anti-infective

Mebadin

dehydroepiandrosterone
Classification:
Androgen (Orphan)

Dehydroepiandrosterone

delaviridine mesylate
Classification:
Antiviral

Rescriptor

demecarium bromide
Classification:
Miotic

Humorsol

demeclocycline HCl
Classification:
Antibiotic, tetracycline

Declomycin

GENERIC NAME	BRAND NAME

deoxynojirimycin, n-butyl
Classification:
Antiviral (Investigational)

Deoxynojirimycin, n-butyl

desflurane
Classification:
General anesthetic

Suprane

desipramine HCl
Classification:
Antidepressant, tricyclic

Desipramine HCl
Norpramin

desmopressin acetate
Classification:
Posterior pituitary hormone

DDAVP
Desmopressin Acetate
Stimate

desonide
Classification:
Glucocorticoid

Desonide
DesOwen
Tridesilon

desoximetasone
Classification:
Glucocorticoid

Desoximetasone
Topicort
Topicort LP

desoxyephedrine
Classification:
Nasal decongestant

Vicks Inhaler

dexamethasone
Classification:
Glucocorticoid

Aeroseb-Dex
Decadron
Dexameth
Dexamethasone
Dexamethasone Intensol
Dexone
Hexadrol

dexamethasone, ophthalmic
Classification:
Ophthalmic glucocorticoid

Dexamethasone Ophthalmic Suspension
Maxidex

dexamethasone acetate
Classification:
Glucocorticoid

Dalalone D.P.
Dalalone L.A.
Decadron-LA
Decaject-L.A.
Dexamethasone Acetate
Dexasone L.A.
Dexone LA
Solurex LA

*Available in Canada Only

GENERIC NAME	BRAND NAME
dexamethasone sodium phosphate Classification: Glucocorticoid	Dalalone Decadron Phosphate Decaject Dexamethasone Sodium Phosphate Dexasone Dexone Hexadrol Phosphate Solurex
dexamethasone sodium phosphate, nasal Classification: Glucocorticoid	Dexacort Phosphate Turbinaire
dexamethasone sodium phosphate, ophthalmic Classification: Ophthalmic glucocorticoid	AK-Dex Decadron Phosphate Dexamethasone Sodium Phosphate
dexchlorpheniramine maleate Classification: Antihistamine	Dexchlor Dexchlorpheniramine Maleate Polaramine
dexpanthenol Classification: Gastrointestinal stimulant	Dexpanthenol Ilopan
dexpanthenol with choline bitartrate Classification: Gastrointestinal stimulant	Ilopan-Choline
dexrazoxane Classification: Antineoplastic adjuvant; cardioprotective	Zinecard
dextran 1 Classification: Plasma volume expander	Promit
dextran 40 Classification: Plasma volume expander	Dextran 40 Gentran 40 LMD 10% Rheomacrodex
dextran 70/75 Classification: Plasma volume expander	Dextran 70 Dextran 75 Gendex 75 Gentran 75 Macrodex

*Available in Canada only

GENERIC NAME	BRAND NAME

dextran sulfate inhalation
Classification:
Mucolytic (Orphan)

Uendex

dextranomer
Classification:
Debriding agent

Debrisan

dextroamphetamine sulfate
Classification:
CNS stimulant

Dexedrine
Dexedrine Spansules
Dextroamphetamine Sulfate
Dextrostat
Oxydess II
Spancap No. 1

dextromethorphan
Classification:
Non-narcotic antitussive

Benylin Adult
Benylin DM
Benylin Pediatric
Children's Hold
Creo-Terpin
Delsym
Dextromethorphan
Drixoral Cough Liquid Caps
Hold DM
Pertussin CS
Pertussin ES
Robitussin Cough Calmers
Robitussin Pediatric
Scot-Tussin DM Cough Chasers
Silphen DM
St. Joseph Cough Suppressant
Sucrets 4-Hour Cough
Sucrets Cough Control
Suppress
Vicks Dry Hacking Cough

dextrose (d-glucose)
Classification:
Caloric

Dextrose (d-Glucose)

dextrothyroxine sodium
Classification:
Antilipemic

Choloxin

dezocine
Classification:
Opioid agonist-antagonist analgesic

Dalgan

GENERIC NAME	BRAND NAME
DHEA (EL10) Classification: Biologic response modifier (Investigational)	DHEA (EL10)
diatrizoate meglumine 18% Classification: Radiopaque agent	Cystografin Dilute
diatrizoate meglumine 28.5% and diatrizoate sodium 29.1% Classification: Radiopaque agent	Renovist II
diatrizoate meglumine 30% Classification: Radiopaque agent	Cystografin Hypaque-Cysto Hypaque Meglumine 30% Reno-M-30 Reno-M-Dip Urovist Cysto Urovist Meglumine DIU/CT
diatrizoate meglumine 34.3% and diatrizoate sodium 35% Classification: Radiopaque agent	Renovist
diatrizoate meglumine 50% and diatrizoate sodium 25% Classification: Radiopaque agent	Hypaque-M 75%
diatrizoate meglumine 52% and diatrizoate sodium 8% Classification: Radiopaque agent	Angiovist 292 MD-60 Renografin-60
diatrizoate meglumine 52.7% and iodipamide meglumine 26.8% Classification: Radiopaque agent	Sinografin
diatrizoate meglumine 60% Classification: Radiopaque agent	Angiovist 282 Hypaque Meglumine 60% Reno-M-60

*Available in Canada only

GENERIC NAME	BRAND NAME

diatrizoate meglumine 60% and diatrizoate 30%
Classification:
Radiopaque agent

Hypaque-M 90%

diatrizoate meglumine 66% and diatrizoate sodium 10%
Classification:
Radiopaque agent

Angiovost 370
Gastrografin
Hypaque-76
MD-76
MD-Gastroview
Renografin-76

diatrizoate meglumine 76%
Classification:
Radiopaque agent

Diatrizoate Meglumine 76%

diatrizoate sodium
Classification:
Radiopaque agent

Hypaque Sodium

diatrizoate sodium 20%
Classification:
Radiopaque agent

Hypaque Sodium 20%

diatrizoate sodium 25%
Classification:
Radiopaque agent

Hypaque Sodium 25%

diatrizoate sodium 41.66%
Classification:
Radiopaque agent

Hypaque Sodium

diatrizoate sodium 50%
Classification:
Radiopaque agent

Hypaque Sodium 50%
Urovist Sodium 300

diazepam
Classification:
Antianxiety; benzodiazepine

D-Tran*
Diazemuls*
Diazepam
Diazepam Intensol
Dizac
E-Pam*
Meval*
Novodipam*
Stress-Pam*
Valium
Valium Roche Oral*
Vivol*
Zetran

*Available in Canada Only

GENERIC NAME	BRAND NAME
diazepam rectal gel Classification: Anticonvulsant; benzodiazepine	Diastat
diazoxide, oral Classification: Glucose elevating agent	Proglycem
diazoxide, parenteral Classification: Antihypertensive; vasodilator	Hyperstat IV
dibromodulcitol Classification: Antineoplastic (Orphan)	Dibromodulcitol
dibucaine HCl, topical Classification: Local anesthetic	Dibucaine Nupercainal
dichloroacetic acid Classification: Cauterizing agent	Dichloroacetic Acid
dichlorphenamide Classification: Diuretic; carbonic anhydrase inhibitor	Daranide
diclofenac potassium Classification: Nonsteroidal anti-inflammatory	Cataflam
diclofenac sodium Classification: Nonsteroidal anti-inflammatory	Diclofenac Sodium Voltaren Voltaren Papide* Voltaren-SR* Voltaren-XR
diclofenac sodium, ophthalmic Classification: Ophthalmic nonsteroidal anti-inflammatory	Voltaren
dicloxacillin sodium Classification: Antibiotic; penicillinase-resistant penicillin	Dicloxacillin Sodium Dycill Dynapen Pathocil

GENERIC NAME	BRAND NAME

dicyclomine HCl
Classification:
Antispasmodic

Antispas
Bentyl
Bentylol*
Byclomine
Dibent
Dicyclomine HCl
Di-Spaz
Formulex*
Or-Tyl

didanosine (ddI, dideoxyinosine)
Classification:
Antiviral; nucleoside

Videx

dienestrol
Classification:
Estrogen

Ortho Dienestrol

diethylcarbamazie citrate
Classification:
Anthelmintics

Hetrazan

diethyldithiocarbamate
Classification:
Biologic response modifier
(Investigational)

Imuthiol

diethylpropion HCl
Classification:
CNS stimulant; anorexiant

Diethylpropion HCl
Tenuate
Tenuate Dospan

diethylstilbestrol (DES)
Classification:
Estrogen

DES
Honvol*
Stilboestrol*
Stilphostrol

diflorasone diacetate
Classification:
Glucocorticoid

Florone
Florone E
Maxiflor
Psorcon

diflunisal
Classification:
Salicylate analgesic

Dolobid
Diflunisal

digitoxin
Classification:
Cardiac glycoside

Crystodigin
Digitaline*
Digitoxin

GENERIC NAME	BRAND NAME
digoxin Classification: Cardiac glycoside	Digoxin Lanoxicaps Lanoxin
digoxin immune fab (ovine) Classification: Antidigoxin antibody	Digibind
dihydroergotamine mesylate Classification: Antimigraine; ergot alkaloid	D.H.E. 45
dihydroergotamine mesylate, nasal Classification: Antimigraine, ergot alkaloid	Migranol
dihydrotachysterol (DHT) Classification: Vitamin, fat soluble	DHT DHT Intensol Solution Hytakerol
dihydrotestosterone Classification: Androgen (Orphan)	Andrdogen-DHT
diloxanide furoate Classification: CDC anti-infective	Furamide
diltiazem HCl Classification: Calcium channel blocker	Cardizem Cardizem CD Cardizem SR Dilacor XR Diltiazem HCl Tiamate Tiazac
dimenhydrinate Classification: Antiemetic; anticholinergic	Children's Dramamine Calm-X Dimenhydrinate Dinate Dramamine Dramanate Dymenate Gravol* Hydrate Marmine Nauseal* Nauseatol*

*Available in Canada only

GENERIC NAME	BRAND NAME

**dimenhydrinate
(cont'd.)**

Nico-Vert
Novodimenate*
Travamine*
Triptone Caplets

dimercaprol
Classification:
Chelating agent

BAL in Oil
British Anti-Lewisite*

dimethyl sulfoxide (DMSO)
Classification:
Anti-inflammatory

Kensol*
Rimso-50

dinoprostone
Classification:
Oxytocic; prostaglandin

Cervidil
Prepidil
Prepidil Gel*
Prostin E2

**dipalmitoylphosphatidylcholine/
glycerol**
Classification:
Lung surfactant (Orphan)

ALEC

diphenhydramine HCl
Classification:
Antihistamine

40 Winks
AllerMax
Banophen
Belix
Benadryl
Benadryl Allergy
Benadryl Dye-Free
Benadryl Dye-Free Allergy Liqui Gels
Benadryl Kapseals
Ben-Allergin-50
Benylin Cough
Compōz
Dermamycin
Diphen Cough
Diphenhist
Diphenhydramine HCl
Dormin
Genahist
Hyrexin-50
Maximum Strength Nytol
Maximum Strength Sleepinal
Maximum Strength Unisom
Miles Nervine Caplets
Nordryl
Nordryl Cough

*Available in Canada Only

GENERIC NAME	BRAND NAME
diphenhydramine HCl (cont'd.)	Nytol Phendry Scot-Tussin Allergy Siladryl Silphen Cough Sleep-eze 3 Sleepwell 2-nite Snooze Fast Sominex Caplets Tusstat Twilite Caplets Uni-Bent Cough
diphenidol Classification: Antiemetic	Vontrol

diphtheria and tetanus toxoids, combined (Td)
Classification:
Toxoid
	Diphtheria and Tetanus Toxoids,
	    Absorbed (for pediatric use)
	Diphtheria and Tetanus Toxoids,
	    Absorbed (for adult use)

diphtheria and tetanus toxoids and whole-cell pertussis vaccine absorbed (DTwP) Classification: Toxoid	Diphtheria and Tetanus Toxoids and Pertussis Vaccine Tri-Immunol DTwP
diphtheria and tetanus toxoids and acellular pertussis vaccine (DTaP) Classification: Toxoid	Acel-Imune Tripedia
diphtheria and tetanus toxoids and whole-cell pertussis and haemophilus influenzae type b conjugate vaccines (DTwP-HIB) Classification: Toxoid	Tetramune
diphtheria antitoxin Classification: Antitoxin	Diphtheria Antitoxin

GENERIC NAME	BRAND NAME

diphtheria equine antitoxin
Classification:
Antitoxin

Diphtheria Equine Antitoxin

dipivefrin HCl
Classification:
Adrenergic agonist

AKPro
Dipivefrin HCl
Propine

dipyridamole
Classification:
Antiplatelet

Dipyridamole
Persantine
Persantine IV

dirithromycin
Classification:
Antibiotic; macrolide

Dynabac

disaccharide tripeptide glycerol dipalmitoyl
Classification:
Antineoplastic (Orphan)

Immther

disodium clodronate
Classification:
Bone resorption inhibitor (Orphan)

Disodium Clodronate

disodium clodronate tetrahydrate
Classification:
Bone resorption inhibitor (Orphan)

Disodium Clodronate Tetrahydrate

disopyramide
Classification:
Antiarrhythmic

Disopyramide Phosphate
Norpace
Norpace CR

disulfiram
Classification:
Antialcoholic

Antabuse
Disulfiram

divalproex sodium
Classification:
Anticonvulsant

Depakote

DMP-450
Classification:
Antiviral (Investigational)

DMP-450

GENERIC NAME	BRAND NAME
dobutamine HCl Classification: Adrenergic agonist	Dobutamine HCl Dobutrex
docetaxel Classification: Antineoplastic, miscellaneous	Taxotere
docusate calcium Classification: Laxative, softener	DC Softgels Docusate Calcium Pro-Cal-Sof Sulfalax Calcium Surfak
docusate potassium Classification: Laxative, softener	Diocto-K Kasof
docusate sodium Classification: Laxative, softener	Colace Correctol Extra Gentle Dialose Diocto Dioeze Disonate Docusate Sodium DOK DOS Softgel D-S-S Modane Soft Regular SS Silace
dolasteron Classification: Antiemetic	Anzemet
donepezil HCl Classification: Cholinesterase inhibitor	Aricept
dopamine HCl Classification: Adrenergic agonist	Dopamine HCl Intropin Revimine*
dorzolamide HCl Classification: Carbonic anhydrase inhibitor, ophthalmic	Trusopt

*Available in Canada only

GENERIC NAME	BRAND NAME

dornase alfa
Classification:
Mucolytic

Pulmozyme

doxacurium chloride
Classification:
Nondepolarizing neuromuscular blocker

Nuromax

doxapram HCl
Classification:
Analeptic

Dopram
Doxapram

doxazosin mesylate
Classification:
Antihypertensive; alpha-adrenergic
blocker

Cardura

doxepin HCl
Classification:
Antianxiety; antidepressant

Doxepin HCl
Sinequan
Sinequan Concentrate
Triadapin*

doxepin, topical
Classification:
Antihistamine

Zonalon

doxorubicin HCl (ADR)
Classification:
Antineoplastic; antibiotic

Adriamycin PFS
Adriamycin RDF
Doxorubicin HCl
Rubex

doxycycline hyclate
Classification:
Antibiotic; tetracycline

Bio-Tab
Doryx
Doxy 100
Doxy 200
Doxy Caps
Doxychel Hyclate
Doxycin*
Doxycycline
Monodox
Vibramycin
Vibramycin IV
Vibra-Tabs

doxylamine succinate
Classification:
Antihistamine

Unisom Nighttime Sleep-Aid

*Available in Canada Only

GENERIC NAME	BRAND NAME
D-penicillamine Classification: Chelating agent	Cuprimine Depen
dronabinol Classification: Antiemetic	Marinol
droperidol Classification: General anesthetic	Droperidol Inapsine
d-xylose Classification: In vivo diagnostic	Xylo-Pfan
dyclonine HCl Classification: Local anesthetic	Dyclone
dynamine Classification: Anti-myasthenia agent (Orphan)	Dynamine
dyphylline (dihydroxypropyl theophylline) Classification: Bronchodilator; xanthine	Dilor Dyphylline Lufyllin Lufyllin-400 Protophylline*

E

echothiophate iodide Classification: Miotic	Phospholine Iodide
econazole nitrate Classification: Antifungal	Spectazole
edetate calcium disodium (calcium EDTA) Classification: Chelating agent	Calcium Disodium Versenate
edetate disodium (EDTA) Classification: Chelating agent	Disotate Edetate Disodium Endrate

*Available in Canada only

GENERIC NAME	BRAND NAME

edrophonium chloride
Classification:
Anticholinesterase

Enlon
Reversol
Tensilon

efavirenz
Classification:
Antiviral (Investigational)

Sustiva

eflornithine HCl (DMFO)
Classification:
Antiprotozoal

Ornidyl

emedastine difumarate
Classification:
Antihistamine, ophthalmic

Emadine

enalaprilat
Classification:
Antihypertensive; angiotensin converting
enzyme inhibitor

Vasotec I.V.

enalapril maleate
Classification:
Antihypertensive; angiotensin converting
enzyme inhibitor

Vasotec

enflurane
Classification:
General anesthetic

Enflurane
Ethrane

enoxacin
Classification:
Fluoroquinolone

Penetrexe

enoxapirin sodium
Classification:
Anticoagulant

Lovenox

enprostil
Classification:
Prostaglandin (Investigational)

Gardrin

ephedrine
Classification:
Adrenergic agonist

Ephedrine
Ephedrine Sulfate

ephedrine, nasal
Classification:
Nasal decongestant

Pretz-D
Kondon's Nasal

*Available in Canada Only

GENERIC NAME	BRAND NAME
epidermal growth factor (human) Classification: Growth hormone, ophthalmic (Orphan)	Epidermal Growth Factor (human)
epinephrine Classification: Adrenergic agonist	Adrenalin Chloride Adrenalin Chloride Solution AsthmaHaler Mist AsthmaNefrin Bronitin Mist Bronkaid Mist Epinephrine Epinephrine HCl Epinephrine Pediatric Epipen Epipen Jr. microNefrin Nephron Inhalant Primatene Mist S-2 Inhalant Sus-Phrine Vaponefrin
epinephrine HCl Classification: Adrenergic agonist	Adrenalin Chloride
epinephrine HCl, ophthalmic Classification: Adrenergic agonist	Epifrin Epinephrine HCl Glaucon
epinephryl borate Classification: Adrenergic agonist	Epinal
epoetin alfa (erythropoietin, EPO) Classification: Hormone; amino acid polypeptide	Epogen Eprex* Procrit
epoetin beta Classification: Hormone; amino acid polypeptide (Orphan)	Marogen
epoprostenol sodium Classification: Antihypertensive	Flolan

GENERIC NAME	BRAND NAME

eprosartan
Classification:
Antihypertensive; angiotension II
antagonist

Teveten

eptifibatide
Classification:
Antiplatelet

Integrilin

ergocalciferol (D$_2$)
Classification:
Vitamin, fat soluble

Calciferol
Calciferol Drops
Drisdol
Drisdol Drops

ergoloid mesylates
Classification:
Ergot alkaloid

Ergoloid Mesylates
Gerimal
Hydergine
Hydergine LC

ergonovine maleate
Classification:
Oxytocic

Ergotrate Maleate

ergotamine tartrate
Classification:
Antimigraine; ergot alkaloid

Ergomar

erwinia asparaginase
Classification:
Antineoplastic (Investigational)

Erwinia Asparaginase

erythromycin base
Classification:
Antibiotic; macrolide

E-Base
E-Mycin
Eryc
Ery-Tab
Erythromycin
Erythromycin Base
Erythromycin Filmtabs
Novorythro*
PCE Dispertab
Robimycin Robitabs

erythromycin estolate
Classification:
Antibiotic; macrolide

Erythromid*
Erythromycin Estolate
Ilosone
Ilosone Pulvules

GENERIC NAME	BRAND NAME
erythromycin ethylsuccinate Classification: Antibiotic; macrolide	E.E.S. 200 E.E.S. 400 EryPed EryPed 200 EryPed 400 Erythromycin Ethylsuccinate
erythromycin IV Classification: Antibiotic; macrolide	Erythromycin Lactobionate Ilotycin Gluceptate
erythromycin, ophthalmic Classification: Antibiotic; macrolide	Erythromycin Ilotycin
erythromycin stearate Classification: Antibiotic; macrolide	Eramycin Erythrocin Stearate Erythromycin Stearate
erythromycin, topical Classification: Anti-acne product	A/T/S Akne-mycin C-Solve 2 Del-Mycin Emgel Erycette Eryderm 2% Erygel Erymax Ery-Sol Erythra-Derm Erythromycin Romycin Staticin Theramycin Z T-Stat
esmolol HCl Classification: Beta-adrenergic blocker	Brevibloc
estazolam Classification: Sedative-hypnotic; benzodiazepine	Estazolam ProSom
estradiol cypionate Classification: Estrogen	depGynogen Depo Estradiol Depogen Estradiol Cypionate Estro-Cyp

*Available in Canada only

GENERIC NAME	BRAND NAME
estradiol vaginal ring Classification: Estrogen	Estring
estradiol, oral Classification: Estrogen	Estrace
estradiol, transdermal system Classification: Estrogen	Climara Estraderm FemPatch Vivelle
estradiol valerate Classification: Estrogen	Delestrogen Dioval 40 Dioval XX Estradiol Valerate Estra-L 20 Estra-L 40 Gynogen L.A. "20" Valergen 20 Valergen 40
estramustine phosphate sodium Classification: Antineoplastic; hormone	Emcyt
estrogenic substance or estrogens aqueous suspension Classification: Estrogen	Estrogenic Substance Aqueous
estrogens, conjugated Classification: Estrogen	C.E.S.* Premarin Premarin Intravenous
estrogens, esterified Classification: Estrogen	Climestrone* Estratab Menest Neo-Estrone*
estrone Classification: Estrogen	Aquest Estrone Aqueous Estrone-5 Femogen Forte* Kestrone-5

*Available in Canada Only

GENERIC NAME	BRAND NAME
estropipate Classification: Estrogen	Estropipate Ogen Ortho-Est
ethacrynate sodium/ethacrynic acid Classification: Loop diuretic	Edecrin Edecrin Sodium
ethambutol HCl Classification: Antitubercular	Etibi* Myambutol
ethanolamine oleate Classification: Sclerosing agent	Ethamolin
ethchlorvynol Classification: Sedative-hypnotic; nonbarbiturate	Placidyl
ethinyl estradiol Classification: Estrogen	Estinyl
ethiodized oil Classification: Radiopaque agent	Ethiodol
ethionamide Classification: Antitubercular	Trecator-SC
ethosuximide Classification: Anticonvulsant; succinimide	Ethosuximide Zarontin
ethotoin Classification: Anticonvulsant; hydantoin	Peganone
etidocaine HCl Classification: Local anesthetic	Duranest Duranest MPF
etidronate disodium, oral Classification: Bone resorption inhibitor	Didronel

GENERIC NAME	BRAND NAME

etidronate disodium, parenteral
Classification:
Bone resorption inhibitor

Didronel IV

etiocholanedione
Classification:
Blood modifier (Orphan)

Etiocholanedione

etodolac
Classification:
Nonsteroidal anti-inflammatory

Etodolac
Lodine
Lodine XL

etomidate
Classification:
General anesthetic

Amidate

etoposide (VP-16-213)
Classification:
Antineoplastic; mitotic inhibitor

Etopophos
Etoposide
Toposar
VePesid

etretinate
Classification:
Antipsoriatic

Tegison

examestane
Classification:
Antineoplastic (Orphan)

Exemestane

F

factor IX complex (human)
Classification:
Hemostatic

AlphaNine SD
Benefix
Hemonyne
Konyne 80
Mononine
Profilnine SD
Proplex T

factor VIIIa (Recombinant, DNA origin)
Classification:
Hemostatic (Orphan)

Factor VIIIa (recombinant, DNA origin)

factor XIII (plasma derived)
Classification:
Hemostatic (Orphan)

Fibrogammin P

GENERIC NAME	BRAND NAME
famiciclovir Classification: Antiviral	Famvir
famotidine Classification: Histamine H_2 receptor antagonist	Pepcid Pepcid AC Acid Controller Pepcid IV
fampridine Classification: Anti-multiple sclerosis agent (Orphan)	Neurelan
fat emulsions Classification: Caloric, fat	Intralipid 10% Intralipid 20% Liposyn II 10% Liposyn II 20% Liposyn III 10% Liposyn III 20%
felbamate Classification: Anticonvulsant	Felbatol
felodipine Classification: Calcium channel blocker	Plendil
fenofibrate Classification: Antilipemic	Tricor
fenoldopam Classification: Antihypertensive	Corlopam
fenoprofen calcium Classification: Nonsteroidal anti-inflammatory	Fenoprofen Nalfon
fenretinide Classification: Retinoid (Investigational)	Fenretinide
fentanyl citrate Classification: Opioid analgesic	Fentanyl Sublimaze
fentanyl transdermal Classification: Opioid analgesic	Duragesic-25 Duragesic-50 Duragesic-75 Duragesic-100

*Available in Canada only

GENERIC NAME	BRAND NAME

fentanyl transmucosal system
Classification:
Opioid analgesic

Fentanyl Oralet

ferrous fumarate
Classification:
Iron preparation

Femiron
Feostat
Ferrets
Ferrous Fumarate
Fumasorb
Fumerin
Hemocyte
Ircon
Nephro-Fer
Span-FF

ferrous gluconate
Classification:
Iron preparation

Fergon
Ferralet
Ferralet Slow Release
Ferrous Gluconate
Simron

ferrous sulfate
Classification:
Iron preparation

Fe^{50}
Feosol
Feratab
Fer-In-Sol
Fer-Iron
Fero-Gradumet
Ferospace
Ferralyn Lanacaps
Ferra-TD
Ferrous Sulfate
Mol-Iron
Slow-Fe

fexofenadine HCl
Classification:
Antihistamine

Allegra

fiacitabine (FIAC)
Classification:
Antiviral (Investigational)

Fiacitabine (FIAC)

fialuridine (FIAU)
Classification:
Antiviral (Investigational)

Fialuridine (FIAU)

fibrinogen (human)
Classification:
Hemostatic (Orphan)

Fibrinogen (human)

GENERIC NAME	BRAND NAME

filgrastim (granulocyte colony stimulating factor, G-CSF)
Classification:
Biologic modifier

Neupogen

finasteride
Classification:
Androgen inhibitor

Propecia
Proscar

fire ant venom, allergenic extract, imported
Classification:
Biologic response modifier (Orphan)

Fire Ant Venom, Allergenic Extract,
Imported

FK-565
Classification:
Biologic response modifier
(Investigational)

FK-565

flavoxate HCl
Classification:
Urinary antispasmodic

Urispas

flecainide acetate
Classification:
Antiarrhythmic

Tambocor

flexible hydroactive dressings and granules
Classification:
Debriding agent

Duoderm
Shur-Clens
Sorbsan

floxuridine
Classification:
Antineoplastic; antimetabolite

Floxuridine
FUDR

fluconazole
Classification:
Antifungal; bis-triazole

Diflucan

flucytosine
Classification:
Antifungal; pyrimidine

Ancobon
Ancotil*

fludarabine
Classification:
Antineoplastic; antimetabolite

Fludara

fludrocortisone acetate
Classification:
Mineralocorticoid

Florinef Acetate

*Available in Canada only

GENERIC NAME	BRAND NAME

flumazenil
Classification:
Benzodiazepine antagonist

Romazicon

flumecinol
Classification:
Anti-hyperbilirubinemia agent (Orphan)

Zixoryn

flunarizine
Classification:
Calcium channel blocker (Orphan)

Sibelium

flunisolide
Classification:
Glucocorticoid

AeroBid
AeroBid-M
Bronalide*

flunisolide, nasal
Classification:
Glucocorticoid

Nasalide
Nasarel
Rhinalar*

fluocinolone acetonide
Classification:
Glucocorticoid

Derma-Smoothe/FS
Fluincinolone
Fluonid
Flurosyn
FS Shampoo
Synalar
Synalar-HP
Synemol

fluocinonide
Classification:
Glucocorticoid

Fluocinonide
Fluocinonide "E" Cream
Fluonex
Lidemol*
Lidex
Lidex-E

fluorescein sodium
Classification:
Ophthalmic diagnostic

AK-Fluor
Fluorescein Sodium
Fluorescite
Fluorets
Fluor-I-Strip
Fluor-I-Strip-A.T.
Ful-Glo
Funduscein-10
Funduscein-25
Ophthifluor

fluorexon
Classification:
Ophthalmic diagnostic

Fluoresoft

*Available in Canada Only

GENERIC NAME	BRAND NAME

fluoride
(See sodium fluoride)

fluorometholone
Classification:
Ophthalmic glucocorticoid

Flarex
Fluor-Op
FML
FML Forte
FML S.O.P.

fluorothymidine (FLT)
Classification:
Antiviral (Investigational)

Flurothymidine (FLT)

fluorouracil (5-fluorouracil;
5-FU)
Classification:
Antineoplastic; antimetabolite

Adrucil
Fluorouracil

fluorouracil, topical
Classification:
Antineoplastic

Efudex
Fluoroplex

fluoxetine
Classification:
Antidepressant

Prozac

fluoxymesterone
Classification:
Androgen

Fluoxymesterone
Halotestin

fluphenazine HCl
Classification:
Antipsychotic

Fluphenazine HCl
Permitil
Prolixin

fluphenazine enanthate and
decanoate
Classification:
Antipsychotic

Fluphenazine Decanoate
Prolixin Decanoate
Prolixin Enanthate

flurandrenolide
Classification:
Glucocorticoid

Cordran
Cordran SP
Cordran Tape
Drenison ¼*
Drenison Tape*
Flurandrenolide

flurazepam HCl
Classification:
Sedative-hypnotic; benzodiazepine

Dalmane
Flurazepam
Somnol*

GENERIC NAME	BRAND NAME

flurbiprofen
Classification:
Nonsteroidal anti-inflammatory

Ansaid
Flurbiprofen

flurbiprofen sodium
Classification:
Ophthalmic nonsteroidal anti-inflammatory

Flurbiprofen Sodium Ophthalmic
Ocufen

flutamide
Classification:
Antineoplastic; antiandrogen

Euflex*
Eulexin

fluticasone propionate, nasal
Classification:
Glucocorticoid

Flonase

fluticasone propionate
Classification:
Glucocorticoid

Flovent
Flovent Rotadisk

fluticasone propionate, topical
Classification:
Glucocorticoid

Cutivate

fluvastatin
Classification:
Antilipemic

Lescol

fluvoxamine maleate
Classification:
Antidepressant

Luvox

folic acid (folacin, folate)
Classification:
Vitamin B complex group

Folic Acid
Folvite
Novofolacid*

follitropin alpha
Classification:
Ovulation stimulant

Gonal-F

follitropin beta
Classification:
Ovulation stimulant

Follistim

fomepizole
Classification:
Antidote

Antizol

foscarnet sodium
Classification:
Antiviral

Foscavir

*Available in Canada Only

GENERIC NAME	BRAND NAME

fosfomycin tromethamine
Classification:
Urinary anti-infective

Monurol

fosinopril sodium
Classification:
Antihypertensive, angiotensin converting
enzyme inhibitor

Monopril

fosphenytoin sodium
Classification:
Anticonvulsant; hydantoin

Cerebyx

furazolidone
Classification:
Antibiotic, broad spectrum

Furoxone

furosemide
Classification:
Loop diuretic

Furosemide
Lasix
Novosemide*
Uritol*

G

gabapentin
Classification:
Anticonvulsant

Neurontin

**gadopentetate dimeglumine
46.9%**
Classification:
Radiopaque agent

Magnevist

gadoteridol
Classification:
Radiopaque agent

ProHance

gallium nitrate
Classification:
Bone resorption inhibitor

Ganite

gamma-hydroxybutyrate
Classification:
CNS stimulant (Orphan)

Gamma-hydroxybutyrate

gammalinolenic acid
Classification:
Antirheumatic (Orphan)

Gammalinolenic Acid

GENERIC NAME	BRAND NAME

ganaxolone
Classification:
Antispasmodic (Orphan)

Ganaxolone

ganciclovir sodium (DHPG)
Classification:
Antiviral

Cytovene
Vitrasert

gelsolin, recombinant human
Classification:
Respiratory agent (Orphan)

Gelsolin, recombinant human

gemcitabine HCl
Classification:
Antineoplastic, miscellaneous

Gemzar

gemfibrozil
Classification:
Antilipemic

Apo-Gemfibrozil*
Gemfibrozil
Lopid
Novo-Gemfibrozil*

genevax-HIV-Px
Classification:
Vaccine (Investigational)

Genevax-HIV-Px

**gentamicin impregnated
PMMA beads**
Classification:
Antibiotic; aminoglycoside (Orphan)

Septopal

gentamicin liposome
Classification:
Antibiotic; aminoglycoside (Orphan)

Maitec

gentamicin sulfate
Classification:
Aminoglycoside

Alcomicin*
Cidomycin*
Garamycin
Garamycin Intrathecal
Garamycin Pediatric
Gentamicin Sulfate
Jenamicin
Pediatric Gentamicin Sulfate

gentamicin sulfate, ophthalmic
Classification:
Aminoglycoside

Garamycin
Genoptic
Genoptic S.O.P.
Gentacidin
Gentak
Gentamicin Ophthalmic

*Available in Canada Only

GENERIC NAME	BRAND NAME
gentamicin sulfate, topical Classification: Aminoglycoside	G-myticin Garamycin Gentamicin
gepirone HCl Classification: Antianxiety (Investigational)	Gepirone HCl
glatiramer acetate Classification: Biologic response modifier	Copaxone
glimepiride Classification: Antidiabetic; sulfonylurea	Amaryl
glipizide Classification: Antidiabetic; sulfonylurea	Glipizide Glucotrol Glucotrol XL
glucagon Classification: Glucose elevating agent	Glucagon
glucocerebrosidase, recombinant retroviral Classification: Enzyme (Orphan)	Glucocerebrosidase, redcombinant retriviral
glucose Classification: Glucose elevating agent	B-D Glucose Dex4 Glucose Glutose Insta-Glucose Insulin Reaction
glucose, ophthalmic Classification: Hyperosmolar preparation	Glucose-40
glutamic acid HCl Classification: Gastric acidifier	Glutamic Acid HCl
glutaraldehyde Classification: Germicidal	Cidex Cidex-7 Cidex Plus 28
glutethimide Classification: Sedative-hypnotic; nonbarbiturate	Glutethimide

*Available in Canada only

GENERIC NAME	BRAND NAME
glyburide Classification: Antidiabetic; sulfonylurea	DiaBeta Glyburide Glynase Prestab Micronase Micronized Glyburide
glycerin (glycerol) Classification: Hyperosmotic	Fleet Babylax Glycerin USP Osmoglyn Sani-Supp
glycerin ophthalmic Classification: Hyperosmolar preparation	Ophthalgan
glycopyrrolate Classification: Anticholinergic	Glycopyrrolate Robinul Robinul Forte
gold sodium thiomalate Classification: Gold compound	Aurolate
gonadorelin acetate Classification: Gonadotrophin releasing hormone	Lutrepulse
gonadorelin HCl Classification: Hormone	Factrel
goserelin acetate Classification: Antineoplastic; hormone	Zoladex
gossypol Classification: Antineoplastic (Orphan)	Gossypol
gp 120 vaccine Classification: Vaccine (Investigational)	Remune
gp 160 vaccine Classification: Vaccine (Investigational)	gp 160 Vaccine
granisetron Classification: Antiemetic	Kytril

*Available in Canada Only

GENERIC NAME	BRAND NAME

grepafloxacin
Classification:
Antibiotic; fluoroquinolone

Raxar

griseofulvin microsize
Classification:
Antifungal

Fulvicin U/F
Grifulvin V
Grisactin
Grisactin 500

griseofulvin ultramicrosize
Classification:
Antifungal

Fulvicin P/G
Grisactin Ultra
Gris-PEG
Ultramicrosize Griseofulvin

guaifenesin
Classification:
Expectorant

Anti-Tuss
Balminil*
Breonesin
Diabetic Tussin EX
Duratuss-G
Fenesin
Gee-Gee
Genatuss
GG-Cen
Glyate
Glycotuss
Glytuss
Guaifenesin
Guaifenex LA
Guiatuss
Halotussin
Humibid Sprinkle
Humibid L.A.
Hytuss
Hytuss 2X
Liquibid
Monafed
Muco-Fen-LA
Mytussin
Naldecon Senior EX
Organidin NR
Pneumomist
Respa-GF
Resyl*
Robitussin
Scot-tussin Expectorant
Siltussin
Sinumist-SR
Touro Ex

*Available in Canada only

GENERIC NAME	BRAND NAME

**guaifenesin
(cont'd.)**

Tusibron
Uni-tussin

guanabenz acetate
Classification:
Antihypertensive, centrally acting

Guanabenz Acetate
Wytensin

guanadrel sulfate
Classification:
Antihypertensive

Hylorel

guanethidine monosulfate
Classification:
Antihypertensive

Ismelin

guanfacine HCl
Classification:
Antihypertensive, centrally acting

Tenex

guanidine HCl
Classification:
Cholinergic muscle stimulant

Guanidine HCl

gusperimus
Classification:
Immunosuppressive (Orphan)

Gusperimus

H

halazepam
Classification:
Antianxiety; benzodiazepine

Paxipam

halcinonide
Classification:
Glucocorticoid

Halog
Halog-E

halobetasol propionate
Classification:
Glucocorticoid

Ultravate

halofantrine
Classification:
Antimalarial (Orphan)

Halofantrine

haloperidol
Classification:
Antipsychotic

Haldol
Haloperidol

GENERIC NAME	BRAND NAME
haloperidol decanoate Classification: Antipsychotic	Haldol Decanoate 50 Haldol Decanoate 100
haloprogin Classification: Antifungal	Halotex
halothane Classification: General anesthetic	Fluothane Halothane
hamamelis water (witch hazel) Classification: Astringent	A-E-R Tucks Witch Hazel
heme arginate Classification: Blood modifier (Orphan)	Normosang
hemin Classification: Antiporphyrial	Panhematin
hemophilus b conjugate vaccine Classification: Vaccine	ActHIB HibTITER OmniHIB Pedvax HIB ProHIBiT
heoxprenaline sulfate Classification: Tocolytic (Investigational)	Delaprem
heparin calcium Classification: Anticoagulant	Calcilean* Hepalean*

heparin sodium and sodium chloride
Classification:
Anticoagulant
	Heparin Sodium and 0.45% Sodium
	    Chloride
	Heparin Sodium and 0.90% Sodium
	    Chloride

heparin sodium injection, USP Classification: Anticoagulant	Heparin Lock Flush Heparin Sodium Hep-Lock
hepatitis A vaccine, inactivated Classification: Vaccine	Havrix VAQTA

GENERIC NAME	BRAND NAME

hepatitis B immune globulin (HBIG)
Classification:
Immune serum

H-BIG
Hep-B-Gammagee
HyperHep

hepatitis B immune globulin, intravenous
Classification:
Immune serum (Orphan)

H-BIGIV

hepatitis B vaccine
Classification:
Vaccine

Engerix-B
Recombivax HB

hetastarch
Classification:
Plasma volume expander

Hespan

hexchlorophene
Classification:
Germicidal

pHisoHex
Septisol Foam

histoplasmin
Classification:
In vivo diagnostic

Histolyn-CYL
Histoplasmin, Diluted

histrelin acetate
Classification:
Gonadotropin-releasing hormone

Supprelin

HIV vaccine
Classification:
Vaccine (Investigational)

Apollon
Genevax
HIV Vaccine

homatropine hydrobromide, ophthalmic
Classification:
Mydriatic

AK-Homatropine
Homatropine HBr
Isopto Homatropine

human immunodeficiency virus immune globulin
Classification:
Immune serum (Orphan)

Hivig

hyaluronidase
Classification:
Enzyme

Wydase

hydralazine HCl
Classification:
Antihypertensive, vasodilator

Apresoline
Hydralazine HCl

GENERIC NAME	BRAND NAME
hydrochlorothiazide Classification: Thiazide diuretic	Diuchlor H* Esidrix Ezide Hydro-Par Hydrochlorothiazide HydroDIURIL Hydrozide* Microzide Neo-Codema* Novohydrazide* Oretic Urozide*
hydrocortisone (cortisol) Classification: Glucocorticoid	Cortamed* Cortef Hydrocortisone Hydrocortone
hydrocortisone acetate Classification: Glucocorticoid	Anucort-HC Anumed HC Anusol-HC Anusol HC-1 CaldeCort CaldeCort Light with Aloe Cort-Dome High Potency Cortaid with Aloe Cortef Feminine Itch Corticaine Gynecort-5 Gynecort 10 Hemorrhoidal HC Hemril-HC Uniserts Hydrocortisone Acetate Hydrocortone Acetate Lanacort 5 Lanacort 10 Maximum Strength Cortaid U-Cort
hydrocortisone acetate intrarectal foam Classification: Glucocorticoid	Cortifoam
hydrocortisone buteprate Classification: Glucocorticoid	Pandel

*Available in Canada only

GENERIC NAME	BRAND NAME

hydrocortisone butyrate
Classification:
Glucocorticoid

Locoid

hydrocortisone cypionate
Classification:
Glucocorticoid

Cortef

hydrocortisone retention enema
Classification:
Glucocorticoid

Cortenema

hydrocortisone sodium phosphate
Classification:
Glucocorticoid

Hydrocortone Phosphate

hydrocortisone sodium succinate
Classification:
Glucocorticoid

A-Hydrocort
Solu-Cortef

hydrocortisone, topical
Classification:
Glucocorticoid

1% HC
Acticort 100
Aeroseb-HC
Ala-Cort
Ala-Scalp
Anusol-HC 2.5%
Bactine Hydrocortisone
CaldeCort Anti-Itch
Cetacort
Cortaid
Cortaid Intensive Therapy
Cort-Dome
CortaGel
Cortizone-5
Cortizone-10
Dermacort
Dermol-HC
Dermolate
Dermtex HC With Aloe
Extra Strength CortaGel
Hi-Cor 1.0
Hi-Cor 2.5
Hycort
Hydrocort
Hydrocortisone
HydroTex
Hytone

GENERIC NAME	BRAND NAME
hydrocortisone, topical (cont'd.)	LactiCare-HC
	Maximum Strength Bactine
	Maximum Strength Cortaid Spray
	Maximum Strength Corticaine
	Nutracort
	Penecort
	Proctocort
	ProtoCream-HC
	Scalpicin
	S-T Cort
	Synacort
	Tegrin-HC
	Texacort
	T/Scalp

hydrocortisone valerate
Classification:
Glucocorticoid

Westcort

hydroflumethiazide
Classification:
Thiazide diuretic

Diucardin
Hydroflumethiazide
Saluron

hydromorphone HCl
Classification:
Opioid analgesic

Dilaudid
Dilaudid-5
Dilaudid-HP
Hydromorphone HCl
HydroStat IR

hydroquinone
Classification:
Depigmentation agent

Ambi Skin Tone
Eldopaque
Eldopaque-Forte
Eldoquin
Eldoquin-Forte
Esoterica Facial
Esoterica Fortified
Esoterica Regular
Esoterica Sensitive Skin Formula
Esoterica Sunscreen
Melanex
Porcelana
Porcelana with Sunscreen
Solaquin
Solaquin Forte

hydroxyamphetamine HBr
Classification:
Ophthalmic vasoconstrictor

Paredrine

GENERIC NAME	BRAND NAME

hydroxychloroquine sulfate
Classification:
Antimalarial

Hydroxychloroquine Sulfate
Plaquenil Sulfate

hydroxycobalamin (vitamin B$_{12a}$)
Classification:
Vitamin, water soluble

Acti-B$_{12}$*
Hydro Cobex
Hydro-Crysti 12
Hydroxycobalamin
LA-12

hydroxyethylcellulose
Classification:
Gonioscopic aid

Gonioscopic

hydroxyprogesterone caproate
Classification:
Progestin

Hylutin
Hydroxyprogesterone Caproate

hydroxypropylmethylcellulose
Classification:
Ophthalmic viscoelastic

Gonak
Goniosol
Ocucoat

hydroxyurea
Classification:
Antineoplastic, miscellaneous

Droxia
Hydrea

hydroxyzine
Classification:
Antianxiety

Anxanil
Atarax
Atarax 100
E-Vista
Hydroxyzine HCl
Hydroxyzine Pamoate
Hyzine-50
Quiess
Vistacon
Vistaril
Vistazine 50

hylan G-F 20
Classification:
Viscoelastic; intra-articular

Synvisc

hyoscyamine sulfate
Classification:
GI anticholinergic

A-Spas S/L
Anaspaz
Cystospaz
Cystospaz-M
Donnamar
ED-SPAZ
Gastrosed
Hyoscyamine Sulfate

GENERIC NAME	BRAND NAME
hyoscyamine sulfate (cont'd.)	Levbid Levsin Levsin Drops Levsin S/L Levsinex Timecaps Neoquess
hypericin Classification: Antiviral (Investigational)	VIMRxyn
hysteroscopy fluid Classification: In vivo diagnostic	Hyskon

I

I-123 murine monoclonal antibody to alpha-fetoprotein Classification: In vivo diagnostic (Orphan)	I-123 murine monoclonal antibody to alpha-fetoprotein
I-123 murine monoclonal antibody to hCG Classification: In vivo diagnostic (Orphan)	I-123 murine monoclonal antibody hCG
I-131 6B-iodomethyl-19-norcholesterol Classification: In vivo diagnostic (Orphan)	I-131 6B-iodomethyl-19-norcholesterol
I-131 murine monoclonal antibody IgG2a to B cell Classification: In vivo diagnostic (Orphan)	I-131 murine monoclonal antibody IgG2a to B cell
I-131 murine monoclonal antibody to alpha-fetoprotein Classification: In vivo diagnostic (Orphan)	I-131 murine monoclonal antibody to alpha-fetoprotein
I-131 murine monoclonal antibody to hCG Classification: In vivo diagnostic (Orphan)	I-131 murine monoclonal antibody to hCG
I-131 radiolabeled B1 monoclonal antibody Classification: Antineoplastic (Orphan)	I-131 radiolabeled B1 monoclonal antibody

*Available in Canada only

GENERIC NAME	BRAND NAME

ibuprofen
Classification:
Nonsteroidal anti-inflammatory

Advil
Advil Junior Strength
Bayer Select Pain Relief Formula
Children's Advil
Children's Motrin
Dynafed IB
Genpril
Haltran
IBU
Ibuprin
Ibuprofen
Ibuprohm
Menadol
Midol IB
Motrin
Motrin IB
Motrin Junior Strength
Nuprin
Saleto-200
Saleto-400
Saleto-600
Saleto-800

ibutilide fumarate
Classification:
Antiarrhythmic

Corvert

idarubicin HCl
Classification:
Antineoplastic; antibiotic

Idamycin
Idamycin PFS

idoxuridine
Classification:
Antineoplastic (Orphan)

Idoxuridine

ifosfamide
Classification:
Antineoplastic; alkylating agent

Ifex

IgG monoclonal anti-CD4 (M-T412)
Classification:
Biologic response modifier (Orphan)

IgG monoclonal anti-CD4 (M-T412)

IgG monoclonal anti-TNF antibody (cA2)
Classification:
Biologic response modifier (Orphan)

IgG monoclonal anti-TNF antibody (cA2)

*Available in Canada Only

GENERIC NAME	BRAND NAME
imiciromab pentetate Classification: In vivo diagnostic (Orphan)	Myoscint
imiglucerase Classification: Enzyme	Cerezyme
imipenem-cilastatin Classification: Antibiotic; carbapenem	Primaxin I.M. Primaxin I.V.
imipramine HCl Classification: Antidepressant	Imipramine HCl Impril* Novopramine* Tofranil
imipramine pamoate Classification: Antidepressant	Tofranil-PM
imiquimod Classification: Biologic response modifier	Aldara
immune globulin, intravenous (IGIV) Classification: Immune serum	Gamimune N Gammagard S/D Gammar P.I.V. Iveegam Polygam S/D Sandoglobulin Venoglobulin-I
immune globulin, intramuscular (IG; gamma globulin; ISG) Classification: Immune serum	Immune Globulin, Intramuscular
imreg-1 Classification: Biologic response modifier (Investigational)	Imreg-1
indapamide Classification: Thiazide diuretic	Indipamide Lozide* Lozol
indigotin disulfonate sodium injection Classification: In vivo diagnostic	Indigo Carmine Solution

*Available in Canada only

GENERIC NAME	BRAND NAME

indinavir sulfate
Classification:
Antiviral; protease inhibitor

Crixivan

indocyanine green
Classification:
In vivo diagnostic

Cardio-Green

indomethacin
Classification:
Nonsteroidal anti-inflammatory

Indocin
Indocin SR
Indochron E-R
Indomethacin
Indomethacin SR

indomethacin sodium trihydrate
Classification:
Nonsteroidal anti-inflammatory

Indocin I.V.

infliximab
Classification:
Biologic response modifier
(Investigational)

Avakine

influenza virus vaccine
Classification:
Vaccine

Fluogen
FluShield
Fluvirin
Fluviral*
Fluzone

inosine pranobex
Classification:
Biologic response modifier (Orphan)

Isoprinosine

insulin injection
Classification:
Antidiabetic

Humulin R
Humulin-R*
Iletin*
Iletin II*
Novolin ge Toronto*
Novolin R
Novolin R Penfill
Pork Regular Iletin II
Regular Iletin I
Regular Insulin
Regular Purified Pork Insulin
Velosulin Human

insulin injection concentrated iletin
Classification:
Antidiabetic

Iletin II U-500 Regular (Concentrated)

GENERIC NAME	BRAND NAME
insulin lispro Classification: Antidiabetic	Humalog
insulin, isophane suspension (NPH) Classification: Antidiabetic	Humulin N Iletin NPH* Iletin II NPH* Novolin ge NPH* Novolin N Novolin N Penfill NPH Iletin I NPH Insulin NPH-N Pork NPH Iletin II
insulin, isophane suspension and insulin injection Classification: Antidiabetic	Humulin 30/70* Humulin 50/50 Humulin 70/30 Novolin ge 30/70* Novolin ge 50/50* Novolin 70/30 Novolin 70/30 PenFill
insulin, protamine zinc suspension (PZI) Classification: Antidiabetic	Iletin PZI*
insulin, zinc suspension extended (ultralente) Classification: Antidiabetic	Humulin-U* Humulin U Ultralente Iletin Ultralente* Novolin ge Ultralente*
insulin, zinc suspension (lente) Classification: Antidiabetic	Humulin L Iletin L* Iletin II L* Lentard Monotard* Lente Iletin I Lente Iletin II Lente Insulin Novolin ge Lente* Novolin L
insulin-like growth factor-I Classification: Growth hormone (Orphan)	Myotrophin

GENERIC NAME	BRAND NAME
insulin-like growth factor-I (recombinant human) Classification: Growth hormone (Orphan)	IGF-I
interferon alfacon-1 Classification: Biologic response modifier	Infergen
interferon alfa-2a (rIFN-A; IFLrA) Classification: Antineoplastic; biologic response modifier	Roferon-A
interferon alfa-2b (IFN-alpha 2; rIFN- 2; 2-interferon) Classification: Antineoplastic; biologic response modifier	Intron A
interferon alfa-n1 Classification: Biologic response modifier (Orphan)	Wellferon
interferon alfa-n3 Classification: Antineoplastic; biologic response modifier	Alferon LDO Alferon N
interferon beta-1A Classification: Biologic response modifier	Avonex
interferon beta-lB (rIFN-B) Classification: Biologic response modifier	Betaseron
interferon beta (recombinant human) Classification: Antineoplastic; biologic response modifier (Orphan)	Interferon beta (recombinant human)
interferon beta (recombinant) Classification: Antineoplastic; biologic response modifier (Orphan)	R-IFN-beta

*Available in Canada Only

GENERIC NAME	BRAND NAME
interferon beta-1a Classification: Antimultiple sclerosis agent (Investigational)	Rebif
interferon gamma-1B Classification: Biologic response modifier	Actimmune
interleukin-1 receptor antagonist (recombinant human) Classification: Biologic response modifier (Orphan)	Antril
interleukin-2 PEG Classification: Biologic response modifier (Investigational)	Interleukin-2 PEG
interleukin-2, recombinant liposome encapsulated Classification: Antineoplastic; biologic response modifier (Orphan)	Interleukin-2, recombinant liposome encapsulated
interleukin-3, recombinant human Classification: Biologic response modifier (Investigational)	Interleukin-3, recombinant human
intravascular perfluoro-chemical emulsion Classification: Perfluorochemical emulsion	Fluosol
inulin Classification: In vivo diagnostic	Inulin Injection
iobenguane sulfate I-131 Classification: In vivo diagnostic (Orphan)	Iobenguane sulfate I-131
iocetamic acid Classification: Radiopaque agent	Cholebrine
iodamide meglumine 24% Classification: Radiopaque agent	Renovue-Dip

*Available in Canada only

GENERIC NAME	BRAND NAME

iodamide meglumine 65%
Classification:
Radiopaque agent

Renovue-65

iodinated glycerol
Classification:
Expectorant

Iophen
Organidin
Par Glycerol
R-Gen

iodine products
Classification:
Antithyroid

Iodine Tincture
Iodine Topical Solution
Idopen
Iodotope
Pima
Potassium Iodide
Sodium Iodide
SSKI
Strong Iodine Solution (Lugol's
   Solution)
Strong Iodine Tincture
Thyro-Block

**iodipamide meglumine 10.3%
and 52%**
Classification:
Radiopaque agent

Cholografin Meglumine

iodixanol
Classification:
Radiopaque agent

Visipaque

iodochlorhydroxyquin
Classification:
Antifungal

Vioform

iodoquinol (diiodohydroxyquin)
Classification:
Amebicide

Diodoquin*
Yodoxin

iohexol
Classification:
Radiopaque agent

Omnipaque

iopamidol 26%
Classification:
Radiopaque agent

Isovue-128

iopamidol 41%
Classification:
Radiopaque agent

Isovue-200
Isovue-M 200

*Available in Canada Only

GENERIC NAME	BRAND NAME
iopamidol 61% Classification: Radiopaque agent	Isovue-300 Isovue-M 300
iopamidol 76% Classification: Radiopaque agent	Isovue-370
iopanoic acid Classification: Radiopaque agent	Telepaque
iopromide Classification: Radiopaque agent	Ultravist
iothalamate meglumine 17.2% Classification: Radiopaque agent	Cysto-Conray II
iothalamate meglumine 30% Classification: Radiopaque agent	Conray-30
iothalamate meglumine 43% Classification: Radiopaque agent	Conray 43 Cysto-Conray
iothalamate meglumine 60% Classification: Radiopaque agent	Conray
iothalamate meglumine 52% and iothalamate sodium 26% Classification: Radiopaque agent	Vascoray
iothalamate sodium 54.3% Classification: Radiopaque agent	Conray 325
iothalamate sodium 66.8% Classification: Radiopaque agent	Conray 400
iothalamate sodium 80% Classification: Radiopaque agent	Angio Conray
ioversol 34% Classification: Radiopaque agent	Optiray 160

*Available in Canada only

GENERIC NAME	BRAND NAME
ioversol 51% Classification: Radiopaque agent	Optiray 240
ioversol 68% Classification: Radiopaque agent	Optiray 320
ioversol 74% Classification: Radiopaque agent	Optiray 350
ioxaglate meglumine 39.3% and ioxaglate sodium 19.6% Classification: Radiopaque agent	Hexabrix
ipecac syrup Classification: Emetic	Ipecac Syrup
ipodate calcium Classification: Radiopaque agent	Oragrafin Calcium
ipodate sodium Classification: Radiopaque agent	Oragrafin Sodium
ipratropium bromide Classification: Anticholinergic	Atrovent Ipratropium Bromide
irbesartan Classification: Antihypertensive; angiotensin II antagonist	Avapro
irinotecan HCl Classification: Antineoplastic; hormone	Camptosar
iron dextran Classification: Iron preparation	DexFerrum InFeD
iscador Classification: Antiviral (Investigational)	Iscador

GENERIC NAME	BRAND NAME
isobutyramide Classification: Blood modifier (Orphan)	Isobutyramide
isoetharine HCl Classification: Bronchodilator; beta-adrenergic agonist	Arm-a-Med Isoetharine HCl Beta-2 Bronkometer Bronkosol Isoetharine Hcl
isoflurane Classification: General anesthetic	Forane Isoflurane
isoniazid (INH) Classification: Antitubercular	Isoniazid Isotamine* Laniazid Laniazid C.T. Nydrazid PMS-Isoniazid*
isophane insulin suspension and insulin injection Classification: Antidiabetic	Humulin 70/30 Humulin 50/50 Novolin 70/30 Novolin 70/30 Penfill
isoproterenol Classification: Adrenergic agonist	Isuprel Isoproterenol HCl Isuprel Mistometer Medihaler-Iso
isosorbide Classification: Osmotic diuretic	Ismotic
isosorbide dinitrate, oral Classification: Antianginal	Coronex* Dilatrate-SR Isordil Tembids Isordil Titradose Isosorbide Dinitrate Sorbitrate Sorbitrate SA
isosorbide dinitrate sublingual and chewable Classification: Antianginal	Isordil Isosorbide Dinitrate Sorbitrate
isosorbide mononitrate Classification: Antianginal	Imdur ISMO Monoket

*Available in Canada only

GENERIC NAME	BRAND NAME
isosulfan blue Classification: Radiopaque agent	Lymphazurin 1%
isotretinoin (13-cis-Retinoic Acid) Classification: Anti-acne product	Accutane
isoxsuprine HCl Classification: Peripheral vasodilator	Isoxsuprine HCl Vasodilan Voxsuprine
isradipine Classification: Calcium channel blocker	DynaCirc
itraconazole Classification: Antifungal; triazole	Sporanox
ivermectin Classification: Anthelmintic	Stromectol

K

GENERIC NAME	BRAND NAME
kanamycin sulfate Classification: Aminoglycoside	Anamid* Kanamycin Sulfate Kantrex
ketamine HCl Classification: General anesthetic	Ketalar
ketoconazole Classification: Antifungal; imidazole	Nizoral
ketoconazole, topical Classification: Antifungal; imidazole	Nizoral
ketoprofen Classification: Nonsteroidal anti-inflammatory	Actron Ketoprofen Orudis Orudis KT Oruvail

*Available in Canada Only

GENERIC NAME	BRAND NAME

ketorolac tromethamine
Classification:
Nonsteroidal anti-inflammatory

Ketorolac Tromethamine
Toradol

ketorolac tromethamine, ophthalmic
Classification:
Ophthalmic nonsteroidal anti-inflammatory

Acular
Acular PF

KL4-surfactant
Classification:
Lung surfactant (Orphan)

KL4-surfactant

L

L-2-oxothiazolidine-4-carboxylic acid
Classification:
Amino acid (Orphan)

Procysteine

L-5 hydroxytryptophan
Classification:
Muscle stimulant (Orphan)

L-5 hydroxytryptophan

labetalol HCl
Classification:
Antihypertensive

Normodyne
Trandate

lacidipine
Classification:
Calcium channel blocker (Investigational)

Lacipil

lactase enzyme
Classification:
Food modifier

Dairy Ease
LactAid
Lactrase
SureLac

lactobacillus
Classification:
Antidiarrheal

Bacid
Kala
Lactinex
MoreDophilus
Pro-Bionate
Superdophilus

lactose
Classification:
Food modifier

Lactose

GENERIC NAME	BRAND NAME
lactulose Classification: Laxative	Cephulac Cholac Chronulac Constilac Constulose Duphalac Enulose Evalose Heptalac Lactulose
lamivudine (3TC) Classification: Antiviral; nucleoside	Epivir
lamotrigine Classification: Anticonvulsant	Lamictal
lansoprazole Classification: Antisecretory; benzimidazoles	Prevacid
latanoprost Classification: Prostaglandin	Xalatan
L-baclofen Classification: Skeletal muscle relaxant (Orphan)	Neuralgon
L-cycloserine Classification: Amino acid (Orphan)	L-cycloserine
L-cysteine Classification: Amino acid (Orphan)	L-cysteine
lentinan Classification: Biologic response modifier (Investigational)	Lentinan
lepirudin Classification: Thrombin inhibitor	Refludan
letrozole Classification: Antineoplastic; anti-estrogen	Femara

*Available in Canada Only

GENERIC NAME	BRAND NAME
leucovorin calcium (citrovorum factor; folinic acid) Classification: Folic acid antagonist	Leucovorin Calcium Wellcovorin
leuprolide acetate Classification: Antineoplastic; hormone	Lupron Lupron Depot Lupron Depot 3 Month Lupron Depot 4 Month Lupron Depot-Ped
levamisole HCl Classification: Antineoplastic, miscellaneous	Ergamisol
levobunolol HCl Classification: Beta-adrenergic blocker	AKBeta Betagan Liquifilm Levobunolol HCl
levocabastine HCl Classification: Ophthalmic antihistamine	Livostin
levocarnitine Classification: Amino acid	Carnitor L-Carnitine VitaCarn
levodopa Classification: Anti-Parkinson agent	Dopar Larodopa
levodopa/carbidopa Classification: Anti-Parkinson agent	Levodopa & Carbidopa Sinemet-10/100 Sinemet-25/100 Sinemet-25/250 Sinemet CR
levofloxacin Classification: Antibiotic; fluoroquinolone	Levaquin
levomethadyl acetate HCl Classification: Opioid agonist	ORLAAM
levonorgestrel implant Classification: Progestin, synthetic	Norplant System

GENERIC NAME	BRAND NAME
levorotatory alkaloids of belladonna Classification: Anticholinergic	Bellafoline
levorphanol tartrate Classification: Opioid analgesic	Levo-Dromoran
levothyroxine sodium (T4; L-thyroxine) Classification: Thyroid hormone	Eltroxin Levo-T Levothroid Levothyroxine Sodium Levoxine Levoxyl Synthroid
L-glutathione (reduced) Classification: Amino acid (Orphan)	Cachexon
lidocaine HCl Classification: Antiarrhythmic	Lidopen Auto-Injector

lidocaine HCl IV
Classification:
Antiarrhthymic
	Lidocaine HCl IV for Cardiac
	   Arrhythmias
	Xylocaine HCl IV for Cardiac
	   Arrhythmias

lidocaine HCl, local Classification: Local anesthetic	Dilocaine Duo-Trach Kit Lidocaine HCl Lidoject-1 Lidoject-2 Nervocaine 1% Octocaine HCl Xylocaine Xylocaine MPF
lidocaine HCl, topical Classification: Local anesthetic	Anestacon DermaFlex Lidocaine HCl Lidocaine Viscous Solarcaine Xylocaine Xylocaine Oral Xylocaine Viscous Zilactin-L

*Available in Canada Only

GENERIC NAME	BRAND NAME

lincomycin HCl
Classification:
Antibiotic; lincosamide

Lincocin
Lincorex

lindane (gamma benzene hexachloride)
Classification:
Scabicide; pediculicide

gBh*
G-well
Kwellada*
Lindane
Scabene

liposomal prostaglandin E1
Classification:
Prostaglandin (Orphan)

Liposomal prostaglandin E1

liothyronine sodium (T3)
Classification:
Thyroid hormone

Cytomel
Liothyronine Sodium
Triostat

liotrix
Classification:
Thyroid hormone

Thyrolar

lisinopril
Classification:
Antihypertensive; angiotensin converting enzyme inhibitor

Prinivil
Zestril

lithium carbonate
Classification:
Antimanic

Carbolith*
Eskalith
Eskalith CR
Lithane
Lithium Carbonate
Lithonate
Lithotabs

lithium citrate
Classification:
Antimanic

Lithium Citrate

liver derivative complex
Classification:
Anti-inflammatory

Kutapressin

L-leucovorin
Classification:
Folic acid antagonist (Orphan)

Isovorin

lobeline
Classification:
Smoking deterrent

Bantron

GENERIC NAME	BRAND NAME

lodoxamide tromethamine
Classification:
Ophthalmic mast cell stabilizer

Alomide

lomefloxacin HCl
Classification:
Antibiotic; fluoroquinolone

Maxaquin

lomustine (CCNU)
Classification:
Antineoplastic; alkylating agent

CeeNu

loperamide
Classification:
Antidiarrheal

Imodium
Imodium A-D
Imodium A-D Caplet
Kaopectate II Caplets
Loperamide
Maalox Anti-Diarrheal Caplets
Neo-Diaral
Pepto Diarrhea Control

loracarbef
Classification:
Antibiotic; cephalosporin

Lorabid

loratidine
Classification:
Antihistamine

Claritin

lorazepam
Classification:
Antianxiety; benzodiazepine

Ativan
Lorazepam
Lorazepam Intensol
Novolorazem*

losartan potassium
Classification:
Antihypertensive; angiotensin II
antagonist

Cozaar

loteprednol
Classification:
Ophthalmic glucocorticoid

Lotemax

lovastatin
Classification:
Antilipemic

Mevacor

loxapine succinate/loxapine HCl
Classification:
Antipsychotic

Loxapax*
Loxapine Succinate
Loxitane IM
Loxitane
Loxitane C Concentrate

*Available in Canada Only

GENERIC NAME	BRAND NAME
L-threonine Classification: Amino acid (Orphan)	Threostat
lutenizing hormone **(recombinant human)** Classification: Hormone (Orphan)	Lutenizing Hormone (recombinant human)
lyme borreliosis vaccine Classification: Vaccine (Investigational)	Lyme Borreliosis Vaccine
lymphocyte immune globulin, **anti-thymocyte globulin** **(equine)** Classification: Immune serum	Atgam
lypressin (8-lysine vasopressin) Classification: Posterior pituitary hormone	Diapid
lysine Classification: Amino acid	Enisyl L-Lysine

M

mafenide acetate Classification: Antibacterial; sulfonamide	Sulfamylon
mafenide acetate Classification: Antibacterial (Orphan)	Sulfamylon Solution
magaldrate (hydroxy **magnesium aluminate)** Classification: Antacid	Lowsium Riopan
magnesia (magnesium **hydroxide)** Classification: Antacid; laxative	Concentrated Phillip's Milk of Magnesia Milk of Magnesia Phillip's Milk of Magnesia
magnesium chloride Classification: Electrolyte replacement	Slow-Mag

GENERIC NAME	BRAND NAME

magnesium citrate
Classification:
Laxative, saline

Citrate of Magnesia

magnesium gluconate
Classification:
Electrolyte replacement

Almora
Magonate
Magtrate

magnesium lactate
Classification:
Electrolyte replacement

Mag-Tab SR

magnesium oxide
Classification:
Electrolyte replacement

Mag-200
Mag-Ox 400
Maox 420
Uro-Mag

magnesium salicylate
Classification:
Salicylate analgesic

Backache Maximum Strength Relief
Bayer Select Maximum Strength
  Backache
Doan's Pills
Magan
Mobidin

magnesium sulfate
Classification:
Laxative, saline

Epsom Salt
Magnesium Sulfate
Magnesium Sulfate Concentrated

malathion
Classification:
Scabicide; pediculicide

Ovide

mangafodipir
Classification:
In vivo diagnostic

Teslascan

manganese
Classification:
Trace element

Chelated Manganese
Manganese
Manganese Chloride
Manganese Sulfate

mannitol
Classification:
Osmotic diuretic

Mannitol
Osmitrol
Resectisol

maprotiline HCl
Classification:
Antidepressant, tetracyclic

Ludiomil
Maprotiline HCl

marimastat
Classification:
Antineoplastic (Investigational)

Marimastat

*Available in Canada Only

GENERIC NAME	BRAND NAME
masoprocol Classification: Antikeratotic	Actinex
matrix metalloproteinase inhibitor Classification: Ophthalmic (Orphan)	Galardin
mazindol Classification: CNS stimulant; anorexiant	Mazanor Sanorex
measles, mumps, and rubella virus vaccine, live Classification: Vaccine	M-M-R-II
measles (Rubeola) virus vaccine, live, attenuated Classification: Vaccine	Attenuvax
measles (Rubeola) and rubella virus vaccine, live Classification: Vaccine	M-R-Vax II
mebendazole Classification: Anthelmintics	Vermox
mecamylamine HCl Classification: Antihypertensive; ganglionic blocker	Inversine
mecasermin Classification: Biologic response modifier (Orphan)	Mecasermin
mechlorethamine HCl (nitrogen mustard; HN$_2$) Classification: Antineoplastic; alkylating agent	Mustargen
meclizine Classification: Antiemetic, anticholinergic	Antivert Antivert/25 Antivert/50 Antrizine Bonamine* Bonine Dizmiss

GENERIC NAME	BRAND NAME
meclizine (cont'd.)	Dramamine II Meclizine HCl Meni-D Ru-Vert-M Vergon
meclocyline sulfosalicylate Classification: Anti-acne product	Meclan
meclofenamate sodium Classification: Nonsteroidal anti-inflammatory	Meclofenamate
medium chain triglycerides Classification: Modular supplement	MCT Oil
medroxyprogesterone acetate Classification: Progestin	Amen Curretab Cycrin Depo-Provera Medroxyprogesterone Acetate Provera
medrysone Classification: Ophthalmic glucocorticoid	HMS
mefenamic acid Classification: Nonsteroidal anti-inflammatory	Ponstel
mefloquine HCl Classification: Antimalarial	Lariam
megestrol acetate Classification: Progestin	Megace Megestrol Acetate
melanoma cell vaccine Classification: Vaccine (Orphan)	Melanoma Cell Vaccine
melanoma vaccine Classification: Vaccine (Orphan)	Melacine
melarsoprol Classification: CDC anti-infective	Arsobal

*Available in Canada Only

GENERIC NAME	BRAND NAME
melphalan (L-Pam; phenylalanine mustard; L-sarcolysin) Classification: Antineoplastic; alkylating agent	Alkeran
menadiol sodium diphosphate (vitamin K$_4$) Classification: Vitamin K	Synkayvite*
menadione/menadiol sodium diphosphate (vitamin K$_3$) Classification: Vitamin K	Synkavite*
meningococcal polysaccharide vaccine Classification: Vaccine	Menomune-A/C/Y/W-135
menotropins Classification: Gonadotropin	Humegon Pergonal
mepenzolate bromide Classification: Anticholinergic	Cantil
meperidine HCl Classification: Opioid analgesic	Demerol HCl Meperidine HCl
mephentermine sulfate Classification: Adrenergic agonist	Wyamine Sulfate
mephenytoin Classification: Anticonvulsant; hydantoin	Mesantoin
mephobarbital Classification: Sedative-hypnotic; barbiturate	Mebaral
mepivacaine HCl Classification: Local anesthetic	Carbocaine Carbocaine with Neo-Cobefrin Isocaine HCl Mepivicane HCl Polocaine Polocaine MPF

GENERIC NAME	BRAND NAME

meprobamate
Classification:
Antianxiety

Equanil
Meditran*
Meprobamate
Miltown
Miltown 600
Neo-Tran*
Novomepro*

merbromin
Classification:
Antiseptic

Mercurochrome

mercaptopurine (6-MP; 6-mercaptopurine)
Classification:
Antineoplastic; antimetabolite

Purinethol

meropenem
Classification:
Antibiotic; carbapenem

Merrem IV

mesalamine
Classification:
GI anti-inflammatory

Asacol
Pentasa
Rowasa

mesna
Classification:
Antineoplastic adjuvant; cytoprotective

Mesnex

mesoridazine besylate
Classification:
Antipsychotic

Serentil

metaproterenol sulfate
Classification:
Bronchodilator; beta-adrenergic agonist

Alupent
Arm-A-Med Metaproterenol Sulfate
Metaprel
Metaproterenol Sulfate

metaraminol
Classification:
Adrenergic agonist

Aramine

metaxalone
Classification:
Skeletal muscle relaxant, centrally acting

Skelaxin

metformin HCl
Classification:
Antidiabetic; biguanides

Glucophage

GENERIC NAME	BRAND NAME
methacholine chloride Classification: Cholinergic	Provocholine
methadone HCl Classification: Opioid analgesic	Dolophine HCl Methadone HCl Methadone HCl Diskets Methadone HCl Intensol Methadose
methamphetamine HCl Classification: CNS stimulant	Desoxyn Desoxyn Gradumets
methantheline bromide Classification: Anticholinergic	Banthine
methazolamide Classification: Diuretic; carbonic anhydrase inhibitor	GlaucTabs Methazolamide Neptazane
methenamine hippurate Classification: Urinary anti-infective	Hiprex Hip-Rex* Urex
methenamine mandelate Classification: Urinary anti-infective	Methenamine Mandelate
methicillin sodium Classification: Antibiotic; penicillinase-resistant penicillin	Staphcillin
methimazole Classification: Antithyroid agent	Tapazole
methionine Classification: Amino acid	M-Caps Methionine Pedameth Uracid
methionyl neutrotrophic factor (brain-derived) Classification: Anti-amyotrophic lateral sclerosis agent (Orphan)	Methionyl Neutrotrophic Factor (brain-derived)

*Available in Canada only

GENERIC NAME	BRAND NAME

methocarbamol
Classification:
Skeletal muscle relaxant, centrally acting

Methocarbamol
Robaxin
Robaxin-750
Tresortil*

methohexital sodium
Classification:
General anesthetic; barbiturate

Brevital Sodium
Brietal Sodium*

**methotrexate sodium
(amethopterin, MTX)**
Classification:
Antineoplastic; antimetabolite

Folex PFS
Methotrexate
Methotrexate LPF
Rheumatrex Dose Pack

methotrimeprazine HCl
Classification:
Analgesic

Levoprome
Nozinan*

methoxamine HCl
Classification:
Adrenergic agonist

Vasoxyl

**methoxsalen, oral
(8-methoxypsoralen, 8-MOP)**
Classification:
Psoralen

8-MOP
Oxsoralen-Ultra

**methoxsalen, topical
(8-methoxypsoralen, 8-MOP)**
Classification:
Psoralen

Oxsoralen

methoxyflurane
Classification:
General anesthetic

Penthrane

methscopolamine bromide
Classification:
Anticholinergic

Pamine

methsuximide
Classification:
Anticonvulsant; succinimide

Celontin Kapseals

methyclothiazide
Classification:
Thiazide diuretic

Aquatensen
Enduron
Methyclothiazide

methyl salicylate
Classification:
Counterirritant

Exocaine Plus
Exocaine Medicated
Analgesic Balm

*Available in Canada Only

GENERIC NAME	BRAND NAME

methylcellulose
Classification:
Laxative, bulk-producing

Citrucel

methyldopa/methyldopate HCl
Classification:
Antihypertensive, centrally acting

Aldomet
Amodopa
Dopamet*
Medimet*
Methyldopa/Methyldopate HCl
Novomedopa*

methylene blue
Classification:
Urinary anti-infective

Methblue 65
Methylene Blue
Urolene Blue

methylergonovine maleate
Classification:
Oxytocic

Methergine
Methylergobasine*

methylnaltrexone
Classification:
Narcotic antagonist (Orphan)

Methylnaltrexone

methylphenidate HCl
Classification:
CNS stimulant

Methylphenidate HCl
Ritalin
Ritalin SR

methylprednisolone
Classification:
Glucocorticoid

Medrol
Methylprednisolone

methylprednisolone acetate
Classification:
Glucocorticoid

Adlone
Depoject
Depopred-40
Depo-Medrol
Depopred-80
depMedalone 40
depMedalone 80
Duralone-40
Duralone-80
M-Prednisol-40
M-Prednisol-80
Medralone 40
Medralone 80
Methylprednisolone Acetate

**methylprednisolone sodium
succinate**
Classification:
Glucocorticoid

A-Methapred
Methylprednisolone Sodium Succinate
Solu-Medrol

GENERIC NAME	BRAND NAME

methyltestosterone
Classification:
Androgen

Android-10
Android-25
Methyltestosterone
Oreton Methyl
Testred
Virilon

methysergide maleate
Classification:
Serotonin antagonist

Sansert

metipranolol HCl
Classification:
Beta-adrenergic blocker

OptiPranolol

metoclopramide
Classification:
Antidopaminergic

Clopra
Maxeran*
Maxolon
Metoclopramide
Metoclopramide HCl
Metoclopramide Intensol
Octamide PFS
Reclomide
Reglan

metocurine iodide
Classification:
Nondepolarizing neuromuscular blocker

Metubine Iodide

metolazone
Classification:
Thiazide-like diuretic

Mykrox
Zaroxolyn

metoprolol
Classification:
Antihypertensive; beta-adrenergic blocker

Betaloc*
Lopresor*
Lopressor
Metoprolol Tartrate
Toprol XL

metrizamide
Classification:
Radiopaque agent

Amipaque

metronidazole
Classification:
Antibacterial; amebicide

Apo-Metronidazole*
Flagyl
Flagyl 375
Flagyl ER
Flagyl I.V.
Flagyl I.V. RTU
Metro I.V.

*Available in Canada Only

GENERIC NAME	BRAND NAME
metronidazole (cont'd.)	Metronidazole Neo-Tric* Novonidazole* PMS-Metronidazole* Protostat Trikacide*
metronidazole, topical Classification: Anti-acne product	MetroGel
metronidazole, vaginal Classification: Antibacterial; amebicide	MetroGel-Vaginal
metyrapone Classification: In vivo diagnostic	Metopirone
metyrosine Classification: Antihypertensive	Demser
mexiletine HCl Classification: Antiarrhythmic	Mexiletine HCl Mexitil
mezlocillin sodium Classification: Antibiotic; extended spectrum penicillin	Mezlin
mibefradil dihydrochloride Classification: Antihypertensive; calcium channel blocker	Posicor
miconazole Classification: Antifungal; imidazole	Monistat i.v.
miconazole nitrate, topical Classification: Antifungal; imidazole	Absorbine Antifungal Food Powder Breeze Mist Antifungal Fungoid Creme Fungoid Tincture Lotrimin AF Maximum Strength Desenex Antifungal Micatin Miconazole Nitrate Micatin Liquid Monistat-Derm Ory-Clear Zeasorb-AF

*Available in Canada only

GENERIC NAME	BRAND NAME

miconazole nitrate, vaginal
Classification:
Antifungal

Femizol-M
M-Zole 7-Dual Pack
Miconazole Nitrate
Monistat 3
Monistat 7
Monistat 7 Combination Pack
Monistat-Derm
Monistat Dual-Pak

microfibrillar collagen hemostat
Classification:
Hemostatic

Avitene Hemostat
Hemopad
Hemotene

midazolam HCl
Classification:
General anesthetic; benzodiazepine

Versed

midodrine HCl
Classification:
Adrenergic agonist

ProAmatine

milrinone lactate
Classification:
Cardiac inotropic agent

Primacor

miglitol
Classification:
Antidiabetic

Glyset

mineral oil
Classification:
Laxative; emollient

Fleet Mineral Oil Enema
Kondremul Plain
Milkinoil
Neo-Cultol

minocycline HCl
Classification:
Antibiotic; tetracycline

Dynacin
Minocin
Minocin IV
Minocycline HCl
Vectrin

minoxidil
Classification:
Antihypertensive; vasodilator

Loniten
Minoxidil

minoxidil, topical
Classification:
Antihypertensive; vasodilator

Minoxidil for Men
Rogaine

mirtazapine
Classification:
Antidepressant, tetracyclic

Remeron

GENERIC NAME	BRAND NAME
misoprostol Classification: Prostaglandin	Cytotec
mitoguazone Classification: Antineoplastic (Orphan)	Mitoguazone
mitomycin (mitomycin-c; MTC) Classification: Antineoplastic; antibiotic	Mutamycin
mitotane (o,p-DDD) Classification: Antineoplastic, miscellaneous	Lysodren
mitoxantrone Classification: Antineoplastic; antibiotic	Novantrone
mivacurium chloride Classification: Nondepolarizing neuromuscular blocker	Mivacron
mixed respiratory vaccine Classification: Vaccine	MRV
modafinil Classification: Centrally acting alpha agonist	Provigil
moexipril HCl Classification: Antihypertensive; angiotensin converting enzyme inhibitor	Univasc
molgramostim Classification: Biologic response modifier (Investigational)	Leucomax
molindone HCl Classification: Antipsychotic	Moban
molybdenum Classification: Trace element	Ammonium Molybdate Molypen
mometasone furoate Classification: Glucocorticoid	Elocon

*Available in Canada only

GENERIC NAME	BRAND NAME

mometasone furoate, nasal
Classification:
Glucocorticoid

Nasonex

monobenzone
Classification:
Depigmentation agent

Benoquin

monochloroacetic acid
Classification:
Cauterizing agent

Mono-Chlor

monoclonal antibody (human), hepatitis B virus
Classification:
Biologic response modifier (Orphan)

Monoclonal Antibody (human), Hepatitis B Virus

monoclonal antibody 17-1A
Classification:
Biologic response modifier (Orphan)

Monoclonal Antibody 17-1A

monoclonal antibody PM-81
Classification:
Biologic response modifier (Orphan)

Monoclonal Antibody PM-81

monoclonal antibody to CD4,5a8
Classification:
Biologic response modifier (Orphan)

Monoclonal Antibody to CD4,5a8

monoclonal antibody, lupus nephritis
Classification:
Biologic response modifier (Orphan)

Monoclonal Antibody, Lupus Nephritis

monoclonal antiidotype melanoma-associate antigen
Classification:
Biologic response modifier (Orphan)

Melimmune

monoclonal factor IX
Classification:
Hemostatic

Mononine

monoctanoin
Classification:
Antilithic

Moctanin

monoplaurin
Classification:
Dermatological (Orphan)

Glylorin

*Available in Canada Only

GENERIC NAME	BRAND NAME
montelukast sodium Classification: Bronchodilator; leukotriene receptor antagonist	Singular
moricizine HCl Classification: Antiarrhythmic	Ethmozine
morphine sulfate Classification: Opioid analgesic	Astramorph PF Duramorph Infumorph 200 Infumorph 500 Kadian Morphine Sulfate MS Contin MS/L MS/L-Concentrate MS/S MSIR OMS Concentrate Oramorph SR RMS Roxanol Roxanol 100 Roxanol Rescudose Roxanol SR
morrhuate sodium Classification: Sclerosing agent	Morrhuate Sodium Scleromate
mumps skin test antigen Classification: In vivo diagnostic	MSTA
mumps virus vaccine, live Classification: Vaccine	Mumpsvax
mupirocin Classification: Topical antibacterial	Bactroban Bactroban Nasal
muromonab-CD3 Classification: Immunosuppressive	Orthoclone OKT3
mycophenolate mofetil Classification: Immunosuppressive	CellCept

*Available in Canada only

GENERIC NAME	BRAND NAME

mylein
Classification:
Anti-multiple sclerosis agent (Orphan)

Myelin

N

nadolol HCl
Classification:
Beta-adrenergic blocker

Corgard
Nadolol HCl

nafarelin acetate
Classification:
Gonadotropin-releasing hormone

Synarel

nafcillin sodium
Classification:
Antibiotic; penicillinase-resistant
penicillin

Nafcil
Nafcillin Sodium
Nallpen
Unipen

naftifine HCl
Classification:
Antifungal

Naftin

nalbuphine HCl
Classification:
Opioid agonist-antagonist analgesic

Nalbuphine HCl
Nubain

nalidixic acid
Classification:
Urinary anti-infective

NegGram
NegGram Caplets

nalmefene HCl
Classification:
Narcotic antagonist

Revex

naloxone HCl
Classification:
Narcotic antagonist

Naloxone HCl
Narcan

naltrexone HCl
Classification:
Narcotic antagonist

ReVia
Trexan (Orphan)

nambumetone
Classification:
Nonsteroidal anti-inflammatory

Relafen

nandrolone decanoate
Classification:
Anabolic steroid

Androlone-D 200
Deca-Durabolin
Hybolin Decanoate-50
Hybolin Decanoate-100

*Available in Canada Only

GENERIC NAME	BRAND NAME
nandrolone decanoate (cont'd.)	Nandrolone Decanoate Neo-Durabolic
nandrolone phenpropionate Classification: Anabolic steroid	Durabolin Hybolin Improved Nandrolone Phenproprionate
naphazoline HCl, nasal Classification: Nasal decongestant	Privine
naphazoline HCl, ophthalmic Classification: Ophthalmic vasoconstrictor	AK-Con Allerest Eye Drops Albalon Clear Eyes Clear Eyes ACR Comfort Eye Drops Degest 2 Maximum Strength Allergy Drops Nafazair Naphazoline HCl Naphcon Naphcon Forte VasoClear Vasocon Regular
naproxen Classification: Nonsteroidal anti-inflammatory	EC-Naprosyn Naprelan Napron X Naprosyn Naproxen
naproxen sodium Classification: Nonsteroidal anti-inflammatory	Aleve Anaprox Anaprox DS Naproxen Sodium
naratriptan Classification: Antimigraine	Amerge
natamycfin Classification: Opththalmic antifungal	Natacyn
nebacumab Classification: Biologic response modifier (Orphan)	Centoxin

GENERIC NAME	BRAND NAME

nedocromil sodium
Classification:
Antiasthmatic

Tilade

nefazadone HCl
Classification:
Antidepressant

Serazone

nelfinavir mesylate
Classification:
Antiviral; protease inhibitor

Viracept

neomycin sulfate
Classification:
Aminoglycoside

Mycifradin Sulfate
Neo-fradin
Neomycin Sulfate
Neo-Tabs

neomycin sulfate, topical
Classification:
Aminoglycoside

Myciguent
Neomycin

neostigmine
Classification:
Anticholinesterase

Neostigmine
Neostigmine Methylsulfate
Prostigmin

netilmicin sulfate
Classification:
Aminoglycoside

Netromycin

neurotrophin-1
Classification:
Anti-amyotrophic lateral sclerosis agent
(Orphan)

Neurotrophin-1

nevirapine
Classification:
Antiviral; non-nucleoside

Viramune

NGD 91-2
Classification:
Antianxiety (Investigational)

NGD 91-2

niacin (vitamin B₃, nicotinic acid)
Classification:
Vitamin, water soluble

Nia-Bid
Niacor
Nico-400
Nicobid Tempules
Nicolar
Nicotinex
Nicotinic Acid
Novoniacin*
Slo-Niacin

*Available in Canada Only

GENERIC NAME	BRAND NAME
niacin, sustained release Classification: Antilipemic	Niaspan
nicardipine HCl Classification: Calcium channel blocker	Cardene Cardene I.V. Cardene SR Nicardipine HCl
nicotinamide (niacinamide) Classification: Vitamin, water soluble	Niacinamide Nicotinamide
nicotine, inhaler Classification: Smoking deterrent	Nicotrol
nicotine, nasal Classification: Smoking deterrent	Nicotrol NS
nicotine polacrilex Classification: Smoking deterrent	Nicorette Nicorette DS
nicotine transdermal system Classification: Smoking deterrent	Habitrol Nicoderm Nicotrol ProStep
nifedipine Classification: Calcium channel blocker	Adalat Adalat CC Nifedipine Procardia Procardia XL
nifurtimox Classification: CDD anti-infective	Lampit
nilutamide Classification: Antineoplastic; antiandrogen	Anandron* Nilandron
nimodipine Classification: Calcium channel blocker	Nimotrop
nisoldipine Classification: Calcium channel blocker	Sular

*Available in Canada only

GENERIC NAME	BRAND NAME

nitrofurantoin
Classification:
Urinary anti-infective

Furadantin
Nephronex*
Novofuran*

nitrofurantoin macrocrystals
Classification:
Urinary anti-infective

Macrobid
Macrodantin .
Nitrofurantoin Macrocrystals

nitrofurazone
Classification:
Antibacterial

Furacin
Nitrofurazone

nitroglycerin, intravenous
Classification:
Antianginal

Nitro-Bid IV
Nitroglycerin
Tridil

nitroglycerin, sublingual
Classification:
Antianginal

Nitrostat

nitroglycerin, sustained release
Classification:
Antianginal

Nitro-Time
Nitroglycerin
Nitroglyn
Nitrong

nitroglycerin, topical
Classification:
Antianginal

Nitro-Bid
Nitroglycerin
Nitrol

nitroglycerin, transdermal systems
Classification:
Antianginal

Deponit
Minitran
Nitrek
Nitrodisc
Nitro-Dur
Nitroglycerin Transdermal
Transdermal-Nitro

nitroglycerin, translingual
Classification:
Antianginal

Nitrolingual

nitroglycerin, transmucosal
Classification:
Antianginal

Nitrogard

nitroprusside sodium
Classification:
Antihypertensive; vasodilator

Nitropress
Sodium Nitroprusside

nizatidine
Classification:
Histamine H_2 receptor antagonist

Axid
Axid AR

*Available in Canada Only

GENERIC NAME	BRAND NAME
nonoxynol Classification: Spermicide	Advantage 24 Because Delfen Contraceptive Conceptrol Emko Emko-Pre-Fil Encare Gynol II K-Y Plus Koromex Ramses Semicid Shur-Seal Gel
norastemizole Classification: Antihistimine (Investigational)	Norastemizole
norepinephrine injection (levarterenol) Classification: Adrenergic agonist	Levophed
norethindrone Classification: Progestin	Micronor Nor-Q.D.
norethindrone acetate Classification: Progestin	Aygestin
norfloxacin Classification: Antibiotic; fluoroquinolone	Noroxin
norfloxacin, ophthalmic Classification: Antibiotic; fluoroquinolone	Chibroxin
norgestrel Classification: Progestin	Ovral* Ovrette
nortriptyline HCl Classification: Antidepressant	Aventyl Nortriptyline HCl Pamelor
novapren Classification: Antiviral (Investigational)	Novapren

GENERIC NAME	BRAND NAME

novobiocin
Classification:
Antibacterial

Albamycin

N-trifluoroacetyladriamycin-14-valerate
Classification:
Antineoplastic (Orphan)

N-trifluoroacetyladriamycin-14-valerate

nystatin, oral
Classification:
Antifungal

Mycostatin
Mycostatin Pastilles
Nadostine*
Nilstat
Nystatin

nystatin, topical
Classification:
Antifungal

Mycostatin
Nilstat
Nystatin
Nystex

nystatin, vaginal
Classification:
Antifungal

Mycostatin
Nystatin

O

octreotide acetate
Classification:
Somatostatin analog

Sandostatin

octaflurorpropane and human albumin microspheres
Classification:
Radiopaque agent

Optison

ocular lubricants
Classification:
Ophthalmic lubricant

Akwa Tears
Artificial Tears
Dry Eyes
Duratears Naturale
HypoTears
Lacri-Lube NP
Lacri-Lube S.O.P.
LubriTears
Puralube
Refresh PM
Stye
Tears Renewed

*Available in Canada Only

GENERIC NAME	BRAND NAME
ofloxacin Classification: Antibiotic; fluoroquinolone	Floxin Floxin I.V.
ofloxacin, ophthalmic Classification: Antibiotic; fluoroquinolone	Ocuflox
ofloxacin, otic Classification: Antibiotic; fluoroquinolone	Floxin Otic
olanzapine Classification: Antipsychotic	Zyprexa
olopatidine Classification: Antihistamine, ophthalmic	Patanol
olsalazine sodium Classification: GI anti-inflammatory	Dipentum
OM 401 Classification: Blood modifier (Orphan)	Drepanol
omeprazole Classification: Antisecretory; benzimidazoles	Prilosec
oncorad Ov103 Classification: Antineoplastic (Orphan)	Oncorad Ov103
ondansetron HCl Classification: Antiemetic	Zofran
opium Classification: Opioid analgesic	Opium Tincture Deodorized Paregoric Paregorique*
oprelvekin Classification: Biologic response modifier	Neumega
orgotein Classification: Anti-amyotrophic lateral sclerosis agent (Orphan)	Orgotein

*Available in Canada only

GENERIC NAME	BRAND NAME

orlistat
Classification:
Antilipemic

Xenical

orphenadrine citrate
Classification:
Skeletal muscle relaxant, centrally acting

Banflex
Flexoject
Flexon
Myolin
Norflex
Orphenadrine Citrate

oxacillin sodium
Classification:
Antibiotic; penicillinase-resistant
penicillin

Bactocill
Oxacillin Sodium
Prostaphlin

oxaliplatin
Classification:
Antineoplastic (Orphan)

Oxaliplatin

oxamniquine
Classification:
Anthelmintic

Vansil

oxandrolone
Classification:
Anabolic steroid

Oxandrin

oxaprozin
Classification:
Nonsteroidal anti-inflammatory

Daypro

oxazepam
Classification:
Antianxiety; benzodiazepine

Apo-Oxazepam*
Novoxapam*
Oxazepam
Serax

oxcarbazeprine
Classification:
Anticonvulsant (Investigational)

Trileptal

oxiconazole nitrate
Classification:
Antifungal

Oxistat

oxidized cellulose
Classification:
Hemostatic

Oxycel
Surgicel

oxtriphylline
Classification:
Bronchodilator; xanthine

Choledyl SA
Novotriphyl*
Oxtriphylline

*Available in Canada Only

GENERIC NAME	BRAND NAME
oxybutynin chloride Classification: Urinary antispasmodic	Ditropan Oxybutynin Chloride
oxychlorosene sodium Classification: Germicidal	Clorpactin WCS-90
oxycodone HCl Classification: Opioid analgesic	OxyContin OxyIR Roxicodone Roxicodone Intensol Supeudol*
oxymetazoline HCl, nasal Classification: Nasal decongestant	4-Way Long Acting Nasal 12-Hour Nasal 12-Hour Sinarest Afrin Afrin Childrens' Nose Drops Afrin Sinus Allerest 12-Hour Nasal Cherocol Nasal Chlorphed-LA Dristan 12-Hour Nasal Dristan Long Lasting Duramist Plus Duration Genasal Nafrine* Neo-Synephrine 12 Hour Nōstrilla NTZ Long-Acting Nasal Oxymetazoline HCl Vicks Sinex Long-Acting
oxymetazoline HCl, ophthalmic Classification: Ophthalmic vasoconstrictor	OcuClear Visine L.R.
oxymetholone Classification: Anabolic steroid	Anadrol-50 Anapolon 50*
oxymorphone HCl Classification: Opioid analgesic	Numorphan Numorphan H.P.
oxytetracycline HCl Classification: Antibiotic; tetracycline	Oxytetracycline HCl Terramycin Terramycin IM

*Available in Canada only

GENERIC NAME	BRAND NAME
oxytocin, parenteral Classification: Oxytocic	Oxytocin Pitocin Syntocinon
oxytocin, synthetic, nasal Classification: Oxytocic	Syntocinon

P

paclitaxel Classification: Antineoplastic, miscellaneous	Taxol
pamidronate disodium Classification: Bone resorption inhibitor	Aredia
panavir Classification: Antiviral (Investigational)	Panavir
pancreatin Classification: Digestive enzyme	4X Pancreatin 600 mg 8X Pancreatin 900 mg Donnazyme Pancrezyme 4X Hi-Vegi-Lip
pancrelipase Classification: Digestive enzyme	Cotazym Capsules Cotazym-S Capsules Creon Creon 10 Creon 20 Ilozyme Tablets Ku-Zyme HP Capsules Pancrease Capsules Pancrease MT4 Pancrease MT10 Pancrease MT 16 Pancrease MT 20 Pancrelipase Protilase Ultrase MT 12 Ultrase MT 20 Viokase Powder Viokase Tablets Zymase

*Available in Canada Only

GENERIC NAME	BRAND NAME
pancuronium bromide Classification: Nondepolarizing neuromuscular blocker	Pancuronium Bromide Pavulon
panretin oral Classification: Biologic response modifier (Investigational)	Panretin Oral
papaverine HCl Classification: Peripheral vasodilator	Papaverine HCl Pavabid Plateau Caps Pavagen TD Pavatine
para-aminobenzoic acid (PABA) Classification: Vitamin, water soluble	Para-Aminobenzoic Acid Potaba
paraldehyde Classification: Anticonvulsant	Paral Paraldehyde
paromomycin sulfate Classification: Aminoglycoside	Humatin
paroxetine Classification: Antidepressant	Paxil
PEG-glucocerebrosidase Classification: Enzyme (Orphan)	Lysodase
pegademase bovine Classification: Enzyme replacement	Adagen
pegaspargase (PEG-L-asparaginase) Classification: Antineoplastic, miscellaneous	Oncaspar
pemoline Classification: CNS stimulant	Cylert
penbutolol Classification: Antihypertensive; beta-adrenergic blocker	Levatol

*Available in Canada only

GENERIC NAME	BRAND NAME

penciclovir
Classification:
Antiviral

Denavir

penicillamine
Classification:
Chelating agent

Cuprimine
Depen

penicillin G (aqueous), parenteral
Classification:
Antibiotic; penicillin

Penicillin G Potassium
Penicillin G Sodium
Pfizerpen

penicillin G benzathine, parenteral
Classification:
Antibiotic; penicillin

Bicillin L-A
Megacillin*
Permapen

penicillin G benzathine and procaine combined
Classification:
Antibiotic; penicillin

Bicillin C-R
Bicillin C-R 900/300

penicillin G procaine, aqueous (APPG)
Classification:
Antibiotic; penicillin

Crysticillin 300 A.S.
Crysticillin 600 A.S.
Wycillin

penicillin V potassium
Classification:
Antibiotic; penicillin

Apo-Pen-VK*
Beepen-VK
Betapen-VK
Novopen-VK*
PVFK*
Penicillin VK
Pen-V
Pen-Vee K
Robicillin-VK
V-Cillin K
Veetids 125
Veetids 250
Veetids 500

pentagastrin
Classification:
Gastrointestinal function test

Peptavlon

pentamidine isethionate
Classification:
Antiprotazoal

NebuPent
Pentacarinat
Pentam 300
Pentamidine Isethionate

GENERIC NAME	BRAND NAME
pentazocine Classification: Opioid agonist-antagonist analgesic	Talwin
pentobarbital sodium Classification: Sedative-hypnotic; barbiturate	Nembutal Sodium Nova-Rectal* Pentobarbital Sodium Pentogen*
pentosan polysulfate sodium Classification: Urinary tract analgesic	Elmiron
pentostatin (DCF; 2-deoxycoformycin) Classification: Antineoplastic; antibiotic	Nipent
pentoxifylline Classification: Hemorrheologic agent	Pentoxifylline Trental
pergolide mesylate Classification: Antiparkinson agent	Permax
penindopril erbumine Classification: Antihypertensive; angiotensin converting enzyme inhibitor	ACEON
permethrin Classification: Scabicide; pediculicide	Elimite Nix
perphenazine Classification: Antipsychotic	Trilafon Perphenazine
phenazopyridine HCl Classification: Urinary analgesic	Azo-Standard Baridium Geridium Phenazo* Phenazopyridine HCl Prodium Pyridiate Pyridium Urodine
phendimetrazine tartrate Classification: CNS stimulant; anorexiant	Adipost Bontril PDM Bontril Slow-Release

*Available in Canada only

GENERIC NAME	BRAND NAME

phendimetrazine tartrate (cont'd.)

Dital
Dyrexan-OD
Melfiat-105 Unicelles
Phendimetrazine Tartrate
Plegine
Prelu-2
Rexigen Forte

phenelzine sulfate
Classification:
Monoamine oxidase inhibitor

Nardil

phenformin
Classification:
Antidiabetic; biguanide (Investigational)

Phenformin

phenindamine tartrate
Classification:
Antihistamine

Nolahist

phenobarbital/phenobarbital sodium
Classification:
Sedative-hypnotic; barbiturate

Luminal Sodium
Phenobarbital
Phenobarbital Sodium
Solfoton

phenolphthalein
Classification:
Laxative; irritant

Alophen Pills
Espotabs
Evac-U-Gen
Evac-U-Lax
Feen-a-mint
Feen-a-mint Gum
Lax Pills
Modane
Phenolax
Prulet

phenoxybenzamine HCl
Classification:
Antihypertensive; alpha-adrenergic
blocker

Dibenzyline

phensuximide
Classification:
Anticonvulsant; succinimide

Milontin Kapseals

phentermine HCl
Classification:
CNS stimulant; anorexiant

Adipex-P
Fastin
Ionamin
Obe-Nix 30
OBY-CAP

GENERIC NAME	BRAND NAME
phentermine HCl **(cont'd.)**	Phentermine Resin Phentermine HCl Zantryl
phentolamine Classification: Antihypertensive; alpha-adrenergic blocker	Regitine Rogitine*
phentolamine Classification: Vasodilator	Vasomax
phenylalanine ammonia-lyase Classification: Enzyme (Orphan)	Phenylase
phenylephrine HCl Classification: Adrenergic agonist	AH-Chew D Neo-Synephrine Phenylephrine HCl
phenylephrine HCl, nasal Classification: Nasal decongestant	Alconefrin Alconefrin-12 Alconefrin-25 Children's Nōstril Neo-Synephrine Nōstril Phenylephrine HCl Rhinall Sinex
phenylephrine HCl, ophthalmic Classification: Ophthalmic vasoconstrictor	AK-Dilate AK-Nefrin Neo-Synephrine 2.5% Neo-Synephrine 10% Neo-Synephrine Viscous Phenoptic Phenylephrine HCl Prefrin Liquifilm Relief Mydfrin 2.5%
phenylpropanolamine HCl Classification: Alpha-adrenergic agonist	Acutrim II Maximum Strength Acutrim Late Day Acutrim 16 Hour Control Dexatrim Dexatrim Pre-Meal Maximum Strength Dexatrim Phenoxine

*Available in Canada only

GENERIC NAME	BRAND NAME

phenylpropanolamine HCl (cont'd.)

Phenylpropanolamine HCl
Propagest
Spray-U-Thin
Unitrol

phenytoin
Classification:
Anticonvulsant; hydantoin

Dilantin Infatab
Dilantin-125

phenytoin sodium, extended
Classification:
Anticonvulsant; hydantoin

Dilantin Kapseals
Phenytoin Sodium

phenytoin sodium, parenteral
Classification:
Anticonvulsant; hydantoin

Dilantin
Phenytoin Sodium

phenytoin sodium, prompt
Classification:
Anticonvulsant; hydantoin

Phenytoin Sodium

phosphorated carbohydrate solution
Classification:
Antiemetic

Emecheck
Emetrol
Nausea Relief
Nausetrol

phosphorous (replacement products)
Classification:
Electrolyte replacement

K-Phos-Neutral
Neutra-Phos
Neutra-Phos-K
Uro-KP Neutral

physostigmine, ophthalmic
Classification:
Miotic

Eserine Sulfate

physostigmine salicylate
Classification:
Anticholinesterase

Antilirium

phytonadione (Vitamin K$_1$)
Classification:
Vitamin K

AquaMEPHYTON
Konakion
Mephyton

pilocarpine HCl
Classification:
Miotic

Adsorbocarpine
Akarpine
Isopto Carpine
Milocarpine*
Ocu-Carpine
Pilocar
Pilocarpine HCl
Pilopine-HS

*Available in Canada Only

GENERIC NAME	BRAND NAME
pilocarpine HCl **(cont'd.)**	Piloptic-1/2 Piloptic-1 Piloptic-2 Piloptic-3 Piloptic-4 Piloptic 6 Pilpto-Carpine Pilostat
pilocarpine nitrate Classification: Miotic	Pilagan
pilocarpine ocular therapeutic **system** Classification: Miotic	Ocusert Pilo-20 Ocusert Pilo-40
pilocarpine, oral Classification: Cholinergic	Salagen
pimozide Classification: Antipsychotic	Orap
pindolol Classification: Antihypertensive; beta-adrenergic blocker	Pindolol Visken
pipecuronium bromide Classification: Nondepolarizing neuromuscular blocker	Arduan
piperacillin sodium Classification: Antibiotic; extended spectrum penicillin	Pipracil
piperacillin sodium and **tazobactam sodium** Classification: Antibiotic; extended spectrum penicillin	Zosyn
piracetam Classification: Muscle stimulant (Orphan)	Nootropil
pirbuterol acetate Classification: Bronchodilator; beta-adrenergic agonist	Maxair

*Available in Canada only

GENERIC NAME	BRAND NAME

piroxicam
Classification:
Nonsteroidal anti-inflammatory

Feldene
Piroxicam

plague vaccine
Classification:
Vaccine

Plague Vaccine

plasma protein fraction
Classification:
Blood derivative

PPF
Plasmanate
Plasma-Plex
Plasmatein
Protenate

plicamycin (mithramycin)
Classification:
Antineoplastic; antibiotic

Mithracin

PMEA
Classification:
Antiviral (Investigational)

PMEA

pneumococcal vaccine, polyvalent
Classification:
Vaccine

Pneumovax 23
Pnu-Imune 23

podofilox
Classification:
Keratolytic

Condylox

podophyllum resin
Classification:
Keratolytic

Pod-Ben-25
Podocon-25
Podofilm*
Podofin

poliovirus vaccine, live, oral, trivalent (TOPV: SABIN)
Classification:
Vaccine

Orimune

poliovirus vaccine, inactivated (IPV:SALK)
Classification:
Vaccine

IPOL

poloxamer 188
Classification:
Blood modifier (Orphan)

RheothRx copolymer

*Available in Canada Only

GENERIC NAME	BRAND NAME
poloxamer 331 Classification: Antimalarial (Orphan)	Protox
polycarbophil Classification: Laxative, bulk-producing	Equalactin Fiberall FiberCon Fiber-Lax FiberNorm Konsyl Fiber Mitrolan
polydimethylsiloxane (silicone oil) Classification: Retinal tamponade	AdatoSil 5000
polyethylene glycol-electrolyte solution Classification: Bowel evacuant	Co-Lav Colovage CoLyte Go-Evac GoLYTELY NuLytely OCL
polymyxin B sulfate, ophthalmic Classification: Antibiotic; polymyxin	Polymyxin B Sulfate Sterile
polymyxin B sulfate, parenteral Classification: Antibiotic; polymyxin	Polymyxin B Sulfate
polysaccharide iron complex Classification: Iron preparation	Hytinic Niferex Niferex-150 Nu-Iron Nu-Iron 150
polythiazide Classification: Thiazide diuretic	Renese
porcine islet preparation, encapsulated Classification: Antidiabetic (Orphan)	BetaRx
porfimer sodium Classification: Antineoplastic, miscellaneous	Photofrin

*Available in Canada only

GENERIC NAME	BRAND NAME

porfiromycin
Classification:
Antineoplastic (Orphan)

Porfiromycin

potassium acetate
Classification:
Electrolyte replacement; potassium

Potassium Acetate

potassium acid phosphate
Classification:
Urinary acidifier

K-Phos Original

**potassium acid phosphate and
sodium acid phosphate**
Classification:
Urinary acidifier

K-Phos M.F.
K-Phos No. 2

**potassium bicarbonate/acetate/
citrate**
Classification:
Electrolyte replacement; potassium

Klor-Con/EF
K-Lyte
K-Lyte DS
Klorvess
Tri-K
Twin-K

potassium chloride
Classification:
Electrolyte replacement; potassium

Cena-K
Gen-K
K+10
K+Care
K-Dur 10
K-Dur 20
K-Lor
K-Lease
K-Lyte/Cl
K-Norm
K-Tab
Kaon-Cl
Kaon-Cl-10
Kaon-Cl 20%
Kaochlor 10%
Kaochlor S-F
Kay Ciel
Klor-Con
Klor-Con 8
Klor-Con 10
Klor-Con/25
Klortrix
Klorvess
Micro-K
Micro-K 10

GENERIC NAME	BRAND NAME
potassium chloride **(cont'd.)**	Micro-K LS Potasalan Potassium Chloride Rum-K Slow-K Ten-K
potassium citrate Classification: Urinary alkalinizer	K-Lyte* Urocit-K
potassium citrate and citric acid Classification: Urinary alkalinizer	Citrolith Polycitra Polycitra-K Polycitra-LC
potassium gluconate Classification: Electrolyte replacement; potassium	Kaon Kaylixir K-G Elixir Potassium Gluconate
potassium iodide Classification: Antithyroid agent	Pima Potassium Iodide Solution SSKI Thyro-Block
potassium perchlorate Classification: Radiopaque agent	Perchloracap
povidone-iodine Classification: Antiseptic; germicidal	ACU-dyne Aerodine Betadine Betadine 5% Sterile Ophthalmic Prep Solution Betagen Biodine Topical 1% Efodine Iodex Iodex-p Mallisol Minidyne Operand Polydine Povidine Povidone-Iodine Proviodine*

GENERIC NAME	BRAND NAME

pralidoxime chloride (2-PAM)
Classification:
Cholinesterase reactivator

Pralidoxime Chloride
Protopam Chloride

pramipexole dihydrochloride
Classification:
Antiparkinson agent

Mirapex

pramoxine HCl, topical
Classification:
Local anesthetic

Itch-X
PrameGel
Prax
ProctoFoam NS
Tronolane
Tronothane HCl

pravastin sodium
Classification:
Antilipemic

Pravachol

prazepam
Classification:
Antianxiety; benzodiazepine

Prazepam

praziquantel
Classification:
Anthelmintics

Biltricide

prazosin
Classification:
Antihypertensive; alpha-adrenergic
blocker

Minipress
Prazosin

prednicarbate
Classification:
Glucocorticoid

Dermatop

prednimustine
Classification:
Antineoplastic (Orphan)

Sterecyt

prednisolone
Classification:
Glucocorticoid

Delta-Cortef
Prednisolone
Prelone

prednisolone acetate
Classification:
Glucocorticoid

Articulose-50
Key-Pred 25
Key-Pred 50
Predalone 50
Predcor-50
Prednisolone Acetate

*Available in Canada Only

GENERIC NAME	BRAND NAME
prednisolone acetate ophthalmic, suspension Classification: Ophthalmic glucocorticoid	Econopred Econopred Plus Pred Forte Pred Mild
prednisolone sodium phosphate ophthalmic, solution Classification: Ophthalmic glucocorticoid	AK-Pred Inflamase Forte Inflamase Mild Prednosolone Sodium Phosphate
prednisolone sodium phosphate Classification: Glucocorticoid	Hydeltrasol Key-Pred-SP Pediapred
prednisolone tebutate Classification: Glucocorticoid	Prednisol TBA Prednisolone Tebutate
prednisone Classification: Glucocorticoid	Deltasone Liqui Pred Meticorten Orasone Panasol-S Prednicen-M Prednisone Prednisone Intensol Concentrate Sterapred Sterapred DS
prilocaine HCl Classification: Local anesthetic	Citanest HCl Citanest HCl Forte
primaquine phosphate Classification: Antimalarial	Primaquine Phosphate
primidone Classification: Anticonvulsant	Mysoline Primidone Sertan*
probenecid Classification: Uricosuric	Benuryl* Probenecid
procainamide HCl Classification: Antiarrhythmic	Procainamide HCl Pronestyl
procainamide, extended release Classification: Antiarrhythmic	Procanabid

*Available in Canada only

GENERIC NAME	BRAND NAME

procainamide, sustained release
Classification:
Antiarrhythmic

Procainamide HCl
Pronestyl-SR

procaine HCl
Classification:
Local anesthetic

Novocain
Procaine HCl

procarbazine HCl
(N-methylhydrazine; MIH)
Classification:
Antineoplastic, miscellaneous

Matulane
Natulan*

prochlorperazine
Classification:
Antipsychotic

Compazine
Compazine Spansules
Prochlorperazine
Stemetil*

procyclidine HCl
Classification:
Anticholinergic

Kemadrin
Procyclid*

progesterone
Classification:
Progestin

Prometrium

progesterone gel
Classification:
Progestin

Crinone

progesterone intrauterine
system
Classification:
Progestin

Progestasert

progesterone powder
Classification:
Progestin

Progesterone

progesterone in oil
Classification:
Progestin

Progesterone in Oil

promazine HCl
Classification:
Antipsychotic

Promanyl*
Promazine HCl
Prozine-50
Sparine

promethazine HCl
Classification:
Antihistamine

Anergan 50
Phenergan
Phenergan Fortis
Phenergan Plain

*Available in Canada Only

GENERIC NAME	BRAND NAME
promethazine HCl (cont'd.)	Promethazine HCl Prothazine Prothazine Plain
propafenone Classification: Antiarrhythmic	Rythmol
propamidine isethionate 0.1%, ophthalmic Classification: Antiprotazoal (Orphan)	Brolene
propantheline bromide Classification: Anticholinergic	Banlin* Pro-Banthine Propantheline Bromide
proparacaine HCl, ophthalmic Classification: Local anesthetic	Alcaine Ophthetic Proparacaine HCl
propiomazine HCl Classification: Sedative-hypnotic; nonbarbiturate	Largon
propiram Classification: Opioid analgesic (Investigational)	Dirame
propofol Classification: General anesthetic	Diprivan
propoxphene HCl Classification: Opioid analgesic	Darvon Pulvules Dolene Propoxyphene HCl
propoxyphene napsylate Classification: Opioid analgesic	Davron-N
propranolol HCl Classification: Beta-adrenergic blocker	Betacron E-R Inderal Inderal LA Inderal 10 Inderal 20 Inderal 40 Inderal 60 Inderal 80 Propranolol HCl Propranolol Intensol

*Available in Canada only

GENERIC NAME	BRAND NAME

propylhexedrine
Classification:
Nasal decongestant

Benzedrex

propyliodone 60%
Classification:
Radiopaque agent

Dionosil Oily

propylthiouracil (PTU)
Classification:
Antithyroid agent

Propylthiouracil
Propyl-Thyracil*

protamine sulfate
Classification:
Heparin antagonist

Protamine Sulfate

protein C concentrate
Classification:
Hemostatic (Orphan)

Protein C Concentrate

protirelin
Classification:
Thyroid function test

Thypinone
Thyrel-TRH

protriptyline HCl
Classification:
Antidepressant, tricyclic

Protriptyline HCl
Vivactil

pseudoephedrine HCl
Classification:
Nasal decongestant

Allermed
Cenafed
Cenafed Syrup
Children's Congestion Relief
Children's Silfedrine
Children's Sudafed
Congestin Relief
Decofed Syrup
DeFed-60
Dorcol Children's Decongestant
Dynafed Pseudo
Efidac/24
Eltor*
Genaphed
Halofed
Mini Thin Pseudo
PediaCare Infant's Decongestant
Pseudoephedrine HCl
Pseudo-Gest
Pseudo
Seudotabs
Sinustop Pro

GENERIC NAME	BRAND NAME
pseudoephedrine HCl **(cont'd.)**	Sudafed Sudafed 12 Hour Caplets Sudex Triaminic AM Decongestant Formula
pseudoephedrine sulfate Classification: Nasal decongestant	Afrin Drixoral Non-Drowsy Formula
pseudomonas hyperimmune **globulin** Classification: Immune serum (Orphan)	MEPIG
psyllium Classification: Laxative, bulk-producing	Alramucil Effer-Syllium Fiberall Fiberall Natural Flavor and Orange Flavor Hydrocil Instant Powder Konsyl Konsyl-D Konsyl-Orange Maalox Daily Fiber Therapy Metamucil Metamucil Instant Mix Lemon Lime Metamucil Instant Mix Orange Metamucil Orange Flavor Metamucil Sugar Free Metamucil Sugar Free Orange Flavor Modane Bulk Mylanta Natural Fiber Supplement Natural Vegetable Perdiem Fiber Prodiem Plain* Reguloid Natural Reguloid Orange Reguloid Sugar Free Orange Reguloid Sugar Free Regular Restore Serutan Syllact V-Lax
pulmonary surfactant **replacement, porcine** Classification: Lung surfactant (Orphan)	Curosurf

*Available in Canada only

GENERIC NAME	BRAND NAME

pyrantel pamoate
Classification:
Anthelmintics

Antiminth
Combantrin*
Pin-Rid
Pin-X
Reese's Pinworm

pyrazinamide
Classification:
Antitubercular

Pyrazinamide
Tebrazid*

pyridostigmine bromide
Classification:
Anticholinesterase

Mestinon
Regonol

pyridoxine HCl (Vitamin B$_6$)
Classification:
Vitamin, water soluble

Nestrex
Pyridoxine HCl
Vitamin B$_6$

pyrimethamine
Classification:
Antimalarial

Daraprim

pyrithione zinc
Classification:
Antiseborrheic

DHS Zinc
Head & Shoulders
Theraplex Z
TVC-2 Dandruff Shampoo
Zincon
ZNP Bar

Q

quazepam
Classification:
Sedative-hypnotic; benzodiazepine

Doral

quetiapine
Classification:
Antipsychotic

Seroquel

quinapril HCl
Classification:
Antihypertensive; angiotensin converting
enzyme inhibitor

Accupril

quinethazone
Classification:
Thiazide diuretic

Hydromox

GENERIC NAME	BRAND NAME

quinidine gluconate
Classification:
Antiarrhythmic

Quinaglute Dura-Tabs
Quinalan
Quinidine Gluconate

quinidine polygalacturonate
Classification:
Antiarrhythmic

Cardioquin

quinidine sulfate
Classification:
Antiarrhythmic

Quinidex Extentabs
Quinidine Sulfate
Quinora

quinine sulfate
Classification:
Antimalarial

Legatrin
Novoquine*
Quinine Sulfate

quinupritin-dalfopristin
Classification:
Antibiotic (Investigational)

Synercid

R

rabies immune globulin, human (RIG)
Classification:
Rabies prophylaxis

Hyperab
Imogam Rabies-HT

rabies vaccine
Classification:
Vaccine

RabAvert

rabies vaccine, human diploid cell cultures (HDCV)
Classification:
Rabies prophylaxis

Imovax Rabies I.D. Vaccine
Imovax Rabies Vaccine

radiopaque polyvinyl chloride
Classification:
Radiopaque agent

Sitzmarks

raloxifene
Classification:
Estrogen receptor modulator

Evista

ramipril
Classification:
Antihypertensive; angiotensin converting enzyme inhibitor

Altace

*Available in Canada only

GENERIC NAME	BRAND NAME

ranitidine
Classification:
Histamine H_2 receptor antagonist

Ranitidine
Zantac
Zantac 75
Zantac EFFERdose
Zantac GELdose

ranitidine bismuth citrate
Classification:
H. pylori agent

Tritec

rauwolfia derivatives-reserpine
Classification:
Antihypertensive

Reserfia*
Reserpine

recombinant vaccinia (human papillomavirus)
Classification:
Antineoplastic (Orphan)

TA-HPV

relaxin (recombinant, human)
Classification:
Anti-multiple sclerosis agent (Orphan)

Relaxin (recombinant, human)

remifentanil HCl
Classification:
Opioid analgesic

Ultiva

repaglinide
Classification:
Antidiabetic; meglitinide

Prandin

respiratory syncytial virus immune globulin IV (human) (RSV-IGIV)
Classification:
Immune serum

RespiGam

retelpase, recombinant
Classification:
Antithrombotic

Retavase

retinoin
Classification:
Antineoplastic (Orphan)

Retinoin

RGG0853,E1A lipid complex
Classification:
Antineoplastic (Orphan)

RGG0853,E1A lipid complex

rhIL-12
Classification:
Biologic response modifier
(Investigational)

rhIL-12

GENERIC NAME	BRAND NAME
Rho (D) immune globulin Classification: Immune serum	Gamulin Rh HypRho-D RhoGAM
Rho (D) immune globulin IV **(human)** Classification: Immune serum	WinRho SD
Rho (D) immune globulin **micro-dose** Classification: Immune serum	HypRho-D Mini-Dose MICRhoGAM Mini-Gamulin Rh
ribavirin Classification: Antiviral	Virazole
riboflavin (B₂) Classification: Vitamin, water soluble	Riboflavin
ricin (blocked) conjugated **murine MCA (anti-b4)** Classification: Antineoplastic (Orphan)	Ricin (blocked) Conjugated Murine MCA (anti-b4)
ricin (blocked) conjugated **murine MCA (anti-my9)** Classification: Antineoplastic (Orphan)	Ricin (blocked) conjugated murine MCA (anti-my9)
ricin (blocked) conjugated **murine MCA (n901)** Classification: Antineoplastic (Orphan)	Ricin (blocked) conjugated murine MCA (n901)
rifabutin Classification: Antitubercular	Mycobutin
rifampin Classification: Antitubercular	Rifadin Ramactine
rifapentine Classification: Antitubercular (Orphan)	Rifapentine
riluzole Classification: Anti-amyotropic lateral sclerosis agent	Rilutek

GENERIC NAME	BRAND NAME

RII retinamide
Classification:
Anti-myelodysplastic agent (Orphan)

RII Retinamide

rimantadine HCl
Classification:
Antiviral

Flumadine

rimexolone
Classification:
Ophthalmic glucocorticoid

Vexol

risperidone
Classification:
Antipsychotic

Risperdal

ritanserin
Classification:
Serotonin S-2 antagonist (Investigational)

Retanserin

ritodrine HCl
Classification:
Uterine relaxant

Ritodrine HCl
Yutopar

ritonavir
Classification:
Antiviral; protease inhibitor

Norvir

rituximab
Classification:
Antineoplastic

Rituxan

rocuronium bromide
Classification:
Nondepolarizing neuromuscular blocker

Zemuron

ropivacaine HCl
Classification:
Local anesthetic

Naropin

ropinirole
Classification:
Antiparkinson agent

Requip

roquinimex
Classification:
Biologic response modifier
(Investigational)

Linomide

rose bengal
Classification:
Ophthalmic diagnostic

Rose Bengal
Rosets

*Available in Canada Only

GENERIC NAME	BRAND NAME

rotavirus vaccine
Classification:
Vaccine

RotaShield

roxatidine acetate
Classification:
Histamine H$_2$ receptor antagonist
(Investigational)

Roxin

**rubella and mumps virus
vaccine, live**
Classification:
Vaccine

Biavax II

rubella virus vaccine, live
Classification:
Vaccine

Meruvax II

R-VIII SQ
Classification:
Hemostatic (Orphan)

REFACTO

S

safflower
Classification:
Modular supplement

Microlipid

salicylic acid, topical
Classification:
Keratolytic

Clear Away
Clear Away Plantar
Compound W
Dr. Scholl's Corn/Callus Remover
Dr. Scholl's Wart Removal Kit
DuoFilm
DuoPlant
Freezone
Gordofilm
Mediplast
Mosco
Occlusal-HP
Off-Ezy Wart Remover
Panscol
Paplex Ultra
Psor-a-set
Sal-Acid
Salactic Film
Sal Plant
Trans-Ver-Sal Adult Patch
Trans-Ver-Sal Pedia Patch

GENERIC NAME	BRAND NAME

salicylic acid, topical (cont'd.)

Trans-Ver-Sal Plantar Patch
Wart-Off
Wart Remover

saline laxatives
Classification:
Laxative

Citrate of Magnesia
Epsom Salt
Fleet
Milk of Magnesia
Milk of Magnesia Concentrated
MOM
Phospho-soda
Sodium Phosphates

saliva substitutes
Classification:
Oral lubricant

Moi-Stir
Moi-Stir Swabsticks
Moi-Stir 10
Optimoist
Salivart
Salix

salmeterol
Classification:
Bronchodilator; beta-adrenergic agonist

Serevent
Serevent Diskus

salsalate
Classification:
Salicylate analgesic

Amigesic
Argesic-SA
Arthra-G
Disalcid
Marthritic
Mono-gesic
Salflex
Salsalate
Salsitab

saquinavir mesylate
Classification:
Antiviral; protease inhibitor

Invirase

sargramostim (granulocyte macrophage colony stimulating factor, GM-CSF)
Classification:
Biologic modifier

Leukine

satumomab pendetide
Classification:
In vivo diagnostic (Orphan)

Oncoscint CR/OV

GENERIC NAME	BRAND NAME
scopolamine hydrobromide Classification: Anticholinergic	Scopace Scopolamine Hydrobromide
scopolamine hydrobromide, ophthalmic Classification: Mydriatic	Isopto Hyoscine
scopolamine, transdermal Classification: Antiemetic; anticholinergic	Transderm-Scōp
secalciferol Classification: Vitamin, fat soluble (Orphan)	Osteo-D
secobarbital sodium Classification: Sedative-hypnotic; barbiturate	Secobarbital Sodium Secogen Sodium* Seconal Sodium Pulvules Seral*
secretin Classification: Gastrointestinal function test	Secretin-Ferring Powder
selegiline HCl (L-deprenyl) Classification: Antiparkinson agent	Carbex Eldepryl Selegline HCl
selenium Classification: Trace element	Selenium Sele-Pak Selepen
selenium sulfide Classification: Antiseborrheic	Exsel Head & Shoulders Intensive Treatment SeleniumSulfide Selsun Selsun Blue Selsun Gold for Women
senna Classification: Laxative; irritant	Black-Draught Dosalex Dr. Caldwell Senna Laxative Fletcher's Castoria Gentlax Senexon Senna-Gen Senokot Senokotxtra Senolax

GENERIC NAME	BRAND NAME

sermorelin acetate
Classification:
Polypeptide; in vivo diagnostic aid

Geref

serretia marcescens extract (polyribosomes)
Classification:
Antineoplastic (Orphan)

Imuvert

sertindole
Classification:
Antipsychotic (Investigational)

Serlect
Sertindole

sertraline HCl
Classification:
Antidepressant

Zoloft

sevoflurane
Classification:
General anesthetic

Ultane

sibutramine HCl monohydrate
Classification:
CNS stimulant; anorexiant

Meridia

sildenafil
Classification:
Smooth muscle relaxant

Viagra

silver nitrate, ophthalmic
Classification:
Ophthalmic antiseptic

Silver Nitrate 1%

silver nitrate, topical
Classification:
Cauterizing agent

Silver Nitrate

silver sulfadiazine
Classification:
Antibacterial

Silvadene
SSD
SSD AF

simethicone
Classification:
Antiflatulent

Degas
Extra Strength Gas-X
Flatulex
Gas Relief
Gas X
Maalox Anti-Gas
Maximum Strength Mylanta Gas
Major-Con
Mylanta Gas
Mylicon

GENERIC NAME	BRAND NAME
simethicone (cont'd.)	Ovol* Phazyme Phazyme 95 Phazyme 125 Simethicone
simvastatin Classification: Antilipemic	Zocor
sincalide Classification: Gastrointestinal function test	Kinevac
skin test antigens, multiple Classification: In vivo diagnostic	Multitest CMI
smallpox vaccine (Vaccinia) Classification: Vaccine	Smallpox Vaccine (Vaccinia)
sodium acetate Classification: Electrolyte replacement	Sodium Acetate
sodium antimony gluconate Classification: CDC anti-infective	Pentustam
sodium ascorbate Classification: Vitamin, water soluble	Cenolate Sodium Ascorbate
sodium bicarbonate Classification: Systemic alkalinizer	Bell/ans Neut Sodium Bicarbonate
sodium chloride Classification: Hyperosmolar preparation	Broncho Saline Slo-Salt Sodium Chloride
sodium chloride, hypertonic Classification: Hyperosmolar preparation	Adsorbonac AK-NaCl Dey-Pak Sodium Chloride 3% and 10% Muro 128 Muroptic-5
sodium chloride, nasal Classification: Nasal decongestant	Afrin Saline Mist Ayr Saline Breathe Free Dristan Saline Spray

*Available in Canada only

GENERIC NAME	BRAND NAME

sodium chloride, nasal (cont'd.)

HuMist Saline Nasal Mist
NāSal
Nasal Moist
Ocean
Pretz
SalineX
SeaMist

sodium citrate/citric acid solution (Shohl's Solution)
Classification:
Urinary alkalinizer

Bicitra
Oracit
PMS-Dicitrate*

sodium dichloroacetate
Classification:
Antilactic acidosis agent (Orphan)

Sodium Dichloroacetate

sodium fluoride
Classification:
Electrolyte replacement; fluoride

ACT
Fluor-A-Day*
Fluoride
Fluoride Loz
Fluorigard
Fluorinse
Fluoritab
Fluotic*
Flura
Flura-Drops
Flura-Loz
Gel-Kam
Gel-Tin
Karidium
Karigel
Karigel-N
Luride
Luride-SF Lozi-Tabs
Luride Lozi-Tabs
Luride 0.25 Lozi-Tabs
Luride 0.5 Lozi-Tabs
Mouth Kote F/R
Minute-Gel
Pediaflor
Pharmaflur 1.1
Pharmaflur
Pharmaflur df
Phos-Flur
Point-Two
Prevident
Sodium Fluoride

*Available in Canada Only

GENERIC NAME	BRAND NAME
sodium fluoride (cont'd.)	Stop Thera-Flur Thera-Flur-N
sodium hyaluronate Classification: Ophthalmic viscoelastic	AMO Vitrax Amvisc Amvisc Plus Healon Healon GV
sodium hyaluronate Classification: Viscoelastic, intra-articular	Hyalgan
sodium hypochlorite Classification: Germicidal	Dakin's Solution
sodium iodide I 123 Classification: Thyroid function test	Sodium Iodide I 123
sodium iodide I 131 Classification: Antithyroid agent	Iodotope Sodium Iodide I 131
sodium lactate Classification: Electrolyte replacement	Sodium Lactate
sodium phenylbutyrate Classification: Blood modifier, urea	Buphenyl
sodium phosphate P 32 Classification: Antineoplastic; radiopharmaceutical	Sodium Phosphate P 32
sodium polystyrene sulfonate Classification: Potassium-removing resin	Kayexalate Sodium Polystyrene Sulfonate SPS
sodium salicylate Classification: Salicylate analgesic	Sodium Salicylate
sodium tetradecyl sulfate Classification: Sclerosing agent	Sotradecol
sodium thiosalicylate Classification: Salicylate analgesic	Rexolate Sodium Thiosalicylate

*Available in Canada only

GENERIC NAME	BRAND NAME

sodium thiosulfate
Classification:
Cyanide antidote

Sodium Thiosulfate

soluble complement receptor (recombinant) type 1
Classification:
Biologic response modifier (Orphan)

Soluble Complement Receptor (recombinant) Type 1

somatostatin
Classification:
Sclerosing agent (Orphan)

Somatostatin

somatropin
Classification:
Growth hormone

Genotropin
Humatrope
Norditropin
Nutropin
Nutropin AQ
Serostim

somatrem
Classification:
Growth hormone

Protropin

sorbitol
Classification:
Genitourinary irrigant

Sorbitol

spectinomycin HCl
Classification:
Antibiotic; aminocyclitol

Trobicin

sotalol
Classification:
Antiarrhythmic; beta-adrenergic blocker

Betapace

sparfloxacin
Classification:
Antibiotic; fluoroquinolone

Zagam

spironolactone
Classification:
Potassium-sparing diuretic

Aldactone
Spironolactone

ST1-RTA immunotoxin (SR 44163)
Classification:
Immune serum (Orphan)

ST1-RTA Immunotoxin (SR 44163)

stanozolol
Classification:
Anabolic steroid

Winstrol

*Available in Canada Only

GENERIC NAME	BRAND NAME
staphage lysate Classification: Vaccine	SPL-Serologic Types I and II
stavudine (d4T) Classification: Antiviral; nucleoside	Zerit
stem cell factor Classification: Biologic response modifier (Investigational)	Stemgen
stimulon Classification: Vaccine (Investigational)	Stimulon
streptococcus immune globulin, group B Classification: Immune serum (Orphan)	Streptoccoccus Immune Globulin, group B
streptokinase Classification: Antithrombotic	Kabikinase Streptase
streptozocin Classification: Antineoplastic; alkylating agent	Zanosar
strontium-89 chloride Classification: Antineoplastic; radiopharmaceutical	Metastron
SU-101 Classification: Antineoplastic (Orphan)	SU-101
succimer Classification: Chelating agent	Chemet
succinylcholine chloride Classification: Depolarizing neuromuscular blocker	Anectine Anectine Flo-Pack Brevidil M* (Bromide Salt) Quelicin Sux-Cert*
sucralfate Classification: Protectant	Carafate Sucralfate Sulcrate*

*Available in Canada only

GENERIC NAME	BRAND NAME
sucrase Classification: Enzyme (Orphan)	Sacarasa
sufentanil citrate Classification: Opioid analgesic	Sufenta Sufentanil Citrate
sulconazole nitrate Classification: Antifungal	Exelderm
sulfacetamide sodium, ophthalmic Classification: Antibiotic; sulfonamide	AK-Sulf Bleph-10 Cetamide Isopto Cetamide Ocusulf-10 Sodium Sulamyd Sodium Sulfacetamide Sulfacetamide Sodium 10% Sulfacetamide Sodium 15% Sulfacetamide Sodium 30% Sulf-10
sulfacetamide sodium, topical Classification: Antiseborrheic	Klaron Sebizon
sulfadiazine Classification: Antibiotic; sulfonamide	Sulfadiazine
sulfamethizole Classification: Antibiotic; sulfonamide	Thiosulfil Forte
sulfamethoxazole Classification: Antibiotic; sulfonamide	Gantanol Sulfamethoxazole Urobak
sulfanilamide Classification: Antibiotic; sulfonamide	AVC
sulfapyridine Classification: Antibiotic; sulfonamide	Dagenan*
sulfasalazine Classification: Anti-inflammatory; sulfonamide	Azulfidine Azulfidine EN-tabs Salazopyrin* Sulfasalazine

*Available in Canada Only

GENERIC NAME	BRAND NAME

sulfinpyrazone
Classification:
Uricosuric

Anturan*
Anturane
Sulfinpyrazone

sulfisoxazole
Classification:
Antibiotic; sulfonamide

Gantrisin
Novosoxazole*

sulfur
Classification:
Anti-acne product

Acne Lotion 10
Bensulfoid
Fostex Medicated
Liquimat
Sulmasque
Sulpho-Lac

sulindac
Classification:
Nonsteroidal anti-inflammatory

Clinoril
Novosudac*
Sulindac

sumatriptan succinate
Classification:
Antimigraine

Imitrex

sumatriptan, nasal
Classification:
Antimigraine

Imitrex Nasal

superoxide dismutase (human)
Classification:
Antioxidant (Orphan)

Superoxide Dismutase (human)

**superoxide dismutase
(recombinant human)**
Classification:
Antioxidant (Orphan)

Superoxide Dismutase (recombinant
human)

suprofen
Classification:
Ophthalmic nonsteroidal anti-
inflammatory

Profenal

suramin
Classification:
CDC anti-infective

Antrypol
Bayer 205
Belganyl
Fourneau 309
Germanin
Moranyl
Naganol
Naphuride

GENERIC NAME	BRAND NAME

surface active extract of saline lavage of bovine lungs
Classification:
Lung surfactant (Orphan)

Infasurf

synsorb Rx
Classification:
Anti-infective (Orphan)

Synsorb Rx

T

T4 endonuclease V, liposome encapsulated
Classification:
Enzyme (Orphan)

T4 Endonuclease V, liposome encapsulated

T4, soluble human, recombinant
Classification:
Antiviral (Investigational)

T4, Soluble Human, recombinant

tacrine HCl
Classification:
Cholinesterase inhibitor

Cognex

tacrolimus (FK506)
Classification:
Immunosuppressive

Prograf

talc, sterile aerosol
Classification:
Pleurodesis agent (Investigational)

Sclerosol

tamoxifen citrate
Classification:
Antineoplastic; hormone

Nolvadex
Tamofen*
Tamone*
Tamoxifen

tamsulosin HCl
Classification:
Alpha-adrenergic blocker

Flomax

tannic acid
Classification:
Protectant

Zilactin Medicated

TAT antagonist
Classification:
Antiviral (Investigational)

TAT Antagonist

GENERIC NAME	BRAND NAME
tazarotene Classification: Anti-acne	Tazorac
technetium Tc-99m antimelanoma monoclonal antibody Classification: In vivo diagnostic (Orphan)	Oncotrac Melanoma Imaging Kit
technetium Tc-99m monoclonal antibody to AFP Classification: In vivo diagnostic (Orphan)	Immuraid, AFP-TC-99m
technetium Tc-99m monoclonal antibody to B cell Classification: In vivo diagnostic (Orphan)	LymphoScan
technetium Tc-99m monoclonal antibody to hCG Classification: In vivo diagnostic (Orphan)	Immuraid, hCG-Tc-99m
telcoplanin Classification: Antibiotic, glycopeptide (Investigational)	Targocid
temazepam Classification: Sedative-hypnotic; benzodiazepine	Restoril Temazepam
tenidap Classification: Anti-inflammatory (Investigational)	Enable
teniposide Classification: Antineoplastic; mitotic inhibitor	Vumon
terazosin Classification: Antihypertensive; alpha-adrenergic blocker	Hytrin
terbinafine HCl Classification: Antifungal	Lamisil

GENERIC NAME	BRAND NAME

terbutaline sulfate
Classification:
Bronchodilator; beta-adrenergic agonist

Brethaire
Brethine
Bricanyl

terconazole
Classification:
Antifungal

Terazol 3
Terazol 7

terfenadine
Classification:
Antihistamine

Terfenadine

teriparatide acetate
Classification:
Hormone

Parathar

terlipressin
Classification:
Posterior pituitary hormone (Orphan)

Glypressin

terpin hydrate
Classification:
Expectorant

Terpin Hydrate

testolactone
Classification:
Antineoplastic; hormone

Teslac

testosterone aqueous suspension
Classification:
Androgen

Histerone 100
Tesamone
Testosterone Aqueous

testosterone cypionate (in oil)
Classification:
Androgen

depAndro 100
depAndro 200
Depotest 100
Depotest 200
Depo-Testosterone
Duratest-100
Duratest-200
Testosterone Cypionate

testosterone enanthate (in oil)
Classification:
Androgen

Andro L.A. 200
Andropository-200
Delatest
Delatestryl
Durathate-200
Everone 200
Testone LA 200
Testosterone Enanthate

*Available in Canada Only

GENERIC NAME	BRAND NAME
testosterone pellet Classification: Androgen	Testopel
testosterone propionate (in oil) Classification: Androgen	Testosterone Propionate
testosterone transdermal Classification: Androgen	Andoderm Testoderm Testoderm TTS
tetanus immune globulin Classification: Immune serum	Hyper-Tet
tetanus toxoid, adsorbed Classification: Toxoid	Tetanus Toxoid, Adsorbed
tetanus toxoid, fluid Classification: Local anesthetic	Tetanus Toxoid, Fluid
tetracaine HCl Classification: Local anesthetic	Pontocaine HCl
tetracaine HCl, topical Classification: Local anesthetic	Pontocaine HCl
tetracaine HCl, ophthalmic Classification: Local anesthetic	Pontocaine HCl Tetracaine HCl
tetracycline HCl Classification: Antibiotic; tetracycline	Cefracycline* Medicycline* Neo-Tetrine* Nor-Tet Novotetra* Panmycin Sumycin 250 Sumycin 500 Sumycin Syrup Teline Teline-500 Tetracap Tetracycline HCl Tetracycline HCl Syrup Tetralean*

*Available in Canada only

GENERIC NAME	BRAND NAME

tetracycline HCl, topical
Classification:
Antibiotic; tetracycline

Actisite
Topicycline

tetrahydrozoline HCl, nasal
Classification:
Nasal decongestant

Tyzine
Tyzine Pediatric Drops

tetrahydrozoline HCl, ophthalmic
Classification:
Ophthalmic vasoconstrictor

Collyrium Fresh Eye Drops
Eyesine
Geneye
Geneye Extra
Mallazine Eye Drops
Murine Plus
Optigene 3
Tetrahydrozoline HCl
Tetrasine
Tetrasine Extra

thalidomide
Classification:
Immunosuppressive agent (Orphan)

Synovir

theophylline
Classification:
Bronchodilator; xanthine

Accurbron
Aerolate III
Aerolate Jr.
Aerolate Sr.
Aquaphyllin
Asmalix
Bronkodyl
Elixomin
Elixophyllin
Lanophyllin
Quibron-T Dividose
Quibron-T/SR Dividose
Respbid
Slo-bid Gyrocaps
Slo-Phyllin
Slo-Phyllin Gyrocaps
Sustaire
Theo-24
Theobid Duracaps
Theochron
Theoclear-80
Theoclear L.A.
Theo-Dur
Theolair
Theolair-SR

GENERIC NAME	BRAND NAME
theophylline **(cont'd.)**	Theophylline Theophylline and 5% Dextrose Theophylline Extended Release Theophylline Oral Theophylline SR Theo-Sav Theospan-SR Theostat 80 Theovent Theo-X T-Phyl Uni-Dur Uniphyl
thiabendazole Classification: Anthelmintic	Mintezol
thiamine HCl (vitamin B$_1$) Classification: Vitamin, water soluble	Betaxin* Thiamilate Thiamine HCl
thiethylperazine maleate Classification: Antiemetic	Torecan
thimerosal Classification: Antiseptic	Aeroaid Mersol Thimerosal
thioguanine (TG;6-thioguanine) Classification: Antineoplastic; antimetabolite	Lanvis* Thioguanine
thiopental sodium Classification: General anesthetic; barbiturate	Pentothal Thiopental Sodium
thioridazine HCl Classification: Antipsychotic	Mellaril Mellaril Concentrate Mellaril-S Novoridazine* Thioridazine HCl Thioridazine HCl Intensol
thiotepa (triethylenethio- **phosphoramide; TSPA;** **TESPA)** Classification: Antineoplastic; alkylating agent	Thioplex

*Available in Canada only

GENERIC NAME	BRAND NAME

thiothixene
Classification:
Antipsychotic

Navane
Thiothixene
Thiothixene HCl Intensol

threonine
Classification:
Amino acid

Threonine

thrombin, topical
Classification:
Hemostatic

Thrombin-JMI
Thrombinar
Thrombogen
Thrombostat

thymic humoral factor
Classification:
Biologic response modifier
(Investigational)

Thymic Humoral Factor

thymopentin
Classification:
Biologic response modifier
(Investigational)

Timunox

thymosin alpha-1
Classification:
Biologic response modifier (Orphan)

Thymosin Alpha-1

thymostimuline (TP-1)
Classification:
Biologic response modifier
(Investigational)

Thymostimuline (TP-1)

thyroid stimulating hormone, human (TSH)
Classification:
In vivo diagnostic (Orphan)

Thyrogen

thyroid USP (desiccated)
Classification:
Thyroid hormone

Armour Thyroid
Cholaxin*
S-P-T
Thyrar
Thyroid USP

thyrotropin (thyroid stimulating hormone, or TSH)
Classification:
Thyroid function test

Thytropar

tiagabine
Classification:
Anticonvulsant

Gabitril

*Available in Canada Only

GENERIC NAME	BRAND NAME
ticarcillin and clavulanate potassium Classification: Antibiotic; extended spectrum penicillin	Timentin
ticarcillin disodium Classification: Antibiotic; extended spectrum penicillin	Ticar Ticaripen*
ticlopidine HCl Classification: Antiplatelet	Ticlid
tiludronate Classification: Bone resorption inhibitor	Skelid
timolol maleate, ophthalmic Classification: Beta-adrenergic blocker	Betimol Timolol Maleate Ophthalmic Timoptic Timoptic-XE
timolol maleate Classification: Antihypertensive; beta-adrenergic blocker	Blocadren Timolol Maleate
timunox thymopentin Classification: Biologic response modifier	Timunox Thymopentin
tioconazole Classification: Antifungal	Vagistat-1
tiopronin Classification: Anticystinuria agent	Thiola
tiratricol Classification: Antineoplastic agent (Orphan)	Triacana
tirilazed mesylate Classification: Antiviral (Investigational)	Tirilazed Mesylate
tizanidine HCl Classification: Skeletal muscle relaxant	Zanaflex

GENERIC NAME	BRAND NAME
T-lymphotropic virus type III Gp 160 antigens (human) Classification: Biologic response modifier (Orphan)	Vaxsyn HIV-1
tobramycin, inhalation Classification: Aminoglycoside	TOBI
tobramycin, ophthalmic Classification: Aminoglycoside	AKTob Tobamycin Opththalmic Tobrex
tobramycin sulfate Classification: Aminoglycoside	Nebcin Tobramycin Sulfate
tocainide HCl Classification: Antiarrhythmic	Tonocard
tolazamide Classification: Antidiabetic; sulfonylurea	Tolazamide Tolinase
tolazoline HCl Classification: Antihypertensive; vasodilator	Priscoline
tolbutamide Classification: Antidiabetic; sulfonylurea	Mobenol* Novobutamide* Orinase Tolbutamide Tolbutone*
tolbutamide sodium Classification: In vivo diagnostic; sulfonylurea	Orinase Diagnostic
tolcapone Classification: Antiparkinson agent	Tasmar
tolmetin sodium Classification: Nonsteroidal anti-inflammatory	Tolectin DS Tolectin 200 Tolectin 600 Tolmetin Sodium
tolnaftate Classification: Antifungal	Absorbine Antifungal Absorbine Athlete's Foot Care Absorbine Jock Itch Absorbine Jr. Antifungal

*Available in Canada Only

GENERIC NAME   BRAND NAME

tolnaftate   Aftate for Athletes Foot
(cont'd.)   Aftate for Jock Itch
                                   Blis-To-Sol
                                   Breeze Mist Antifungal Powder
                                   Desenex Spray Liquid
                                   Dr. Scholl's Athlete's Foot
                                   Dr. Scholl's Maximum Strength Tritan
                                   Genaspor
                                   NP-27
                                   Quinsana Plus
                                   Tinactin
                                   Ting
                                   Tolnaftate
                                   Zeasorb-AF

topiramate   Topamax
Classification:
Anticonvulsant

topotecan HCl   Hycamtin
Classification:
Antineoplastic; hormone

toremifene citrate   Fareston
Classification:
Antineoplastic; anti-estrogen

torsemide   Demadex
Classification:
Loop diuretic

tramadol HCl   Ultram
Classification:
Analgesic

trandolapril   Mavik
Classification: Tarka
Antihypertensive; angiotensin converting
enzyme inhibitor

tranexamic acid   Cyklokapron
Classification:
Hemostatic

tranylcypromine sulfate   Parnate
Classification:
Monoamine oxidase inhibitor

trazodone HCl   Desyrel
Classification: Desyrel Dividose
Antidepressant, tetracyclic   Trazodone HCl

GENERIC NAME	BRAND NAME

tretinoin
Classification:
Antineoplastic, miscellaneous

Vesanoid

tretinoin (vitamin A acid, retinoic acid)
Classification:
Anti-acne product

Acticin
Renova
Retin-A
Retin-A Micro
Vesanoid
Vitinoin*

triamcinolone
Classification:
Glucocorticoid

Aristocort
Atolone
Kenacort
Triamcinolone

triamcinolone acetonide
Classification:
Glucocorticoid

Azmacort
Kenaject-40
Kenalog
Kenalog-10
Kenalog-40
Tac-3
Tac-40
Triam-A
Triamcinolone Acetonide
Triamonide 40
Tri-Kort
Trilog

triamcinolone acetonide, nasal
Classification:
Glucocorticoid

Nasacort
Nasacort AQ

triamcinolone acetonide (Topical-Oral)
Classification:
Glucocorticoid

Kenalog in Orabase
Oralone Dental

triamcinolone acetonide, topical
Classification:
Glucocorticoid

Aristocort
Aristocort A
Delta-Tritex
Flutex
Kenalog
Kenalog-H
Kenonel
Triacet
Triamcinolone Acetonide
Triderm

*Available in Canada Only

GENERIC NAME	BRAND NAME
triamcinolone diacetate Classification: Glucocorticoid	Amcort Aristocort Forte Aristocort Intralesional Articulose L.A. Triamcinolone Triam Forte Triamolone 40 Trilone Trisoject
triamcinolone hexacetonide Classification: Glucocorticoid	Aristospan Intra-articular Aristospan Intralesional
triamterene Classification: Potassium-sparing diuretic	Dyrenium
triazolam Classification: Sedative-hypnotic; benzodiazepine	Halcion Triazolam
tricalciumphosphate Classification: Electrolyte replacement; calcium	Posture
trichlormethiazide Classification: Thiazide diuretic	Diurese Metahydrin Naqua Trichlormethiazide
trichloroacetic acid Classification: Cauterizing agent	Tri-Chlor
trichosanthin Classification: Antiviral (Investigational)	Trichosanthin
triclosan Classification: Germicidal	Septi-Soft Septisol Solution
tridihexethyl chloride Classification: Anticholinergic	Pathilon
trientine HCl Classification: Chelating agent	Syprine

*Available in Canada only

GENERIC NAME	BRAND NAME

trientine HCl
Classification:
Chelating agent (Orphan)

Cuprid

trifluoperazine HCl
Classification:
Antipsychotic

Novoflurazine*
Solazine*
Stelazine
Trifluoperazine HCl

triflupromazine HCl
Classification:
Antipsychotic

Vesprin

trifluridine
Classification:
Ophthalmic antiviral

Viroptic

trihexphenidyl HCl
Classification:
Anticholinergic

Aparkane*
Artane
Artane Sequels
Novohexidyl*
Trihexy-2
Trihexy-5
Trihexyphenidyl HCl

trimeprazine
Classification:
Antihistamine

Panectyl*

trimethadione
Classification:
Anticonvulsant; oxazolidinedione

Tridione

trimethobenzamide HCl
Classification:
Antiemetic; anticholinergic

Arrestin
Pediatric Triban
T-Gen
Tebamide
Ticon
Tigan
Triban
Trimazide
Trimethobenzamide
Trimethobenzamide HCl

trimethoprim (TMP)
Classification:
Antibiotic; folic acid antagonist

Proloprim
Trimethoprim
Trimpex

*Available in Canada Only

GENERIC NAME	BRAND NAME
trimethoprim, sulfamethoxazole (TMP-SMZ) Classification: Antibiotic; sulfonamide	Bactrim Bactrim DS Bactrim IV Cotrim Cotrim D.S. Cotrim Pediatric Septra Septra DS Septra I.V. Sulfatrim Trimethoprim and Sulfamethoxazole Trimethoprim and Sulfamethoxazole DS
trimetrexate glucoronate Classification: Folate antagonist	Neutrexin
trimipramine maleate Classification: Antidepressant	Surmontil
trioxsalen, oral Classification: Psoralen	Trisoralen
tripelennamine HCl Classification: Antihistamine	PBZ PBZ-SR Tripelennamine HCl
triple sulfa, vaginal Classification: Antibiotic; sulfonamide	Dayto-Sulf Gyne-Sulf Sultrin Triple Sulfa Triple Sulfa Trysul V.V.S.
trisaccharides A and B Classification: Biologic response modifier (Orphan)	Biosynject
troglitazone Classification: Antidiabetic	Rezulin
trolamine salicylate Classification: Analgesic	Analgesia Creme Aspercreme Cream Mobisyl Myoflex Sportscreme

*Available in Canada only

GENERIC NAME	BRAND NAME

troleandomycin
Classification:
Antibiotic; macrolide

Tao

tromethamine
Classification:
Systemic alkalinizer

Tham

tropicamide, ophthalmic
Classification:
Mydriatic

Mydriacyl
Opticyl
Tropicacyl
Tropicamide

trospectomycin
Classification:
Antibiotic; aminocyclitol (Investigational)

Spexil

trovafloxacin
Classification:
Antibiotic; fluoroquinolone

Trovan

tryptophan
Classification:
Amino acid

L-Tryptophan

tuberculin (old), multiple puncture devices
Classification:
In vivo diagnostic

Mono Vacc Test (O.T)
Tuberculin, Old, Tine Test

tuberculin PPD multiple puncture device
Classification:
In vivo diagnostic

Aplitest
Tine Test PPD

tuberculin purified protein derivative (mantoux; PPD)
Classification:
In vivo diagnostic

Aplisol
Tubersol

tubocurarine chloride
Classification:
Nondepolarizing neuromuscular blocker

Tubarine*
Tubocurarine

tumor necrosing factor-binding protein I and II
Classification:
Biologic response modifier (Orphan)

Tumor Necrosing Factor-binding Protein I and II

tumor necrosis factor
Classification:
Biologic response modifier
(Investigational)

Tumor Necrosis Factor

*Available in Canada Only

GENERIC NAME	BRAND NAME
tyloxapol Classification: Artificial eye lubricant	Enuclene
tyloxapol Classification: Mucolytic (Orphan)	Tyloxapol
typhoid vaccine Classification: Vaccine	Typhim Vi Typhoid Vaccine (AKD) Typhoid Vaccine (H-P) Vivotif Berna Vaccine
tyropanoate sodium Classification: Radiopaque agent	Bilopaque

U

undecylenic acid Classification: Antifungal	Blis-To-Sol Powder Caldesene Cruex Decylenes Desenex Desenex Maximum Strength Fungoid AF Protectol
urea Classification: Osmotic diuretic	Carbamex* Ureaphil
urea (carbamide), topical Classification: Emollient	Aquacare Carmol 10 Carmol 20 Gordons Urea Gormel Creme Lanaphilic Nutraplus Ultra Mide 25 Ureacin-10 Ureacin-20 Ureacin-40
uridine 5'-triphosphate Classification: Mucolytic (Orphan)	Uridine 5'-triphosphate

GENERIC NAME	BRAND NAME

urofollitropin
Classification:
Ovulation stimulant

Fertinex
Metrodin

urogastrone
Classification:
Ophthalmic (Orphan)

Urogastrone

urokinase
Classification:
Antithrombotic

Abbokinase
Abbokinase Open-Cath

ursodeoxycholic acid
Classification:
Antilithic (Orphan)

Ursofalk

ursodiol
Classification:
Antilithic

Actigall
URSO

V

vaccinia immune globulin (VIG) (human)
Classification:
Immune serum

Vaccinia Immune Globulin (VIG) (human)

valacyclovir HCl
Classification:
Antiviral

Valtrex

valproate sodium
Classification:
Anticonvulsant

Depakene Syrup
Valproic Acid Syrup

valproic acid
Classification:
Anticonvulsant

Depacon
Depakene
Valproic Acid

valsartan
Classification:
Antihypertensive; angiotensin II antagonist

Diovan

vancomycin HCl
Classification:
Antibiotic; tricyclic glycopeptide

Lyphocin
Vancocin
Vancoled
Vancomycin HCl

GENERIC NAME	BRAND NAME
varicella virus vaccine Classification: Vaccine	Varivax
varicella-zoster immune globulin (human) (VZIG) Classification: Immune serum	Varicella-Zoster Immune Globulin (Human)
vasopressin Classification: Posterior pituitary hormone	Pitressin Synthetic
vecuronium bromide Classification: Nondepolarizing neuromuscular blocker	Norcuron
veldona Classification: Biologic response modifier (Investigational)	Veldona
venlafaxine Classification: Antidepressant	Effexor Effexor-XR
verapamil HCl Classification: Calcium channel blocker	Calan Calan SR Covera-HS Isoptin Isoptin SR Verapamil HCl Verelan
vidarabine, ophthalmic Classification: Antiviral	Vira-A Ophthalmic
vigabatrin Classification: Anticonvulsant (Investigational)	Sabril
viloxazine Classification: Antidepressant (Investigational)	Catatrol
vinblastine sulfate (VLB) Classification: Antineoplastic; mitotic inhibitor	Velban Velbe* Vinblastine Sulfate

GENERIC NAME	BRAND NAME

vincristine sulfate (VCR; LCR)
Classification:
Antineoplastic; mitotic inhibitor

Oncovin
Vincasar PFS
Vincristine Sulfate

vinorelbine tartrate
Classification:
Antineoplastic; mitotic inhibitor

Navelbine

vitamin A
Classification:
Vitamin, fat soluble

Aquasol A
Del-Vi-A
Palmitrate-A 5000
Vitamin A

vitamin E
Classification:
Vitamin, fat soluble

Amino-Opti-E
Aquasol E
Daltose*
E-200 I.U. Softgels
E-Complex-600
E-Vitamin Succinate
Tocopherol
Vitamin E
Vita-Plus E Softgells

VX478
Classification:
Antiviral (Investigational)

VX478

W

warfarin sodium
Classification:
Anticoagulant

Coumadin
Warfilone Sodium*
Warnerin*

X

xylometazoline HCl, nasal
Classification:
Nasal decongestant

Otrivin
Otrivin Pediatric Nasal Drops

Y

yellow fever vaccine
Classification:
Vaccine

YF-Vax

*Available in Canada Only

GENERIC NAME	BRAND NAME
yohimbine HCl Classification: Alpha adrenergic blocker	Aphrodyne Dayto-Himbin Yocon Yohimbine HCl Yohimex

Z

zafirlukast Classification: Bronchodilator; leukotriene receptor antagonist	Accolate
zalcitabine (ddC; dideoxycytidine) Classification: Antiviral	Hivid
zileuton Classification: Bronchodilator; 5-lipoxygenase inhibitor	Zyflo
zinc gluconate Classification: Electrolyte replacement; zinc	Zinc Gluconate
zidovudine, formerly azidothymidine or AZT Classification: Antiviral	Retrovir
zinc oxide Classification: Protectant	Zinc Oxide
zinc sulfate Classification: Electrolyte replacement; zinc	Orazinc Verazinc Zinca-Pak Zincate Zinc 15 Zinc-220 Zinc Sulfate
zinc sulfate solution Classification: Ophthalmic astringent	Eye-Sed
zintevir Classification: Antiviral (Investigational)	Zintevir

*Available in Canada only

GENERIC NAME	BRAND NAME
ziprasidone Classification: Antipsychotic (Investigational)	Zeldox
zolmitriptan Classification: Antimigraine	Zomig
zonisamide Classification: Anticonvulsant (Investigational)	Exegran

Section II — Brand to Generic

BRAND NAME	GENERIC NAME

1/2 Halfprin
Classification:
Salicylate analgesic; antipyretic

aspirin

1% HC
Classification:
Glucocorticoid

hydrocortisone, topical

10-Benzagel
Classification:
Anti-acne product

benzoyl peroxide

2.5% Mydfrin Ophthalmic
Classification:
Ophthalmic vasoconstrictor

phenylephrine HCl, ophthalmic

24,25-dihydroxycholecalciferol
Classification:
Vitamin, fat soluble (Orphan)

24,25-dihydroxycholecalciferol

2-Chlorodeoxyadenosine
Classification:
Antineoplastic (Orphan)

2-chlorodeoxyadenosine

3,4-diaminopyridine
Classification:
Anti-myasthenia agent (Orphan)

3,4-diaminopyridine

4X Pancreatin 600 mg
Classification:
Digestive enzyme

pancreatin

40 Winks
Classification:
Antihistamine

diphenhydramine HCl

4-Way Long Acting Nasal
Classification:
Nasal decongestant

oxymetazoline HCl, nasal

5,6-dihydro-5-azacytidine
Classification:
Antineoplastic (Orphan)

5,6-dihydro-5-azacytidine

5-aza-2 deoxycitidine
Classification:
Antineoplastic (Orphan)

5-aza-2 deoxycitidine

*Available in Canada Only

BRAND NAME	GENERIC NAME
5-Benzagel Classification: Anti-acne product	benzoyl peroxide
8X Pancreatin 900 mg Classification: Digestive enzyme	pancreatin
8-Hour Bayer Timed Release Classification: Salicylate analgesic; antipyretic	aspirin
9-[3-pyridylmethyl]-9- deazaguanine Classification: Antineoplastic (Orphan)	9-[3-pyridylmethyl]-9-deazaguanine
9-cis retinoic acid Classification: Antineoplastic (Orphan)	9-cis retinoic acid

A

A/T/S Classification: Anti-acne product	erythromycin, topical
A-Hydrocore Classification: Glucocorticoid	hydrocortisone sodium succinate
A-Methapred Classification: Glucocorticoid	methylprednisolone sodium succinate
A.S.A. Classification: Salicylate analgesic; antipyretic	aspirin
Abacavir Classification: Antiviral (Investigational)	abacavir
Abbokinase Open-Cath Classification: Antithrombotic	urokinase

*Available in Canada only

BRAND NAME	GENERIC NAME
Abbokinase Classification: Antithrombotic	urokinase
Abelcet Classification: Antifungal	amphtericin B, liposomal
Abenol 120 mg* Classification: Analgesic, antipyretic	acetaminophen
Abenol 325 mg* Classification: Analgesic, antipyretic	acetaminophen
Abenol 650 mg* Classification: Analgesic, antipyretic	acetaminophen
Absorbine Antifungal Classification: Antifungal	tolnaftate
Absorbine Antifungal Foot Powder Classification: Antifungal	miconazole nitrate, topical
Absorbine Athlete's Foot Care Classification: Antifungal	tolnaftate
Absorbine Jock Itch Classification: Antifungal	tolnaftate
Absorbine Jr. Antifungal Classification: Antifungal	tolnaftate
Accolate Classification: Bronchodilator; leukotriene receptor antagonist	zafirlukast

*Available in Canada Only

BRAND NAME	GENERIC NAME
Accupril Classification: Antihypertensive; angiotensin converting enzyme inhibitor	quinapril HCl
Accurbron Classification: Bronchodilator; xanthine	theophylline
Accutane Classification: Anti-acne product	isotretinoin (13-cis-Retinoic Acid)
Acebutolol HCl Classification: Beta-adrenergic blocker	acebutolol
Acel-Imune Classification: Toxoid	diphtheria and tetanus toxoids and acellular pertussis vaccine (Dtap)
ACEON Classification: Antihypertensive; angiotensin converting enzyme inhibitor	perindopril erbumine
Acetaminophen Uniserts Classification: Analgesic; antipyretic	acetaminophen
Acetazolamide Classification: Diuretic; carbonic anhydrase inhibitor	acetazolamide
Acetohexamide Classification: Antidiabetic; sulfonylurea	acetohexamide
Acetorphan Classification: Antidiarrheal (Investigational)	acetorphan
Acetylcysteine Classification: Mucolytic	acetylcysteine

*Available in Canada only

BRAND NAME	GENERIC NAME
Aclovate Classification: Glucocorticoid	alclometasone dipropionate
Acne 10 Classification: Anti-acne product	benzoyl peroxide
Acne 5 Classification: Anti-acne product	benzoyl perioxide
Acne Lotion 10 Classification: Anti-acne product	sulfur
Aconiazide Classification: Antitubercular (Orphan)	aconiazide
ACT Classification: Electrolyte replacement; fluoride	sodium fluoride
ACTH-80 Classification: Anterior pituitary hormone	corticotropin injection, repository
ACTH Classification: Anterior pituitary hormone	corticotropin injection
Acthar Classification: Anterior pituitary hormone	corticotropin injection
Act HIB Classification: Vaccine	hemophilius b conjugate vaccine
Acthrel Classification: In vivo diagnostic	corticorelin ovine triflutate
Acti-B$_{12}$* Classification: Vitamin, water soluble	hydroxocobalamin (Vitamin B$_{12}$)

BRAND NAME	GENERIC NAME
Acticin Classification: Anti-acne product	tretinoin (vitamin A acid, retinoic acid)
Acticort 100 Classification: Glucocorticoid	hydrocortisone, topical
Actidose-Aqua Classification: Adsorbent	charcoal, activated
Actidose with Sorbitol Classification: Adsorbent	charcoal, activated
Actigall Classification: Antilithic	ursodiol
Actimmune Classification: Biologic response modifier	interferon gamma-1B
Actinex Classification: Antikeratotic	masoprocol
Actisite Classification: Antibiotic; tetracycline	tetracycline HCl, topical
Activase Classification: Antithrombotic	alteplase, recombinant
Actron Classification: Nonsteroidal anti-inflammatory	ketoprofen
Acu-dyne Classification: Antiseptic; germicidal	povidone-iodine
Acular Classification: Ophthalmic nonsteroidal anti-inflammatory	ketorolac tromethamine, ophthalmic

*Available in Canada only

BRAND NAME	GENERIC NAME

Acular PF
Classification:
Nonsteroidal anti-inflammatory

ketorolac tromethamine, ophthalmic

Acutrim 16 hour
Classification:
Alpha-adrenergic agonist

phenylpropanolamine HCl

Acutrim II Maximum Strength
Classification:
Alpha-adrenergic agonist

phenylpropanolamine HCl

Acutrim Late Day
Classification:
Alpha-adrenergic agonist

phenylpropanolamine HCl

Acyclovir
Classification:
Antiviral

acyclovir

Acyclovir Sodium
Classification:
Antiviral

acyclovir sodium

AD-439
Classification:
Antiviral (Investigational)

AD-439

AD-519
Classification:
Antiviral (Investigational)

AD-519

Adagen
Classification:
Enzyme replacement

pegademase bovine

Adalat
Classification:
Calcium channel blocker

nifedipine

Adalat CC
Classification:
Calcium channel blocker

nifedipine

AdatoSil 5000
Classification:
Retinal tamponade

polydimethylsiloxane (silicone oil)

*Available in Canada Only

BRAND NAME	GENERIC NAME

ADCI
Classification:
Anticonvulsant (Investigational)

ADCI

Adefovir Dipivoxil
Classification:
Antiviral (Investigational)

adefovir dipivoxil

Adenocard
Classification:
Antiarrhythmic

adenosine

Adenoscan
Classification:
In vivo diagnostic aid

adenosine

Adenosine Phosphate
Classification:
Nucleoside

adenosine phosphate (A_5MP)

Adipex-P
Classification:
CNS stimulant; anorexiant

phentermine HCl

Adipost
Classification:
CNS stimulant; anorexiant

phendimetrazine tartrate

Adrenalin Chloride
Classification:
Adrenergic agonist

epinephrine

Adrenalin Chloride
Classification:
Adrenergic agonist

epinephrine HCl

Adrenalin Chloride Solution
Classification:
Adrenergic agonist

epinephrine

Adriamycin PFS
Classification:
Antineoplastic; antibiotic

doxorubicin HCl (ADR)

Adriamycin RDF
Classification:
Antineoplastic; antibiotic

doxorubicin HCl (ADR)

BRAND NAME	GENERIC NAME

Adrucil
Classification:
Antineoplastic; antimetabolite

fluorouracil (5-fluorouracil; 5-FU)

Adsorbocarpine
Classification:
Miotic

pilocarpine HCl

Adsorbonac Ophthalmic Solution
Classification:
Hyperosmolar preparation

sodium chloride, hypertonic

Adsorbotear
Classification:
Ophthalmic lubricant

artificial tears solution

Advanced Formula Tegrin
Classification:
Keratolytic

coal tar

Advantage 24
Classification:
Spermicide

nonoxynol

Advil
Classification:
Nonsteroidal anti-inflammatory

ibuprofen

Advil Junior Strength
Classification:
Nonsteroidal anti-inflammatory

ibuprofen

Aeroaid
Classification:
Antiseptic

thimerosal

AeroBid
Classification:
Glucocorticoid

flunisolide

Aerobid-M
Classification:
Glucocorticoid

flunisolide

Aerolate III
Classification:
Bronchodilator; xanthine

theophylline

*Available in Canada Only

BRAND NAME	GENERIC NAME
Aerolate Jr. Classification: Bronchodilator; xanthine	theophylline
Aerolate Sr. Classification: Bronchodilator; xanthine	theophylline
Aeropin Classification: Anticoagulant (Orphan)	2-O-desulfated heparin
Aeroseb-Dex Classification: Glucocorticoid	dexamethasone
Aeroseb-HC Classification: Glucocorticoid	hydrocortisone, topical
Aerosol talc Classification: Sclerosing agent (Orphan)	aerosol talc (sterile)
Aerozoin Classification: Protectant	benzoin
Afrin Classification: Nasal decongestant	oxymetazoline HCl, nasal
Afrin Children's Nose Drops Classification: Nasal decongestant	oxymetazoline HCl, nasal
Afrin Nasal Mist Classification: Nasal decongestant	sodium chloride, nasal
Afrin Sinus Classification: Nasal decongestant	oymetazoline HCl, nasal
Aftate for Athlete's Foot Classification: Antifungal	tolnaftate

BRAND NAME	GENERIC NAME

Aftate for Jock Itch
Classification:
Antifungal

tolnaftate

Agrylin
Classification:
Antiplatelet

anagrelide HCl

AH-chew D
Classification:
Adrenergic agonist

phenylephrine HCl

Airbron*
Classification:
Mucolytic

acetylcysteine (N-Acetylcysteine)

Airet
Classification:
Bronchodilator; beta-adrenergic agonist

albuterol sulfate

AKBeta
Classification:
Beta-adrenergic blocker

levobunolol HCl

AKPro
Classification:
Adrenergic agonist

dipiverfin HCl

AKTob
Classification:
Aminoglycoside

tobramycin, ophthalmic

AK-Chlor
Classification:
Antibacterial

chloramphenicol, ophthalmic

AK-Con
Classification:
Ophthalmic vasoconstrictor

naphazoline HCl, ophthalmic

AK-Dex
Classification:
Ophthalmic glucocorticoid

dexamethasone, ophthalmic

AK-Dilate
Classification:
Ophthalmic vasoconstrictor

phenylephrine HCl, ophthalmic

BRAND NAME	GENERIC NAME
AK-Fluor Classification: Ophthalmic diagnostic	fluorescein sodium
AK-Homatropine Classification: Mydriatic	homatropine hydrobromide, ophthalmic
AL-721 Classification: Antiviral (Investigational)	AL-721
AK-NaCl Classification: Hyperosmolar preparation	sodium chloride, hypertonic
AK-Nefrin Classification: Ophthalmic vasoconstrictor	phenylephrine HCl, ophthalmic
AK-Pentolate Classification: Mydriatic	cyclopentolate HCl
AK-Pred Classification: Glucocorticoid	prednisolone sodium phosphate ophthalmic solution
AK-Sulf Classification: Antibiotic; sulfonamide	sulfacetamide sodium, ophthalmic
AK-Tracin Classification: Antibacterial	bacitracin, ophthalmic
Akarpine Classification: Miotic	pilocarpine HCl
Akineton Classification: Anticholinergic	biperiden HCl/biperiden lactate
Akne-mycin Classification: Anti-acne product	erythromycin, topical

BRAND NAME	GENERIC NAME
Akwa Tears Classification: Ophthalmic lubricant	artificial tears solution
Akwa Tears Classification: Ophthalmic lubricant	ocular lubricants
Ala-Scalp Classification: Glucocorticoid	hydrocortisone, topical
Ala-Cort Classification: Glucocorticoid	hydrocortisone, topical
Alazine Classification: Antihypertensive; vasodilator	hydralazine HCl
Albalon Liquifilm Ophthalmic Classification: Ophthalmic vasoconstrictor	naphazoline HCl, ophthalmic
Albamycin Classification: Antibacterial	novobiocin
Albenza Classification: Anthelmintics	albendazole
Albuminar-5 Classification: Blood derivative	albumin human 5%
Albuminar-25 Classification: Blood derivative	albumin human 25%
Albunex Classification: Blood derivative	Albumin 5%
Albutein 25% Classification: Blood derivative	albumin human 25%

BRAND NAME	GENERIC NAME

Albutein 5%
Classification:
Blood derivative

albumin human 5%

Albuterol
Classification:
Bronchodilator; beta-adrenergic agonist

albuterol sulfate

Alcaine
Classification:
Local anesthetic

proparacaine HCl, ophthalmic

Alcomicin*
Classification:
Aminoglycoside

gentamicin sulfate

Alconefrin-25
Classification:
Nasal decongestant

phenylephrine HCl, nasal

Alconefrin
Classification:
Nasal decongestant

phenylephrine HCl, nasal

Aldactone
Classification:
Potassium-sparing diuretic

spironolactone

Aldara
Classification:
Biologic response modifier

imiquimod

Aldomet
Classification:
Antihypertensive, centrally acting

methyldopa/methyldopate HCl

ALEC
Classification:
Lung surfactant (Orphan)

dipalmitoylphosphatidycholine/gycerol

Alfenta
Classification:
Opioid analgesic

alfentanil HCl

Alferon LDO
Classification:
Biologic response modifier
(Investigational)

interferon alfa-n3

*Available in Canada only

BRAND NAME	GENERIC NAME

Alferon N
Classification:
Antineoplastic; biologic response
modifier

interferon alfa-n3

Alka-Seltzer
Classification:
Salicylate analgesic; antipyretic

aspirin

Alka-Mints
Classification:
Antacid; calcium supplement

calcium carbonate

Alkeran
Classification:
Antineoplastic; alkylating agent

melphalan (L-Pam; phenylalanine
mustard, L-sarcolysin)

Allegra
Classification:
Antihistamine

fexofenadine HCl

Aller-chlor
Classification:
Antihistamine

chlorpheniramine meleate

Allerest 12-Hour Nasal
Classification:
Nasal decongestant

oxymetazoline HCl, nasal

Allerest Eye Drops
Classification:
Ophthalmic vasoconstrictor

naphazoline HCl, ophthalmic

AllerMax
Classification:
Antihistamine

diphenhydramine HCl

Allopurinol
Classification:
Uricosuric

allopurinol

Almora
Classification:
Electrolyte replacement

magnesium gluconate

Alomide
Classification:
Ophthalmic mast cell stabilizer

lodoxamide tromethamine

*Available in Canada Only

BRAND NAME	GENERIC NAME
Alophen Pills Classification: Laxative; irritant	phenolphthalein
Alpha-1-antitrypsin Classification: Enzyme replacement (Orphan)	alpha-1-antitrypsin (human)
Alphagan Classification: Adrenergic agonist	brimonidine tartrate
AlphaNine Classification: Hemostatic	factor IX complex (human)
AlphaNine SD Classification: Hemostatic	factor IX complex (human)
Alphatrex Classification: Glucocorticoid	betamethasone dipropionate
Alprazolam Intensol Classification: Antianxiety; benzodiazepine	alprazolam
Alramucil Classification: Laxative, bulk-producing	psyllium
Altace Classification: Antihypertensive; angiotensin converting enzyme inhibitor	ramipril
Alternagel Classification: Antacid	aluminum hydroxide gel
Altracin Classification: Antibacterial (Orphan)	bacitracin
Alu-Cap Classification: Antacid	aluminum hydroxide gel

*Available in Canada only

BRAND NAME	GENERIC NAME
Alu-Tab Classification: Antacid	aluminum hydroxide gel
Aluminum Hydroxide Classification: Antacid	aluminum hydroxide gel
Aluminum Hydroxide Gel Classification: Antacid	aluminum hydroxide gel
Alupent Classification: Bronchodilator; beta-adrenergic agonist	metaproterenol sulfate
Alurate Classification: Sedative-hypnotic; barbiturate	aprobarbital
Alvircept Sudotox Classification: Antiviral (Investigational)	alvircept sudotox
Amantadine HCl Classification: Antiviral; antiparkinson agent	amantadine HCl
Amaryl Classification: Antidiabetic; sulfonylurea	glimepiride
Ambi 10 Classification: Anti-acne product	benzoyl peroxide
Ambien Classification: Sedative-hypnotic; nonbarbiturate	zolpidem tartrate
AmBisome Classification: Antifungal	amphotericin B, liposomal
Amcort Classification: Glucocorticoid	triamcinolone diacetate

BRAND NAME	GENERIC NAME
Amen Classification: Progestin	medroxyprogesterone acetate
Amerge Classification: Antimigraine	naratriptan
Americaine Classification: Local anesthetic	benzocaine, topical
Americaine Anesthetic Classification: Local anesthetic	benzocaine, topical
Americaine Anesthetic Lubricant Classification: Local anesthetic	benzocaine, topical
Amicar Classification: Hemostatic	aminocaproic acid
Amidate Classification: General anesthetic	etomidate
Amigesic Classification: Salicylate analgesic	salsalate
Amikacin Classification: Aminoglycoside	amikacin sulfate
Aminess Classification: Nitrogen product	amino acid solution, renal
Amino-Opti-E Classification: Vitamin, fat soluble	vitamin E
Aminocaproic Acid Classification: Hemostatic	aminocaproic acid

*Available in Canada only

BRAND NAME	GENERIC NAME

Aminohippurate Sodium
Classification:
In vivo diagnostic

aminohippurate sodium (PAH)

Aminophylline
Classification:
Bronchodilator; xanthine

aminophylline (theophylline ethylenediamine)

Aminosalicylate Sodium
Classification:
Anti-inflammatory (Orphan)

aminosalicylate sodium

Aminosyn-HBC
Classification:
Nitrogen product

amino acid solution, stress

Aminosyn-RF
Classification:
Nitrogen product

amino acid solution, renal

Aminosyn-PF
Classification:
Nitrogen product

amino acid solution

Aminosyn
Classification:
Nitrogen product

amino acid solution

Aminosyn II
Classification:
Nitrogen product

amino acid solution

Amipaque
Classification:
Radiopaque agent

metrizamide

Amitone
Classification:
Antacid; calcium supplement

calcium carbonate

Amitriptyline HCl
Classification:
Antidepressant

amitriptyline HCl

Ammonium Chloride
Classification:
Systemic acidifier

ammonium chloride

BRAND NAME	GENERIC NAME
Ammonium Molybdate Classification: Trace element	molybdenum
Amodopa Classification: Antihypertensive, centrally acting	methyldopa/methyldopate HCl
AMO Vitrax Classification: Ophthalmic viscoelastic	sodium hyaluronate
Amoxapine Classification: Antidepressant, tricyclic	amoxapine
Amoxican Classification: Antibiotic; aminopenicillin	amoxicillin trihydrate
Amoxicillin Classification: Antibiotic; aminopenicillin	amoxicillin trihydrate
Amoxil Classification: Antibiotic; aminopenicillin	amoxicillin trihydrate
Amoxil Pediatric Drops Classification: Antibiotic; aminopenicillin	amoxicillin trihydrate
Amphetamine Sulfate Classification: CNS stimulant	amphetamine sulfate
Amphojel Classification: Antacid	aluminum hydroxide gel
Amphotec Classification: Antifungal	amphotericin B, cholesteryl
Amphotericin B Classification: Antifungal	amphotericin B

BRAND NAME	GENERIC NAME
Ampicillin Classification: Antibiotic; aminopenicillin	ampicillin, oral
Ampicillin Sodium Classification: Antibiotic, aminopenicillin	ampicillin sodium, parenteral
Ampligen Classification: Biologic response modifier (Investigational)	ampligen
Amvisc Classification: Ophthalmic viscoelastic	sodium hyaluronate
Amvisc Plus Classification: Ophthalmic viscoelastic	sodium hyaluronate
Amyl Nitrite Classification: Antianginal	amyl nitrite
Amyl Nitrite Aspirols Classification: Antianginal	amyl nitrite
Amyl Nitrite Vaporole Classification: Antianginal	amyl nitrite
Amytal Sodium Classification: Sedative-hypnotic; barbiturate	amobarbital sodium
Anadrol-50 Classification: Anabolic steroid	oxymetholone
Anafranil Classification: Antidepressant, tricyclic	clomipramine
Analgesic Creme Classification: Analgesic	trolamine salicylate

BRAND NAME	GENERIC NAME
Anamid* Classification: Aminoglycoside	kanamycin sulfate
Anandron* Classification: Antineoplastic; antiandrogen	nilutamide
Anapolon 50* Classification: Anabolic steroid	oxymethalone
Anaprox Classification: Nonsteroidal anti-inflammatory	naproxen sodium
Anaprox DS Classification: Nonsteroidal anti-inflammatory	naproxen sodium
Anaspaz Classification: GI anticholinergic	hyoscyamine sulfate
Anatrast Classification: Radiopaque agent	barium sulfate
Anacasal* Classification: Salicylate analgesic; antipyretic	aspirin
Analgesic Balm Classification: Counterirritant	methyl salicylate
Ancef Classification: Antibiotic; cephalosporin	cefazolin sodium
Ancobon Classification: Antifungal; pyrimidine	flucytosine
Ancotil* Classification: Antifungal; pyrimidine	flucytosine

BRAND NAME	GENERIC NAME

Androderm
Classification:
Androgen

testosterone transdermal system

Androgel-DHT
Classification:
Androgen (Orphan)

dihydrotestosterone

Android- 25
Classification:
Androgen

methyltestosterone

Android-10
Classification:
Androgen

methyltestosterone

Andro L.A. 200
Classification:
Androgen

testosterone enanthate (in oil)

Androlone- D 200
Classification:
Anabolic steroid

nandrolone decanoate

Anectine
Classification:
Depolarizing neuromuscular blocker

succinylcholine chloride

Anectine Flo-Pack
Classification:
Depolarizing neuromuscular blocker

succinylcholine chloride

Anergan 50
Classification:
Antihistamine

promethazine HCl

Anestacon
Classification:
Local anesthetic

lidocaine HCl, topical

Angio-Conray
Classification:
Radiopaque agent

iothalamate sodium 80%

Angiovist 282
Classification:
Radiopaque agent

diatrizoate meglumine 60%

BRAND NAME	GENERIC NAME
Angiovist 292 Classification: Radiopaque agent	diatrizoate meglumine 52% and diatrizoate sodium 8%
Angiovist 370 Classification: Radiopaquc agent	diatrizoate meglumine 66% and diatrizoate sodium 10%
Anistropine Methylbromide Classification: Anticholinergic	anistropine methylbromide
Ansaid Classification: Nonsteroidal anti-inflammatory	flurbiprofen
Antabuse Classification: Antialcoholic	disulfiram
Anthra-Derm Classification: Antipsoriatic	anthralin (Dithranol)
Anti-Tuss Classification: Expectorant	guaifenesin
Antiepilepsirine Classification: Anticonvulsant (Orphan)	antiepilepsirine
Antihemophilic Factor (Porcine) Hyate: C Classification: Hemostatic	antihemophilic factor (AHF, Factor VIII)
Antihist-1 Classification: Antihistime	clemastine fumarate
Antilirium Classification: anticholinesterase	physostigmine salicylate
Antiminth Classification: Anthelmintics	pyrantel pamoate

BRAND NAME	GENERIC NAME

Antispas
Classification:
Antispasmodic

dicyclomine HCl

Anti-thymocyte Serum
Classification:
Immunosuppressive (Orphan)

anti-thymocyte serum

Antivenin (Crotalidae) Polyvalent
Classification:
Antivenin

antivenin (crotalidae) polyvalent

Antivenin (crotalidae) Purified (avian)
Classification:
Antivenin (Orphan)

antivenin (crotalidae) purified (avian)

Antivenin (Latrodectus mactans)
Classification:
Antivenin

black widow spider species antivenin

Antivenin (Micrurus Fulvius)
Classification:
Antivenin

antivenin (micrurus fulvius)

Antivert/25
Classification:
Antiemetic; anticholinergic

meclizine

Antivert/50
Classification:
Antiemetic; anticholinergic

meclizine

Antivert
Classification:
Antiemetic; anticholinergic

meclizine

Antizol
Classification:
Antidote

fomepizole

Antril
Classification:
Biologic response modifier (Orphan)

interleukin-1 receptor antagonist (recombinant human)

BRAND NAME	GENERIC NAME

Antrizine
Classification:
Antiemetic; anticholinergic

meclizine

Antrypol
Classification:
CDC anti-infective

suramin

Anturan
Classification:
Uricosuric

sulfinpyrazone

Anturane*
Classification:
Uricosuric

sulfinpyrazone

Anucort-HC
Classification:
Glucocorticoid

hydrocortisone acetate

Anumed HC
Classification:
Glucocorticoid

hydrocortisone acetate

Anusol-HC
Classification:
Glucocorticoid

hydrocortisone acetate

Anzemet
Classification:
Antiemetic

dolasteron

Anxanil
Classification:
Antianxiety

hydroxyzine

Apacet
Classification:
Analgesic; antipyretic

acetaminophen

Aparkane*
Classification:
Anticholinergic

trihexyphenidyl HCl

Aphrodyne
Classification:
Alpha-adrenergic blocker

yohimbine HCl

*Available in Canada only

BRAND NAME	GENERIC NAME

Aphthasol
Classification:
Anti-inflammatory

amlexanox

A.P.L.
Classification:
Chorionic gonadotropin

chorionic gonadotropin, human (HCG)

APL 400-200
Classification:
Antineoplastic (Orphan)

APL 400-200

Aplisol
Classification:
In vivo diagnostic

tuberculin purified protein derivative
(mantoux, PPD)

Aplitest
Classification:
In vivo diagnostic

tuberculin PPD multiple puncture device

Apo-Amitriptyline*
Classification:
Antidepressant

amitriptyline HCl

Apo-Atenol*
Classification:
Antihypertensive; beta-adrenergic blocker

atenolol

Apo-Amoxi*
Classification:
Antibiotic; aminopenicillin

amoxicillin trihydrate

Apo-Bisacodyl*
Classification:
Laxative; irritant

bisacodyl

Apo-Carbamazepine*
Classification:
Anticonvulsant

carbamazepine

Apo-Gemfibrozil*
Classification:
Antilipemic

gemfibrozil

Apo-Metronidazole*
Classification:
Antibacterial; amebicide

metronidazole

*Available in Canada Only

BRAND NAME	GENERIC NAME
Apo-Oxazepam* Classification: Antianxiety; benzodiazepine	oxazepam
Apo-Pen-VK* Classification: Antibiotic; penicillin	penicillin V potassium
APO-Sulfatrim* Classification: Sulfonamide	co-trimoxazole (trimethoprim and sulfamethoxazole) [See trimethoprim and sulfamethoxazole]
Apoallopurinol* Classification: Uricosuric	allopurinol
APO Cloxi* Classification: Antibiotic; penicillinase resistant penicillin	cloxacillin sodium
Apollon Classification: Vaccine (Investigational)	HIV vaccine
Apomorphine HCl Classification: Antiparkinson agent (Orphan)	Apomorphine HCl
Apresoline Classification: Antihypertensive; vasodilator	hydralazine HCl
Aquacare Classification: Emollient	urea (carbamide), topical
Aquachloral Supprettes Classification: Sedative-hypnotic; nonbarbiturate	chloral hydrate
AquaMephyton Classification: Vitamin K	phytonadione (vitamin K_1)
Aquaphyllin Classification: Bronchodilator; xanthine	theophylline

*Available in Canada only

BRAND NAME	GENERIC NAME

Aquasol A
Classification:
Vitamin, fat soluble

vitamin A

Aquasol E
Classification:
Vitamin, fat soluble

vitamin E

Aquaphyllin
Classification:
Bronchodilator; xanthine

theophylline

Aquatensen
Classification:
Thiazide diuretic

methyclothiazide

Aquest
Classification:
Estrogen

estrone

AR177
Classification:
Antiviral (Investigational)

AR177

Aralen HCl
Classification:
Antimalarial

chloroquine HCl

Aralen Phosphate
Classification:
Antimalarial

chloroquine phosphate

Aramine
Classification:
Adrenergic

metaraminol

Arcitumomab
Classification:
In vivo diagnostic (Orphan)

arcitumomab

Arduan
Classification:
Nondepolarizing neuromuscular blocker

pipecuronium bromide

Aredia
Classification:
Bone resorption inhibitor

pamidronate disodium

BRAND NAME	GENERIC NAME
Argesic-SA Classification: Salicylate analgesic	salsalate
Argine Butyrate Classification: Blood modifier (Orphan)	arginine butyrate
Aricept Classification: Cholinesterase inhibitor	donepizil HCl
Arimidex Classification: Antineoplastic	anastrazole
Aristocort Classification: Glucocorticoid	triamcinolone
Aristocort Classification: Glucocorticoid	triamcinolone acetonide, topical
Aristocort A Classification: Glucocorticoid	triamcinolone acetonide, topical
Aristocort Forte Classification: Glucocorticoid	triamcinolone diacetate
Aristocort Intralesional Classification: Glucocorticoid	triamcinolone diacetate
Aristospan Intra-Articular Classification: Glucocorticoid	triamcinolone hexacetonide
Aristospan Intralesional Classification: Glucocorticoid	triamcinolone hexacetonide
Arm-a-Med Metaproterenol Sulfate Classification: Bronchodilator; beta-adrenergic agonist	metaproterenol sulfate

BRAND NAME	GENERIC NAME

Arm-a-Med Isoetharine HCl
Classification:
Bronchodilator; beta-adrenergic agonist

isoetharine HCl

Armour Thyroid
Classification:
Thyroid hormone

thyroid USP (desiccated)

Arnica Tincture
Classification:
Irritant

arnica

Aromatic Ammonia
Classification:
Ammonia inhalant

aromatic ammonia spirit

Aromatic Ammonia Aspirols
Classification:
Ammonia inhalant

aromatic ammonia spirit

Aromatic Ammonia Spirit
Classification:
Ammonia inhalant

aromatic ammonia spirit

Aromatic Ammonia Vaporole
Classification:
Ammonia inhalant

aromatic ammonia spirit

Arrestin
Classification:
Antiemetic; anticholinergic

trimethobenzamide HCl

Arsobal
Classification:
CDC anti-infective

melarsoprol

Artane
Classification:
Anticholinergic

trihexyphenidyl HCl

Artane Sequels
Classification:
Anticholinergic

trihexyphenidyl HCl

Arthra-G
Classification:
Salicylate analgesic

salsalate

BRAND NAME	GENERIC NAME
Arthritis Foundation Pain Reliever Classification: Salicylate analgesic; antipyretic	aspirin
Arthritis Pain Formula Classification: Salicylate analgesic; antipyretic	aspirin
Arthritis Pain Formula Classification: Analgesic; antipyretic	acetaminophen
Arthropan Classification: Salicylate analgesic	choline salicylate
Articulose-50 Classification: Glucocorticoid	prednisolone acetate
Articulose L.A. Classification: Glucocorticoid	triamcinolone diacetate
Artificial Tears Solution Classification: Ophthalmic lubricant	artificial tears solution
Arvin Classification: Antithrombotic (Orphan)	ancrod
AS-101 Classification: Biologic response modifier (Investigational)	AS-101
A-Spas S/L Classification: GI anticholinergic	hyoscyamine sulfate
Asacol Classification: GI anti-inflammatory	mesalamine

BRAND NAME	GENERIC NAME
Ascorbic Acid Classification: Vitamin, water soluble	ascorbic acid (vitamin C)
Ascorbicap Classification: Vitamin, water soluble	ascorbic acid (vitamin C)
Ascriptin A/D Classification: Salicylate analgesic; antipyretic	aspirin
Ascriptin Extra Strength Classification: Salicylate analgesic; antipyretic	aspirin
Asendin Classification: Antidepressant	amoxapine
Asmalix Classification: Bronchodilator; xanthine	theophylline
Aspercreme Cream Classification: Analgesic	trolamine salicylate
Aspergum Classification: Salicylate analgesic; antipyretic	aspirin
Aspirin* Classification: Salicylate analgesic; antipyretic	aspirin
Aspirin Free Classification: Analgesic; antipyretic	acetaminophen
Aspirin Free Pain Relief Classification: Analgesic; antipyretic	acetaminophen
Aspirmox Classification: Salicylate analgesic; antipyretic	aspirin

BRAND NAME	GENERIC NAME
Aspirmox Extra Protection for Arthritis Pain Classification: Salicylate analgesic; antipyretic	aspirin
Astelin Classification: Antihistamine	azelastine
AsthmaMist Haler Classification: Adrenergic agonist	epinephrine
AsthmaNefrin Classification: Adrenergic agonist	epinephrine
Astramorph PF Classification: Opioid analgesic	morphine sulfate
Atarax 100 Classification: Antianxiety	hydroxyzine
Atasol* Classification: Analgesic; antipyretic	acetaminophen
Atenolol Classification: Antihypertensive; beta-adrenergic blocker	atenolol
Ateviridine Mesylate Classification: Antiviral (Investigational)	ateviridine mesylate
Atgam Classification: Immune serum	lymphocyte immune globulin; anti-thymocyte globulin (equine)
Ativan Classification: Antianxiety; benzodiazepine	lorazepam
ATnativ Classification: Antithrombin	antithrombin III, human

*Available in Canada only

BRAND NAME	GENERIC NAME

Atolone
Classification:
Glucocorticoid

triamcinolone

Atromid-S
Classification:
Antilipemic

clofibrate

Atropine Care Ophthalmic
Classification:
Mydriatic

atropine sulfate, ophthalmic

Atropine Sulfate
Classification:
Anticholinergic

atropine sulfate

Atropine Sulfate Ophthalmic
Classification:
Mydriatic

atropine sulfate, ophthalmic

Atropisol
Classification:
Mydriatic

atropine sulfate, ophthalmic

Atrovent
Classification:
Anticholinergic

ipratropium bromide

Attenuvax
Classification:
Vaccine

measles, (rubeola) virus vaccine, live attenuated

Auriculin
Classification:
Renal allograft function (Orphan)

anaritide acetate

Augmentin
Classification:
Antibiotic; aminopenicillin

amoxcillin and potassium clavulanate

Auro Ear Drops
Classification:
Emulsifier

carbamide peroxide, otic

Aurolate
Classification:
Gold compound

gold sodium thiomalate

BRAND NAME	GENERIC NAME
Autoplex T Classification: Hemostatic	anti-inhibitor coagulant complex
Avakine Classification: Biologic response modifier (Investigational)	infliximab
Avapro Classification: Antihypertensive; angiotensin II antagonist	irbesartan
AVC Classification: Antibiotic; sulfonamide	sulfanilamide
Aventyl Classification: Antidepressant	nortriptyline HCl
Avita Classification: Anti-acne product	tretinoin (vitamin A acid, retinoic acid)
Avitene Hemostat Classification: Hemostatic	microfibrillar collagen hemostat
Avlosulfon* Classification: Leprostatic	dapsone (DDS)
Axid Classification: Histamine H_2 receptor antagonist	nizatidine
Axid AR Classification: Histamine H_2 receptor antagonist	nizatidine
Aygestin Classification: Progestin	norethindrone acetate

*Available in Canada only

BRAND NAME	GENERIC NAME
Ayr Saline Classification: Nasal decongestant	sodium chloride, nasal
Azactam Classification: Antibiotic; monobactam	aztreonam
Azathioprine Sodium Classification: Immunosuppressive	azathioprine
Azelex Classification: Anti-acne product	azelic acid
AzdU Classification: Antiviral (Investigational)	azidouridine
Azmacort Classification: Glucocorticoid	triamcinolone acetonide
Azo-Standard Classification: Urinary analgesic	phenazopyridine HCl
Azulfidine Classification: Anti-inflammatory; sulfonamide	sulfasalazine
Azulfidine EN-tabs Classification: Anti-inflammatory; sulfonamide	sulfasalazine

B

BRAND NAME	GENERIC NAME
B-D Glucose Classification: Glucose elevating agent	glucose
Baby Anbesol Classification: Local anesthetic	benzocaine, oral

BRAND NAME	GENERIC NAME
Baby Orajel Classification: Local anesthetic	benzocaine, oral
Bacid Classification: Antidiarrheal	lactobacillus
Baciguent Classification: Antibacterial	bacitracin, topical
Bacitin Classification: Antibacterial	bacitracin, topical
Bacitracin Classification: Antibacterial	bacitracin, topical
Bacitracin Classification: Antibacterial	bacitracin, ophthalmic
Bacitracin U.S.P. Classification: Antibacterial	bacitracin, intramuscular
Backache Maximum Strength Relief Classification: Salicylate analgesic	magnesium salicylate
Baclofen Classification: Skeletal muscle relaxant, direct acting	baclofen
Bactine Hydrocortisone Classification: Glucocorticoid	hydrocortisone, topical
Bactocill Classification: Antibiotic; penicillinase-resistant penicillin	oxacillin sodium

BRAND NAME	GENERIC NAME

Bactopen
Classification:
Antibiotic; penicillinase-resistant
penicillin

cloxacillin sodium

BactoShield
Classification:
Germicidal

chlorhexidine gluconate, topical

Bactrim
Classification:
Antibiotic; sulfonamide

trimethroprim and sulfamethoxazole
(TMP-SMZ)

Bactrim DS
Classification:
Antibiotic; sulfonamide

trimethoprim and sulfamethoxazole
(TMP-SMZ)

Bactrim IV
Classification:
Antibiotic; sulfonamide

trimethoprim and sulfamethoxazole
(TMP-SMZ)

Bactroban
Classification:
Topical antibacterial

mupirocin

Bactroban Nasal
Classification:
Topical antibacterial

mupirocin

BAL in Oil
Classification:
Chelating agent

dimercaprol

Balminil
Classification:
Expectorant

guaifenesin

Balnetar
Classification:
Keratolytic

coal tar

Bandphen
Classification:
Antihistamine

diphenhydramine HCl

Baniflex
Classification:
Skeletal muscle relaxant, centrally acting

orphenadrine citrate

BRAND NAME	GENERIC NAME

Banlin
Classification:
Anticholinergic

propantheline bromide

Banthine
Classification:
Anticholinergic

methantheline bromide

Bantron
Classification:
Smoking deterrent

lobeline

Barbased
Classification:
Sedative-hypnotic; barbiturate

butabarbital sodium

Baridium
Classification:
Urinary analgesic

phenazopyridine HCl

Barium Sulfate U.S.P.
Classification:
Radiopaque agent

barium sulfate

Baro-Cat
Classification:
Radiopaque agent

barium sulfate

Baroflave
Classification:
Radiopaque agent

barium sulfate

**Barosperse 110 Powder for
Suspension**
Classification:
Radiopaque agent

barium sulfate

**Barosperse Powder for
Suspension**
Classification:
Radiopaque agent

barium sulfate

Basaljel
Classification:
Antacid

aluminum hydroxide gel

BRAND NAME	GENERIC NAME

Basaljel
Classification:
Antacid

aluminum carbonate gel

Baycol
Classification:
Antilipemic

cervistatin sodium

Bayer 205
Classification:
CDC anti-infective

suramin

Bayer
Classification:
Salicylate analgesic; antipyretic

aspirin

Bayer Children's Aspirin
Classification:
Salicylate analgesic; antipyretic

aspirin

Bayer Low Adult Strength
Classification:
Salicylate analgesic; antipyretic

aspirin

**Bayer Select Maximum
Strength Backache**
Classification:
Salicylate analgesic

magnesium salicylate

Beano
Classification:
Food modifier

alpha-D-galactosidase enzyme

Because
Classification:
Spermicide

nonoxynol

Becloflorte Inhaler*
Classification:
Glucocorticoid

beclomethasone dipropionate

Beclovent
Classification:
Glucocorticoid

beclomethasone dipropionate

Beconase AQ Nasal
Classification:
Glucocorticoid

beclomethasone dipropionate, nasal

BRAND NAME	GENERIC NAME
Beconase Inhalation Classification: Glucocorticoid	beclomethasone dipropionate, nasal
Bedoz* Classification: Vitamin, water soluble	cyanocobalamin (Vitamin B_{12})
Beepen-VK Classification: Antibiotic; penicillin	penicillin V potassium
Belganyl Classification: CDC anti-infective	suramin
Belix Classification: Antihistamine	diphenhydramine HCl
Bell/ans Classification: System alkalinizer	sodium bicarbonate
Belladonna Tincture Classification: Anticholinergic	belladonna
Bellafoline Classification: Anticholinergic	belladonna alkaloids
Bellafoline Classification: Anticholinergic	levorotatory alkaloids of belladonna
Ben-Allergin-50 Classification: Antihistamine	diphenhydramine HCl
Benadryl Kapseals Classification: Antihistamine	diphenhydramine HCl
Benefix Classification: Hemostatic	factor IX complex (human)

BRAND NAME	GENERIC NAME
Benoquin Classification: Depigmentation agent	monobenzone
Bensulfoid Classification: Anti-acne product	sulfur
Bentyl Classification: Antispasmodic	dicyclomine HCl
Bentylol* Classification: Antispasmodic	dicyclomine HCl
Benuryl* Classification: Uricosuric	probenecid
Benylin Adult Classification: Non-narcotic antitussive	dextromethorphan
Benylin Cough Classification: Antihistamine	diphenhydramine HCl
Benylin DM Classification: Non-narcotic antitussive	dextromethorphan
Benylin Pediatric Classification: Non-narcotic antitussive	dextromethorphan
Benza Classification: Antiseptic	benzalkonium chloride
Benzac 5 Classification: Anti-acne product	benzoyl peroxide
Benzac 10 Classification: Anti-acne product	benzoyl peroxide

BRAND NAME	GENERIC NAME

Benzac AC 10
Classification:
Anti-acne product

benzoyl peroxide

Benzac AC 2 1/2
Classification:
Anti-acne product

benzoyl peroxide

Benzac AC 5
Classification:
Anti-acne product

benzoyl peroxide

Benzac AC Wash 10
Classification:
Anti-acne product

benzoyl peroxide

Benzac AC Wash 2 1/2
Classification:
Anti-acne product

benzoyl peroxide

Benzac AC Wash 5
Classification:
Anti-acne product

benzoyl peroxide

Benzachlor-50*
Classification:
Antiseptic

benzalkonium chloride

Benzac W 10
Classification:
Anti-acne product

benzoyl peroxide

Benzac W 2 ½
Classification:
Anti-acne product

benzoyl peroxide

Benzac W 5
Classification:
Anti-acne product

benzoyl peroxide

Benzac W Wash 10
Classification:
Anti-acne product

benzoyl peroxide

Benzac W Wash 5
Classification:
Anti-acne product

benzoyl peroxide

BRAND NAME	GENERIC NAME

Benzalkonium Chloride
Classification:
Antiseptic

benzalkonium chloride

Benzashave
Classification:
Anti-acne product

benzoyl peroxide

Benzedrex
Classification:
Nasal decongestant

propylhexedrine

Benzocaine
Classification:
Local anesthetic

benzocaine, topical

Benzocol
Classification:
Local anesthetic

benzocaine, topical

Benzodent
Classification:
Local anesthetic

benzocaine, oral

Benzonatate Softgels
Classification:
Non-narcotic antitussive

benzonatate

Benzoin Compound
Classification:
Protectant

benzoin

Benzoin Tincture
Classification:
Protectant

benzoin

Benzoyl 10
Classification:
Anti-acne product

benzoyl peroxide

Benzoyl 15
Classification:
Anti-acne product

benzoyl peroxide

Benzoyl Peroxide
Classification:
Anti-acne product

benzoyl peroxide

BRAND NAME	GENERIC NAME

Benzthiazide
Classification:
Thiazide diuretic

benzthiazide

Benztropine Mesylate
Classification:
Anticholinergic

benztropine mesylate

Berna Vaccine
Classification:
Vaccine

typhoid vaccine

Beta-2
Classification:
Bronchodilator; beta-adrenergic

isoetharine HCl agonist

Beta-Val
Classification:
Glucocorticoid

betamethasone valerate

Beta Cort*
Classification:
Glucocorticoid

betamethasone valerate

Betacrone E-R
Classification:
Beta-adrenergic blocker

propranolol HCl

Betaderm
Classification:
Glucocorticoid

betamethasone valerate

Betadine
Classification:
Antiseptic; germicidal

povidone-iodine

**Betadine 5% Sterile
Ophthalmic Prep Solution**
Classification:
Antiseptic; germicidal

povidone-iodine

Betagan Liquifilm
Classification:
Beta-adrenergic blocker

levobunolol HCl

Betaloc*
Classification:
Antihypertensive; beta-adrenergic blocker

metoprolol

BRAND NAME	GENERIC NAME

Betamethasone Dipropionate
Classification:
Glucocorticoid

betamethasone dipropionate

Betamethasone Sodium Phosphate
Classification:
Glucocorticoid

betamethasone sodium phosphate

Betamethasone Sodium Phosphate and Betamethasone Acetate
Classification:
Glucocorticoid

betamethasone sodium phosphate and betamethasone acetate

Betamethasone Valerate
Classification:
Glucocorticoid

betamethasone valerate

Betapace
Classification:
Antiarrhythmic; beta-adrenergic blocker

sotalol HCl

Betapen-VK
Classification:
Antibiotic; penicillin

penicillin V potassium

BetaRx
Classification:
Antidiabetic (Orphan)

porcine islet preparation, encapsulated

Betaseron
Classification:
Biologic response modifier

interferon beta-1b (rIFN-B)

Betatrex
Classification:
Vitamin, water soluble

betamethasone valerate

Betaxin*
Classification:
Glucocorticoid

thiamine HCl (Vitamin B_1)

Bethanechol Chloride
Classification:
Cholinergic stimulant

bethanechol chloride

BRAND NAME	GENERIC NAME
Betimol Classification: Beta-adrenergic blocker	timolol maleate, ophthalmic
Betoptic Classification: Beta-adrenergic blocker	betaxolol HCl
Betoptic S Classification: Beta-adrenergic blocker	betaxolol HCl
Biavax II Classification: Vaccine	rubella and mumps virus vaccine, live
Biaxin Classification: Antibiotic; macrolide	clarithromycin
Bichloracetic Acid Classification: Cauterizing agent	dichloroacetic acid
Bicillin C-R Classification: Antibiotic; penicillin	penicillin G benzathine and procaine combined
Bicillin C-R 900/300 Classification: Antibiotic; penicillin	penicillin G benzathine and procaine combined
Bicillin L-A Classification: Antibiotic; penicillin	penicillin G benzathine, parenteral
Bicitra Classification: Urinary alkalinizer	sodium citrate/citric acid solution (Shohl's Solution)
BiCNU Classification: Antineoplastic; alkylating agent	carmustine (BCNU)
Bicozene Classification: Local anesthetic	benzocaine, topical

BRAND NAME	GENERIC NAME

Bilopaque
Classification:
Radiopaque agent

tyropanoate sodium

Biltricide
Classification:
Antithelmintics

praziquantel

Bio-Tab
Classification:
Antibiotic; tetracycline

doxycycline hyclate

Biocef
Classification:
Antibiotic; cephalosporin

cephalexin monohydrate

Bioclate
Classification:
Hemostatic

antihemophilic factor (AHF, Factor VIII)

Biodine Topical 1%
Classification:
Antiseptic; germicidal

povidone-iodine

Biomox
Classification:
Antibiotic; aminopenicillin

amoxicillin trihydrate

Bion Tears
Classification:
Ophthalmic lubticant

artificial tears solution

Biosynject
Classification:
Biologic response modifier (Orphan)

trisaccharides A and B

Bisacodyl
Classification:
Laxative; irritant

bisacodyl

Bisacodyl Uniserts
Classification:
Laxative; irritant

bisacodyl

Bisco-Lax
Classification:
Laxative; irritant

bisacodyl

BRAND NAME	GENERIC NAME
Bitin Classification: CDC anti-infective	bithionol
Black-Draught Classification: Laxative; irritant	senna
BlemErase Classification: Anti-acne product	benzoyl peroxide
Blenoxane Classification: Antineoplastic; antibiotic	bleomycin sulfate
Bleph-10 Liquifilm Classification: Antibiotic; sulfonamide	sulfacetamide sodium, ophthalmic sodium
Bleph-10 S.O.P Classification: Antibiotic; sulfonamide	sulfacetamide sodium, ophthalmic sodium
Blis-To-Sol Classification: Antifungal	tolnaftate
Blis-To-Sol Powder Classification: Antifungal	undecylenic acid
Blocadren Classification: Antihypertensive; beta-adrenergic blocker	timolol maleate
Bluboro Powder Classification: Astringent	aluminum acetate solution
Boil-Ease Classification: Local anesthetic	benzocaine, topical
Bonamine* Classification: Antiemetic; anticholinergic	meclizine HCl

BRAND NAME	GENERIC NAME

Bonine
Classification:
Antiemetic; anticholinergic

meclizine HCl

Bontril PDM
Classification:
CNS stimulant; anorexiant

phendimetrazine tartrate

Bontril Slow-Release
Classification:
CNS stimulant; anorexiant

phendimetrazine tartrate

Boric Acid
Classification:
Protectant

boric acid ointment

Borofax
Classification:
Protectant

boric acid ointment

Boropak Powder
Classification:
Astringent

aluminum acetate solution

Botox
Classification:
Paralytic (Orphan)

botulinum toxin type A

Botulinum Toxin Type B
Classification:
Paralytic (Orphan)

botulinum toxin type B

Botulinum Toxin Type F
Classification:
Paralytic (Orphan)

botulinum toxin type F

Botulism Immune Globulin
Classification:
Immune serum (Orphan)

botulism immune globulin

Bovine Colostrum
Classification:
Antidiarrheal (Orphan)

bovine colostrum

BranchAmin
Classification:
Nitrogen product

amino acid solution, stress

BRAND NAME	GENERIC NAME
Breathe Free Classification: Nasal decongestant	sodium chloride, nasal
Breeze Mist Antifungal Classification: Antifungal	miconazole nitrate, topical
Breeze Mist Antifungal Powder Classification: Antifungal	tolnaftate
Breonesin Classification: Expectorant	guaifenesin
Brethaire Classification: Bronchodilator; beta-adrenergic agonist	terbutaline sulfate
Brethine Classification: Bronchodilator; beta-adrenergic agonist	terbutaline sulfate
Bretylate* Classification: Antiarrhythmic	bretylium tosylate
Bretylium Tosylate Classification: Antiarrhythmic	bretylium tosylate
Bretylol Classification: Antiarrhythmic	bretylium tosylate
Brevibloc Classification: Beta-adrenergic blocker	esmolol HCl
Brevidil M* (Bromide Salt) Classification: Depolarizing neuromuscular blocker	succinylcholine chloride
Brevital Sodium Classification: General anesthetic; barbiturate	methohexital sodium

BRAND NAME	GENERIC NAME

Brevoxyl
Classification:
Anti-acne product

benzoyl peroxide

Bricanyl
Classification:
Bronchodilator; beta-adrenergic agonist

terbutaline sulfate

Brietal Sodium*
Classification:
General anesthetic; barbiturate

methohexital sodium

British Anti-Lewisite*
Classification:
Chelating agent

dimercaprol

Brolene
Classification:
Antiprotazoal (Orphan)

propamidine isethionate 0.1%, ophthalmic

Bromhexine
Classification:
Mucolytic (Orphan)

bromhexine

Bromodeoxyuridine
Classification:
Antineoplastic adjuvant (Orphan)

bromodeoxyuridine

Bromo Seltzer
Classification:
Analgesic; antipyretic

acetaminophen, buffered

Brompheniramine
Classification:
Antihistamine

brompheniramine maleate

Bronalide*
Classification:
Glucocorticoid

flunisolide

Broncho Saline
Classification:
Diluent

sodium chloride

Bronitin Mist
Classification:
Adrenergic agonist

epinephrine

BRAND NAME	GENERIC NAME
Bronkaid Mist Classification: Adrenergic agonist	epinephrine
Bronkodyl Classification: Bronchodilator; xanthine	theophylline
Bronkometer Classification: Bronchodilator; beta-adrenergic agonist	isoetharine HCl
Bronkosol Classification: Bronchodilator; beta-adrenergic agonist	isoetharine HCl
Bucladin-S Softabs Classification: Antiemetic; anticholinergic	buclizine HCl
Bufferin Classification: Salicylate analgesic; antipyretic	aspirin
Buffex Classification: Salicylate analgesic; antipyretic	aspirin
Bumetanide Classification: Loop diuretic	bumetanide
Bumex Classification: Loop diuretic	bumetanide
Buminate 25% Classification: Blood derivative	albumin human 25%
Buminate Classification: Blood derivative	albumin human 5%
Buphenyl Classification: Blood modifier, urea	sodium phenylbutyrate

BRAND NAME	GENERIC NAME

Bupivacaine HCl
Classification:
Local anesthetic

bupivacaine HCl

Buprenex
Classification:
Opioid agonist-antagonist analgesic

buprenorphine HCl

Burow's Solution
Classification:
Astringent

aluminum acetate solution

BuSpar
Classification:
Antianxiety

buspirone HCl

Butabarbital Sodium
Classification:
Sedative-hypnotic; barbiturate

butabarbital sodium

Butalan
Classification:
Sedative-hypnotic; barbiturate

butabarbital sodium

Butesin Picrate
Classification:
Local anesthetic

butamben picrate

Butisol Sodium
Classification:
Sedative-hypnotic; barbiturate

butabarbital sodium

Butyrycholinesterase
Classification:
Antidote (Orphan)

butyrylcholinesterase

Bycolmine
Classification:
Antispasmodic

dicyclomine HCl

C

C/T/S
Classification:
Anti-acne product

clindamycin, topical

BRAND NAME	GENERIC NAME
C1 inhibitor Classification: Immunosuppressive (Orphan)	C1 inhibitor
C1-esterase-inhibitor Classification: Immunosuppressive (Orphan)	C1-esterase-inhibitor
C-Solve 2 Classification: Anti-acne product	erythromycin, topical
C.E.S.* Classification: Estrogen	estrogens, conjugated
Cachexon Classification: Amino acid (Orphan)	L-glutathione (reduced)
Calanolide A Classification: Antiviral (Investigational)	calanolide A
Caldecort Anti-Itch Classification: Glucocorticoid	hydrocortisone, topical
Caffedrine Classification: Analeptic	caffeine
Caffeine Classification: Analeptic	caffeine
Caffeine and Sodium Benzoate Classification: Analeptic	caffeine
Cal-Guard Classification: Antacid; calcium supplement	calcium carbonate
Cal-Plus Classification: Antacid; calcium supplement	calcium carbonate

*Available in Canada only

BRAND NAME	GENERIC NAME
Cal Carb HD Classification: Antacid; calcium supplement	calcium carbonate
Calan Classification: Calcium channel blocker	verapamil HCl
Calan SR Classification: Calcium channel blocker	verapamil HCl
Calci-Chew Classification: Antacid; calcium supplement	calcium carbonate
Calci-Mix Classification: Antacid; calcium supplement	calcium carbonate
Calcibind Classification: Antihypercalciuria agent	cellulose sodium phosphate
Calciday-667 Classification: Antacid; calcium supplement	calcium carbonate
Calciferol Classification: Vitamin, fat soluble	ergocalciferol D_2
Calciferol Drops Classification: Vitamin, fat soluble	ergocalciferol D_2
Calcijex Classification: Vitamin, fat soluble	calcitriol (1,25- dihydroxycholecal-ciferol)
Calcilean* Classification: Anticoagulant	heparin calcium
Calcimar Classification: Parathyroid agent	calcitonin (salmon)

BRAND NAME	GENERIC NAME
Calcisorb* Classification: Antihypercalcemia agent	cellulose sodium phosphate
Calcium 600 Classification: Antacid; calcium supplement	calcium carbonate
Calcium Ascorbate Classification: Vitamin, water soluble	calcium ascorbate
Calcium Carbonate Classification: Antacid; calcium supplement	calcium carbonate
Calcium Chloride Classification: Electrolyte replacement; calcium	calcium chloride
Calcium Disodium Versenate Classification: Chelating agent	edetate calcium disodium (calcium EDTA)
Calcium Gluceptate Classification: Electrolyte replacement; calcium	calcium gluceptate
Calcium Gluconate Classification: Electrolyte replacement; calcium	calcium gluconate
Calcium Lactate Classification: Electrolyte replacement; calcium	calcium lactate
Calcium Pantothenate Classification: Vitamin, water soluble	calcium pantothenate (B5, Pantothenic Acid)
Caldecort Classification: Glucocorticoid	hydrocortisone acetate
Caldecort Light with Aloe Classification: Glucocorticoid	hydrocortisone acetate

*Available in Canada only

BRAND NAME	GENERIC NAME
Calderol Classification: Vitamin, fat soluble	calcifediol (25-hydroxycholecalciferol)
Caldesene Classification: Antifungal	undecylenic acid
Calm-X Classification: Antiemetic; anticholinergic	dimenhydrinate
Calphron Classification: Electrolyte replacement; calcium	calcium acetate
Caltrate 600 Classification: Antacid; calcium supplement	calcium carbonate
Cama Arthritis Pain Reliever Classification: Salicylate analgesic; antipyretic	aspirin
Campain* Classification: Analgesic; antipyretic	acetaminophen
Camptosar Classification: Antineoplastic; hormone	irinotecan HCl
Canesten* Classification: Antifungal	clotrimazole, vaginal
Cantil Classification: Anticholinergic	mepenzolate bromide
Caompazine Stemetil* Classification: Antipsychotic	prochlorperazine
Capastat Sulfate Classification: Antitubercular	capreomycin sulfate

BRAND NAME	GENERIC NAME
Capitrol Classification: Antiseborrheic	chloroxine
Capoten Classification: Antihypertensive; angiotensin converting enzyme inhibitor	captopril
Capsin Classification: Analgesic	capsaicin
Captopril Classification: Antihypertensive; angiotensin converting enzyme inhibitor	captopril
Capzasin P Classification: Analgesic	capsaicin
Carafate Classification: Protectant	sucralfate
Carbaprost Tromethamine Classification: Oxytocic; prostaglandin	hemabate
Carbatrol Classification: Anticonvulsant	carbamazepine, extended release
Carbex Classification: Antiparkinson agent	selegiline HCl (L-deprenyl)
Carbidopa & Levodopa Classification: Antiparkinson agent	levodopa/carbidopa
Carbmax* Classification: Emollient	urea

*Available in Canada only

BRAND NAME	GENERIC NAME

Carbocaine
Classification:
Local anesthetic

mepivacaine HCl

Carbolith*
Classification:
Antimanic

lithium carbonate

Carboptic
Classification:
Miotic

carbachol, topical

Carbovir
Classification:
Antiviral; protease inhibitor (Orphan)

carbovir

Cardene
Classification:
Calcium channel blocker

nicardipine HCl

Cardene IV
Classification:
Calcium channel blocker

nicardipine HCl

Cardene SR
Classification:
Calcium channel blocker

nicardipine HCl

Cardio-Green
Classification:
In vivo diagnostic

indocyanine green

Cardioquin
Classification:
Antiarrhythmic

quinidine polygalacturonate

Cardizem
Classification:
Calcium channel blocker

diltiazem HCl

Cardizem CD
Classification:
Calcium channel blocker

diltiazem HCl

Cardizem SR
Classification:
Calcium channel blocker

diltiazem HCl

BRAND NAME	GENERIC NAME
Cardura Classification: Antihypertensive; alpha-adrenergic blocker	doxazosin mesylate
Carisoprodol Classification: Skeletal muscle relaxant, centrally acting	carisoprodol
Carmol 10 Classification: Emollient	urea (carbamide), topical
Carmol 20 Classification: Emollient	urea (carbamide), topical
Carnitor Classification: Amino acid	levocarnitine
Carrisyn Classification: Antiviral (Investigational)	acemannan
Cartrol Classification: Beta-adrenergic blocker	carteolol HCl
Cascara Sagrada Classification: Laxative; irritant	cascara sagrada
Cascara Sagrada Aromatic Fluid Extract Classification: Laxative; irritant	cascara sagrada
Casec Classification: Food modifier	calcium caseinate
Casodex Classification: Antineoplastic; hormone	bicalutamide

*Available in Canada only

BRAND NAME	GENERIC NAME

Castor Oil
Classification:
Laxative; irritant

castor oil

Cataflam
Classification:
Nonsteroidal anti-inflammatory

diclofenac potassium

Catapres
Classification:
Antihypertensive, centrally acting

clonidine HCl

Catapres-TTS-1
Classification:
Antihypertensive, centrally acting

clonidine HCl transdermal

Catapres-TTS-2
Classification:
Antihypertensive, centrally acting

clonidine HCl transdermal

Catapres TTS-3
Classification:
Antihypertensive, centrally acting

clonidine HCl transdermal

Catarase 1:5000
Classification:
Enzymes

chymotrypsin

Catatrol
Classification:
Antidepressant (Investigational)

viloxazine

CD4-IgG
Classification:
Immune serum (Investigational)

CD4-IgG

CEA-Scan
Classification:
In vivo diagnostic

arcitumomab-Tc99m sodium
pertechnetatein

Ce-Vi-Sol
Classification:
Vitamin, water soluble

ascorbic acid (Vitamin C)

Cebid Timecelles
Classification:
Vitamin, water soluble

ascorbic acid (Vitamin C)

BRAND NAME	GENERIC NAME

Ceclor
Classification:
Antibiotic; cephalosporin

cefaclor

Ceclor CD
Classification:
Antibiotic; cephalosporin

cefaclor

Cecon
Classification:
Vitamin, water soluble

ascorbic acid (vitamin C)

Cedax
Classification:
Antibiotic; cephalosporin

ceftibutin

CeeNu
Classification:
Antineoplastic; alkylating agent

lomustine (CCNU)

Cefadroxil
Classification:
Antibiotic; cephalosporin

cefadroxil

Cefanex
Classification:
Antibiotic; cephalosporin

cephalexin monohydrate

Cefazolin Sodium
Classification:
Antibiotic; cephalosporin

cefazolin sodium

Cefizox
Classification:
Antibiotic; cephalosporin

ceftizoxime sodium

Cefobid
Classification:
Antibiotic; cephalosporin

cefoperazone sodium

Cefotan
Classification:
Antibiotic; cephalosporin

cefotetan disodium

Cefracycline*
Classification:
Antibiotic; tetracycline

tetracycline HCl

*Available in Canada only

BRAND NAME	GENERIC NAME
Ceftin Classification: Antibiotic; cephalosporin	cefuroxime axetil
Cefuroxime Sodium Classification: Antibiotic; cephalosporin	cefuroxime sodium
Cefzil Classification: Antibiotic; cephalosporin	cefprozil
Cel-U-Jec Classification: Glucocorticoid	betamethasone sodium phosphate
Celestone Classification: Glucocorticoid	betamethasone
Celestone Phosphate Classification: Glucocorticoid	betamethasone sodium phosphate
Celestone Soluspan Classification: Glucocorticoid	betamethasone sodium phosphate and betamethasone acetate
CellCept Classification: Immunosuppressive	mycophenolate mofetil
Cellufresh Classification: Ophthalmic lubricant	artificial tears solution
Celontin Kapseals Classification: Anticonvulsant; succinimide	methsuximide
Cena-K Classification: Electrolyte replacement; potassium	potassium chloride
Cenafed Classification: Nasal decongestant	pseudoephedrine HCl

*Available in Canada Only

BRAND NAME	GENERIC NAME
Cenafed Syrup Classification: Nasal decongestant	pseudoephedrine HCl
Cenolate Classification: Vitamin, water soluble	ascorbic acid (vitamin C)
Cenolate Classification: Vitamin, water soluble	sodium ascorbate
CenTNF Classification: Anitumor necrosing factor (Investigational)	cA2
Centoxin Classification: Biologic response modifier (Orphan)	nebacumab
Cephalexin Classification: Antibiotic; cephalosporin	cephalexin monohydrate
Cephalothin Sodium Classification: Antibiotic; cephalosporin	cephalothin sodium
Cephapirin Sodium Classification: Antibiotic; cephalosporin	cephapirin sodium
Cephradine Classification: Antibiotic; cephalosporin	cephapirin sodium
Cephulac Classification: Laxative	lactulose
Ceporacin* Classification: Antibiotic; cephalosporin	cephalothin sodium
Ceporex* Classification: Antibiotic; cephalosporin	cephalexin monohydrate

*Available in Canada only

BRAND NAME	GENERIC NAME

Ceptaz
Classification:
Antibiotic; cephalosporin

ceftazidime

Cerebyx
Classification:
Anticonvulsant; hydantoin

fosphenytoin sodium

Ceredase
Classification:
Enzyme replacement

alglucerase

Cerezyme
Classification:
Enzyme

imiglucerase

Cervidil
Classification:
Oxytocic; prostaglandin

dinoprostone

Cetacort
Classification:
Glucocorticoid

hydrocortisone, topical

Cetamide
Classification:
Antibiotic; sulfonamide

sulfacetamide sodium, ophthalmic

Cetane
Classification:
Vitamin, water soluble

ascorbic acid (vitamin C)

Cetazol
Classification:
Diuretic; carbonic anhydrase inhibitor

acetazolamide

Cevalin
Classification:
Vitamin, water soluble

ascorbic acid (vitamin C)

Cevi-Bid
Classification:
Vitamin, water soluble

ascorbic acid (vitamin C)

CharcoAid
Classification:
Adsorbent

charcoal activated

*Available in Canada Only

BRAND NAME	GENERIC NAME
CharcoAid 2000 Classification: Adsorbent	charcoal, activated
Charcoal Classification: Antiflatulent	charcoal
Charcoal, Activated Classification: Adsorbent	charcoal activated
CharcoCaps Classification: Antiflatulent	charcoal
Chelated Magnesium Classification: Electrolyte replacement	magnesium gluconate
Chemet Classification: Chelating agent	succimer
Chenix Classification: Antilithic (Orphan)	chenodiol
Cheracol Nasal Classification: Nasal decongestant	oxymetazoline HCl, nasal
Chibroxin Classification: Antibiotic; fluoroquinolone	norfloxacin, ophthalmic
Chigger-tox Classification: Local anesthetic	benzocaine, topical
Children's Advil Classification: Nonsteroidal anti-inflammatory	ibuprofen
Children's Dramamine Classification: Antiemetic; anticholinergic	dimenhydrinate

BRAND NAME	GENERIC NAME

Children's Dynafed Jr.
Classification:
Analgesic; antipyretic

acetaminophen

Children's Feverall
Classification:
Analgesic; antipyretic

acetaminophen

Children's Hold
Classification:
Non-narcotic antitussive

dextromethorphan

Children's Nōstril
Classification:
Nasal decongestant

phenylephrine HCl

Children's Silfedrine
Classification:
Nasal decongestant

pseudoephedrine HCl

Children's Sudafed
Classification:
Nasal decongestant

pseudoephedrine HCl

Chimeric Mab (C2B8) to CD20
Classification:
Biologic response modifier (Orphan)

chimeric Mab (C2B8) to CD20

Chlo-Amine
Classification:
Antihistamine

chlorpheniramine maleate

Chlor-100
Classification:
Antihistamine

chlorpheniramine maleate

Chlor-Pro 10
Classification:
Antihistamine

chlorpheniramine maleate

Chlor-Pro
Classification:
Antihistamine

chlorpheniramine maleate

Chlor-Trimeton
Classification:
Antihistamine

chlorpheniramine maleate

BRAND NAME	GENERIC NAME
Chlor-Trimeton 12 Hour Allergy Classification: Antihistimine	chlorpheniramine maleate
Chlor-Trimeton Allergy Classification: Antihistimine	chlorpheniramine maleate
Chlor-Trimeton Allergy 8 Hour Classification: Antihistimine	chlorpheniramine maleate
Chlor-Trimeton Repetabs Classification: Antihistamine	chlorpheniramine maleate
Chloral Hydrate Classification: Sedative-hypnotic; nonbarbiturate	chloral hydrate
Chloramphenicol Classification: Antibacterial; antirickettsial	chloramphenicol sodium succinate
Chloramphenicol Classification: Antibacterial	chloramphenicol, ophthalmic
Chloramphenicol Sodium Succinate Classification: Antibacterial; antirickettsial	chloramphenicol sodium succinate
Chlorate Classification: Antihistamine	chlorpheniramine maleate
Chlordiazepoxide HCl Classification: Antianxiety; benzodiazepine	chlordiazepoxide HCl
Chloresium Classification: Systemic deodorizer	chlorophyll derivatives

BRAND NAME	GENERIC NAME
Chlorophylin Classification: Systemic deodorizer	chlorophyll derivatives
Chloromycetin Classification: Antibacterial	chloramphenicol, ophthalmic
Chloroptic Classification: Antibacterial	chloramphenicol, ophthalmic
Chloroptic S.O.P. Classification: Antibacterial	chloramphenicol, ophthalmic
Chloroquine Phosphate Classification: Antimalarial	chloroquine phosphate
Chlorothiazide Classification: Thiazide diuretic	chlorothiazide
Chlorphed-LA Classification: Nasal decongestant	oxymetazoline HCl, nasal
Chlorpheniramine Maleate Classification: Antihistamine	chlorpheniramine maleate
Chlorpromanyl* Classification: Antipsychotic	chlorpromazine HCl
Chlorpropamide Classification: Antidiabetic; sulfonylurea	chlorpropamide
Chlorspan-12 Classification: Antihistamine	chlorpheniramine maleate
Chlorthalidone Classification: Thiazide-like diuretic	chlorthalidone

*Available in Canada Only

BRAND NAME	GENERIC NAME
Chlorzoxazone Classification: Skeletal muscle relaxant, centrally acting	chlorzoxazone
Cholac Classification: Laxative	lactulose
Cholan-HMB Classification: Hydrocholeretics	dehydrocholic acid
Cholaxin* Classification: Thyroid hormone	thyroid USP (desiccated)
Cholebrine Classification: Radiopaque agent	iocetamic acid
Choledyl SA Classification: Bronchodilator; xanthine	oxtriphylline
Cholera Vaccine Classification: Vaccine	cholera vaccine
Cholestyramine Classification: Antilipemic	cholestyramine
Choline Classification: Amino acid	choline
Choline Bitartrate Classification: Amino acid	choline
Choline Chloride Classification: Amino acid	choline
Choline Dihydrogen Citrate Classification: Amino acid	choline

*Available in Canada only

BRAND NAME	GENERIC NAME

Choline Magnesium Trisalicylate
Classification:
Salicylate analgesic

choline magnesium trisalicylate

Cholografin Meglumine
Classification:
Radiopaque agent

iodipamide megulumine 10.3% and 52%

Choloxin
Classification:
Antilipemic

dextrothyroxine sodium

Chondroitinase
Classification:
Enzyme (Orphan)

chondroitinase

Chooz
Classification:
Antacid; calcium supplement

calcium carbonate

Chorex-5
Classification:
Chorionic gonadotropin

chorionic gonadotropin, human (HCG)

Chorex-10
Classification:
Chorionic gonadotropin

chorionic gonadotropin, human (HCG)

Chorionic Gonadotropin
Classification:
Chorionic gonadotropin

chorionic gonadotropin (human) (HCG)

Choron 10
Classification:
Chorionic gonadotropin

chorionic gonadotropin, human (HCG)

Chroma-Pak
Classification:
Trace element

chromium

Chromic Chloride
Classification:
Trace element

chromium

Chromium
Classification:
Trace element

chromium

BRAND NAME	GENERIC NAME
Chronulac Classification: Laxative	lactulose
Chymex Classification: Gastrointestinal function test	bentiromide
Chymodiactin Classification: Enzyme	chymopapain
CI-1020 Classification: Antiviral (Investigational)	CI-1020
Cibacalcin Classification: Parathyroid agent	calcitonin (human)
Cidex-7 Classification: Germicidal	glutaraldehyde
Cidex Classification: Germicidal	glutaraldehyde
Cidex Plus Classification: Germicidal	glutaraldehyde
Cidomycin* Classification: Aminoglycoside	gentamicin sulfate
Ciliary Neurotrophic Factor Classification: Anti-amytrophic lateral sclerosis agent (Orphan)	ciliary neurotrophic factor
Ciliary Neurotrophic Factor Recombinant Human Classification: Anti-amyotrophic lateral sclerosis agent (Orphan)	ciliary neurotrophic factor recombinant human

BRAND NAME	GENERIC NAME

Ciloxan
Classification:
Antibiotic; fluoroquinolone

ciprofloxacin, ophthalmic

Cinobac
Classification:
Urinary anti-infective

cinoxacin

Cinoxacin
Classification:
Urinary anti-infective

cinoxacin

Cipro
Classification:
Antibiotic; fluoroquinolone

ciprofloxacin HCl

Cipro I.V.
Classification:
Antibiotic; fluoroquinolone

ciprofloxacin HCl

Citanest HCl
Classification:
Local anesthetic

prilocaine HCl

Citanest HCl Forte
Classification:
Local anesthetic

prilocaine HCl

Citracal
Classification:
Electrolyte replacement; calcium

calcium citrate

Citracal Liquitab
Classification:
Electrolyte replacement; calcium

calcium citrate

Citrate of Magnesia
Classification:
Laxative; saline

magnesium citrate

Citrate of Magnesia
Classification:
Laxative; saline

saline laxatives

Citrolith
Classification:
Systemic alkalinizer

citrate and citric acid

BRAND NAME	GENERIC NAME

Citrolith
Classification:
Urinary alkalinizer

potassium citrate and citric acid

Citrucel
Classification:
Laxative, bulk-producing

methylcellulose

Claforan
Classification:
Antibiotic; cephalosporin

cefotaxime sodium

Claripen*
Classification:
Antilipemic

clofibrate

Claripex*
Classification:
Antilipemic

clofibrate

Claritin
Classification:
Antihistamine

loratidine

Clearasil Maximum Strength
Classification:
Anti-acne product

benzoyl peroxide

Clear Away
Classification:
Keratolytic

salicylic acid, topical

Clear Away Plantar
Classification:
Keratolytic

salicylic acid, topical

Clear By Design
Classification:
Anti-acne product

benzoyl peroxide

Clear Eyes
Classification:
Ophthalmic vasoconstrictor

naphazoline HCl, ophthalmic

Clear Eyes ACR
Classification:
Ophthalmic vasoconstrictor

naphazoline HCl, ophthalmic

*Available in Canada only

BRAND NAME	GENERIC NAME
Clemastine Fumarate Classification: Antihistamine	clemastine fumarate
Cleocin Classification: Antibiotic; lincosamide	clindamycin HCl
Cleocin Pediatric Classification: Antibiotic; lincosamide	clindamycin palmitate HCl
Cleocin Phosphate Classification: Antibiotic; lincosamide	clindamycin phosphate
Cleocin T Classification: Anti-acne product	clindamycin, topical
Climara Classification: Estrogen	estradiol transdermal system
Climestrone* Classification: Estrogen	estrogens, esterified
Clinafloxacin Classification: Antibiotic; fluoroquinolone (Investigational)	clinafloxacin (CI-960)
Clinda-Derm Classification: Anti-acne product	clinadmycin, topical
Clindamycin, HCl Classification: Antibiotic; lincosamide	clindamycin HCl
Clindamycin Phosphate Classification: Antibiotic; lincosamide	clindamycin phosphate
Clindets Classification: Anti-acne product	clindamycin, topical

BRAND NAME	GENERIC NAME
Clinoril Classification: Nonsteroidal anti-inflammatory	sulindac
Cloderm Classification: Glucocorticoid	clorcortolone pivalate
Clomid Classification: Ovulation stimulant	clomiphene citrate
Clomipramine HCl Classification: Antidepressant; tricyclic	clomipramine HCl
Clonidine HCl Classification: Antihypertensive, centrally acting	clonidine HCl
Clopra Classification: Antidopaminergic	metoclopramide
Clorazepate Dipotassium Classification: Antianxiety; benzodiazepine	clorazepate dipotassium
Clorpactin WC S-90 Classification: Germicidal	oxychlorosene sodium
Clostridial Collagenase Classification: Enzyme (Orphan)	clostridial collagenase
Clotrimidazole Classification: Anti-sickle cell disease agent (Orphan)	clotrimidazole
Cloxacillin Sodium Classification: Antibiotic; penicillinase-resistant penicillin	cloxacillin sodium
Clozaril Classification: Antipsychotic	clozapine

*Available in Canada only

BRAND NAME	GENERIC NAME
Clysodrast Classification: Laxative, irritant	bisacodyl tannex
Cobantrin* Classification: Anthelmintics	pyrantel pamoate
Cocaine HCl Classification: Local anesthetic	cocaine
Cocaine Viscous Classification: Local anesthetic	cocaine
Codeine Phosphate Classification: opioid analgesic; antitussive	codeine
Codeine Sulfate Classification: opioid analgesic, antitussive	codeine
Cogentin Classification: Anticholinergic	benztropine mesylate
Cognex Classification: Cholinesterase inhibitor	tacrine HCl
Co-Lav Classification: Bowel evacuant	polyethylene glycol-electrolyte solution
Colace Classification: Laxative, softener	docusate sodium
Colchicine Classification: Antigout	colchicine
Colestid Classification: Antilipemic	colestipol HCl

BRAND NAME	GENERIC NAME
Colloral Classification: Antirheumatic (Orphan)	collagen (purified Type II)
Collyrium Fresh Eye Drops Classification: Ophthalmic vasoconstrictor	tetrahydrozoline HCl, ophthalmic
Colovage Classification: Bowel evacuant	polyethylene glycol-electrolyte solution
Coly-Mycin M Classification: Antibiotic; polymyxin	colistimethate sodium
CoLyte Classification: Bowel evacuant	polyethylene glycol-electrolyte solution
Combantrin* Classification: Anthelmintics	pyrantel
Comfort Eye Drops Classification: Ophthalmic vasoconstrictor	naphazoline HCl, ophthalmic
Compazine Classification: Antipsychotic	prochlorperazine
Compazine Spansules Classification: Antipsychotic	prochlorperazine
Compound W Classification: Keratolytic	salicylic acid, topical
Compōz Classification: Antihistamine	diphenhydramine HCl
Concentrated Aluminum Hydroxide Classification: Antacid	aluminum hydroxide gel

BRAND NAME	GENERIC NAME

Concentrated Phillip's Milk of Magnesia
Classification:
Antacid, laxative

magnesia (magnesium hydroxide)

Conceptrol
Classification:
Spermicide

nonoxynol

Condylox
Classification:
Keratolytic

podofilox

Conray-30
Classification:
Radiopaque agent

iothalamate meglumine 30%

Conray 43
Classification:
Radiopaque agent

iothalamate meglumine 43%

Conray 325
Classification:
Radiopaque agent

iothalamate sodium 54.3%

Conray 400
Classification:
Radiopaque agent

iothalamate sodium 66.8%

Conray
Classification:
Radiopaque agent

iothalamate meglumine 60%

Constilac
Classification:
Laxative

lactulose

Constulose
Classification:
Laxative

lactulose

Control
Classification:
Alpha-adrenergic agonist

phenylpropanolamine HCl

Copaxone
Classification:
Biologic response modifier

glatiramer acetate

BRAND NAME	GENERIC NAME
Cophene-B Classification: Antihistamine	brompheniramine maleate
Copper Classification: Trace element	copper
Cordarone Classification: Antiarrhythmic	amiodarone HCl
Cordran Classification: Glucocorticoid	flurandrenolide
Cordran SP Classification: Glucocorticoid	flurandrenolide
Cordran Tape Classification: Glucocorticoid	flurandrenolide
Coreg Classification: Antihypertensive	carvedilol
Corgard Classification: Beta-adrenergic blocker	nadolol
Coricidin Nasal Mist Classification: Nasal decongestant	oxymetazoline HCl, nasal
Corlopam Classification: Antihypertensive	fenoldopam
Cormax Classification: Glucocorticoid	clobestasol propionate
Coronex* Classification: Antianginal	isosorbide dinitrate, oral

BRAND NAME	GENERIC NAME
Corophyllin* Classification: Bronchodilator; xanthine	aminophylline (theophylline ethylenediamine)
Correctol Extra Gentle Classification: Laxative, softener	docusate sodium
Cort-Dome Classification: Glucocorticoid	hydrocortisone, topical
Cort-Dome High Potency Classification: Glucocorticoid	hydrocortisone, acetate
Cortaid Classification: Glucocorticoid	hydrocortisone acetate
Cortaid Intensive Therapy Classification: Glucocorticoid	hydrocortisone, topical
Cortamed* Classification: Glucocorticoid	hydrocortisone
Cortef Classification: Glucocorticoid	hydrocortisone
Cortef Classification: Glucocorticoid	hydrocortisone cypionate
Cortenema Classification: Glucocorticoid	hydrocortisone retention enema
Corticaine Classification: Glucocorticoid	hydrocortisone acetate
Corticotropin Classification: Anterior pituitary hormone	corticotropin injection

BRAND NAME	GENERIC NAME
Cortifoam Classification: Glucocorticoid	hydrocortisone acetate intrarectal foam
Cortisone Acetate Classification: Glucocorticoid	cortisone
Cortizone-5 Classification: Glucocorticoid	hydrocortisone, topical
Cortizone-10 Classification: Glucocorticoid	hydrocortisone, topical
Cortone Acetate Classification: Glucocorticoid	cortisone
Cortrosyn Classification: Anterior pituitary hormone	cosyntropin
Corvert Classification: Antiarrhythmic	ibutilide fumarate
Cosmegen Classification: Antineoplastic; antibiotic	dactinomycin (actinomycin D; ACT)
Cotazym Capsules Classification: Digestive enzyme	pancrelipase
Cotazym-S Capsules Classification: Digestive enzyme	pancrelipase
Cotrim Classification: Antibiotic; sulfonamide	trimethoprim and sulfamethoxazole (TMP-SMZ)
Cotrim DS Classification: Antibiotic; sulfonamide	trimethoprim and sulfamethoxazole (TMP-SMZ)

BRAND NAME	GENERIC NAME
Cotrim Pediatric Classification: Antibiotic; sulfonamide	trimethoprim and sulfamethoxazole (TMP-SMZ)
Coumadin Classification: Anticoagulant	warfarin sodium
Covera-HS Classification: Calcium channel blocker	verapamil HCl
Cozaar Classification: Antihypertensive; angiotensin II antagonist	losartan potassium
Creamy Tar Classification: Keratolytic	coal tar
Creon Classification: Digestive enzyme	pancrelipase
Creon 10 Classification: Digestive enzyme	pancrelipase
Creon 20 Classification: Digestive enzyme	pancrelipase
Creo-Terpin Classification: Non-narcotic antitussive	dextromethorphan
Crinone Classification: Progestin	progesterone gel
Crixivan Classification: Antiviral; protease inhibitor	indinavir sulfate
Crolom Classification: Anti-inflammatory	cromolyn sodium, ophthalmic

BRAND NAME	GENERIC NAME
Cromolyn Sodium Classification: Antiasthmatic	cromolyn sodium
CroTab Classification: Antivenin (Orphan)	antivenin, polyvalent crotalid
Cruex Classification: Antifungal	undecylenic acid
Cryptosporidium Hyperimmune IgG Concentrate Classification: Immune serum (Orphan)	cryptosporidium hyperimmune IgG concentrate
Cryptosporidium Parvum Bovine Immune Globulin Classification: Immune serum (Orphan)	cryptosporidium parvum bovine immune globulin
Crystamine Classification: Vitamin, water soluble	cyanocobalamin (vitamin B_{12})
Crysti-12 Classification: Vitamin, water soluble	cyanocobalamin (vitamin B_{12})
Crysti 1000 Classification: Vitamin, water soluble	cyanocobalamin (vitamin B_{12})
Crysticillin 300 A.S. Classification: Antibiotic; penicillin	penicillin G procaine, aqueous (APPG)
Crysticillin 600 A.S. Classification: Antibiotic; penicillin	penicillin G procaine, aqueous (APPG)
Crystodigin Classification: Cardiac glycoside	digitoxin

*Available in Canada only

BRAND NAME	GENERIC NAME

Cupric Sulfate
Classification:
Trace element

copper

Cuprid
Classification:
Chelating agent (Orphan)

trientine HCl

Cuprimine
Classification:
Chelating agent

D-penicillamine

Cuprimine
Classification:
Chelating agent

penicillamine

Curdlan Sulfate
Classification:
Antiviral (Investigational)

curdlan sulfate

Curosurf
Classification:
Lung surfactant (Orphan)

pulmonary surfactant replacement, porcine

Curretab
Classification:
Progestin

medroxyprogesterone acetate

Cūtar Bath Oil
Classification:
Keratolytic

coal tar

Cutivate
Classification:
Glucocorticoid

fluticasone propionate, topical

Cyanabin*
Classification:
Vitamin, water soluble

cyanocobalamin (vitamin B_{12})

Cyanoject
Classification:
Vitamin, water soluble

cyanocobalamin (vitamin B_{12})

Cyclobenzaprine HCl
Classification:
Skeletal muscle relaxant, centrally acting

cyclobenzaprine HCl

BRAND NAME	GENERIC NAME
Cyclocort Classification: Glucocorticoid	amcinonide
Cyclogyl Classification: Mydriatic	cyclopentolate HCl
Cyclomen* Classification: Androgen	danazol
Cyclopentolate Classification: Mydriatic	cyclopentolate HCl
Cyclospasmol Classification: Peripheral vasodilator	cyclandelate
Cycrin Classification: Progestin	medroxyprogesterone acetate
Cyklokapron Classification: Hemostatic	tranexamic acid
Cylert Classification: CNS stimulant	pemoline
Cyomine Classification: Vitamin, water soluble	cyanocobalamin (vitamin B_{12})
Cyprohepatadine HCl Classification: Antihistamine	cyprohepatadine
Cystadane Classification: Antihomocystinuria agent	betaine anhydrous
Cystagon Classification: anticystine agent	cysteamine bitartrate

*Available in Canada only

BRAND NAME	GENERIC NAME

Cysteine HCl
Classification:
Nitrogen product

cysteine HCl

Cysto-Conray II
Classification:
Radiopaque agent

iothalamate meglumine 17.2%

Cystografin
Classification:
Radiopaque agent

diatrizoate meglumine 30%

Cystografin dilute
Classification:
Radiopaque agent

diatrizoate meglumine 18%

Cystospaz
Classification:
Anticholinergic

hyoscyamine sulfate

Cystospaz-M
Classification:
Anticholinergic

hyoscyamine sulfate

Cytadren
Classification:
Adrenal steroid inhibitor

aminoglutethimide

Cytarabine
Classification:
Antineoplastic; antimetabolite

cytarabine (Ara-C; cytosine arabinoside)

CytoGam
Classification:
Immune serum

cytomegalovirus immune globulin
intravenous (human) (CMV-IGIV)

Cytolin
Classification:
Immune serum (Investigational)

cytolin

Cytomel
Classification:
Thyroid hormone

liothyronine sodium (T3)

Cytosar-U
Classification:
Antineoplastic; antimetabolite

cytarabine (Ara-C; cytosine arabinoside)

BRAND NAME	GENERIC NAME
Cytotec Classification: Prostaglandin	misoprostol
Cytovene Classification: Antiviral	ganciclovir (DHPG)
Cytoxan Classification: Antineoplastic; alkylating agent	cyclophosphamide

D

D-Tran* Classification: Antianxiety; benzodiazepine	diazepam
D-S-S Classification: Laxative, softener	docusate sodium
D.H.E. 45 Classification: Antimigraine; ergot alkaloid	dihydroergotamine mesylate
Dagenan* Classification: Antibiotic; sulfonamide	sulfapyridine
Dairy Ease Classification: Food modifier	lactase enzyme
Dakin's Solution Classification: Germicidal	sodium hypochlorite
Dalalone D.P. Classification: Glucocorticoid	dexamethasone acetate
Dalalone L.A. Classification: Glucocorticoid	dexamethasone acetate

*Available in Canada only

BRAND NAME	GENERIC NAME

Dalgan
Classification:
Opioid agonist-antagonist analgesic

dezocine

Dalmane
Classification:
Sedative-hypnotic; benzodiazepine

flurazepam HCl

Daltose*
Classification:
Vitamin, fat soluble

vitamin E

Danazol
Classification:
Androgen

danazol

Danocrine
Classification:
Androgen

danazol

Dantrium
Classification:
Skeletal muscle relaxant, direct acting

dantrolene sodium

Dantrium Intravenous
Classification:
Skeletal muscle relaxant, direct acting

dantrolene sodium

Dapcin
Classification:
Analgesic; antipyretic

acetaminophen

Dapsone
Classification:
Leprostatic

dapsone (DDS)

Daranide
Classification:
Diuretic; carbonic anhydrase inhibitor

dichlorphenamide

Daraprim
Classification:
Antimalarial

pyrimethamine

Darvon-N
Classification:
Opioid analgesic

propoxyphene napsylate

BRAND NAME	GENERIC NAME
Darvon Pulvules Classification: Opioid analgesic	propoxyphene HCl
DaunoXome Classification: Antineoplastic; antibiotic	daunorubicin citrate liposomal
Daypro Classification: Nonsteroidal anti-inflammatory	oxaprozin
Dayto-Himbin Classification: Alpha-adrenergic blocker	yohimbine HCl
Dayto-Sulf Classification: Antibiotic; sulfonamide	triple sulfa
Dazamide Classification: Diuretic; carbonic anhydrase inhibitor	acetazolamide
DC Softgels Classification: Laxative, softener	docusate calcium
Debrisan Classification: Debriding agent	dextranomer
Debrox Classification: Emulsifier	carbamide peroxide, otic
Deca-Durabolin Classification: Anabolic steroid	nandrolone decanoate
Decaderm Classification: Glucocorticoid	dexamethasone
Decadron-LA Classification: Glucocorticoid	dexamethasone acetate

BRAND NAME	GENERIC NAME
Decadron Phosphate Classification: Glucocorticoid	dexamethasone sodium phosphate
Decadron Phosphate Classification: Ophthalmic glucocorticoid	dexamethasone, ophthalmic
Decaject-LA Classification: Glucocorticoid	dexamethasone acetate
Decholin Classification: Hydrocholeretics	dehydrocholic acid
Declomycin Classification: Antibiotic; tetracycline	demeclocycline HCl
Decofed Syrup Classification: Nasal decongestant	pseudoephedrine HCl
Decylenes Classification: Antifungal	undecylenic acid
DeFed-60 Classification: Nasal decongestant	pseudoephedrine HCl
Defibrotide Classification: Blood modifier (Orphan)	defibrotide
Degas Classification: Antiflatulent	simethicone
Degest 2 Classification: Ophthalmic vasoconstrictor	naphazoline HCl, ophthalmic
Dehydrex Classification: Ophthalmic (Orphan)	dehydrex

BRAND NAME	GENERIC NAME
Dehydrocholic acid Classification: Hydrocholeretics	dehydrocholic acid
Dehydroepiandrosterone Classification: Androgen (Orphan)	dehydroepiandrosterone
Del-Vi-A Classification: Vitamin, fat soluble	vitamin A
Delaprem Classification: Tocolytic (Investigational)	heoxprenaline sulfate
Del Aqua- 5 Classification: Anti-acne product	benzoyl peroxide
Del Aqua-10 Classification: Anti-acne product	benzoyl peroxide
Delatestryl Classification: Androgen	testosterone enanthate (in oil)
Delatest Classification: Androgen	testosterone enanthate (in oil)
Delestrogen Classification: Estrogen	estradiol valerate
Delfen Contraceptive Classification: Spermicide	nonoxynol
Del-Mycin Classification: Anti-acne product	erythromycin, topical
Delsym Classification: Non-narcotic antitussive	dextromethorphan

BRAND NAME	GENERIC NAME
Delta-Cortef Classification: Glucocorticoid	prednisolone
Delta-D Classification: Vitamin, fat soluble	cholecalciferol
Demadex Classification: Loop diuretic	torsemide
Demerol HCl Classification: Opioid analgesic	meperidine HCl
Demser Classification: Antihypertensive	metyrosine
Denavir Classification: Antiviral	penciclovir
Denorex Classification: Keratolytic	coal tar
Deoxynojirimycin, n-butyl Classification: Antiviral (Investigational)	deoxynojirimycin, n-butyl
Depacon Classification: Anticonvulsant	valproate sodium
Depakene Classification: Anticonvulsant	valproic acid
Depakene Syrup Classification: Anticonvulsant	valproate sodium
Depakote Classification: Anticonvulsant	divalproex sodium

BRAND NAME	GENERIC NAME
depAndro 100 Classification: Androgen	testosterone cypionate (in oil)
depAndro 200 Classification: Androgen	testosterone cypionate (in oil)
Depen Classification: Chelating agent	D-penicillamine
Depen Classification: Chelating agent	penicillamine
depGynogen Classification: Estrogen	estradiol cypionate
depMedalone 40 Classification: Glucocorticoid	methylprednisolone acetate
depMedalone 80 Classification: Glucocorticoid	methylprednisolone acetate
Depo Estradiol Classification: Estrogen	estradiol cypionate
Depo-Medrol Classification: Glucocorticoid	methylprednisolone acetate
Depo-Provera Classification: Progestin	medroxyprogesterone acetate
Depo-Testosterone Classification: Androgen	testosterone cypionate (in oil)
Depogen Classification: Estrogen	estradiol cypionate

BRAND NAME	GENERIC NAME
Depoject Classification: Glucocorticoid	methylprednisolone acetate
Deponit Classification: Antianginal	nitroglycerin, transdermal systems
Depopred-40 Classification: Glucocorticoid	methylprednisolone acetate
Deporpred-80 Classification: Glucocorticoid	methylprednisolone acetate
Depotest-100 Classification: Androgen	testosterone cypionate (in oil)
Depotest-200 Classification: Androgen	testosterone cypionate (in oil)
Derifil Classification: Systemic deodorizer	chlorophyll derivatives
Dermacort Classification: Glucocorticoid	hydrocortisone, topical
Dermamycin Classification: Antihistamine	diphenhydramine HCl
Derma-Smoothe/FS Classification: Glucocorticoid	fluocinolone acetonide
Dermatop Classification: Glucocorticoid	prednicarbate
Dermolate Classification: Glucocorticoid	hydrocortisone, topical

BRAND NAME	GENERIC NAME
Dermoplast Classification: Local anesthetic	benzocaine, topical
Dermtex HC Classification: Glucocorticoid	hydrocortisone, topical
DES Classification: Estrogen	diethylstilbestrol
Desenex Classification: Antifungal	undecylenic acid
Desenex Maximum Strength Classification: Antifungal	undecylenic acid
Deseferal Classification: Chelating agent	deferoxamine mesylate
Desipramine HCl Classification: Antidepressant, tricyclic	desipramine HCl
Desmopressin Acetate Classification: Posterior pituitary hormone	desmopressin acetate
Desonide Classification: Glucocorticoid	desonide
DesOwen Classification: Glucocorticoid	desonide
Desoximetasone Classification: Glucocorticoid	desoximetasone
Desoxyn Classification: CNS stimulant	methamphetamine HCl

*Available in Canada only

BRAND NAME	GENERIC NAME

Desoxyn Gradumets
Classification:
CNS stimulant

methamphetamine HCl

Desquam-E 5
Classification:
Anti-acne product

benzoyl peroxide

Desquam-E 10
Classification:
Anti-acne product

benzoyl peroxide

Desquam-X5
Classification:
Anti-acne product

benzoyl peroxide

Desquam-X10
Classification:
Anti-acne product

benzoyl peroxide

Desquam-X5 Wash
Classification:
Anti-acne product

benzoyl peroxide

Desquam-X10 Wash
Classification:
Anti-acne product

benzoyl peroxide

Desyrel
Classification:
Antidepressant, tetracyclic

trazodone HCl

Desyrel Dividose
Classification:
Antidepressant, tetracyclic

trazodone HCl

Devrom
Classification:
Systemic deodorizer

bismuth subgallate

Dex4 Glucose
Classification:
Glucose elevating agent

glucose

Dexacort Phosphate Turbinaire
Classification:
Glucocorticoid

dexamethasone sodium phosphate

BRAND NAME	GENERIC NAME
Dexamethasone Acetate Classification: Glucocorticoid	dexamethasone acetate
Dexamethasone Ophthalmic Suspension Classification: Ophthalmic glucocorticoid	dexamethasone, ophthalmic
Dexamethasone Sodium Phosphate Classification: Glucocorticoid	dexamethasone sodium phosphate
Dexamethasone Sodium Phosphate Classification: Ophthalmic glucocorticoid	dexamethasone sodium phosphate
Dexasone Classification: Glucocorticoid	dexamethasone sodium phosphate
Dexasone L.A. Classification: Glucocorticoid	dexamethasone acetate
Dexatrim Classification: Alpha-adrenergic agonist	phenylpropanolamine HCl
Dexatrim Maximum Strength Classification: Alpha-adrenergic agonist	phenylpropanolamine HCl
Dexatrim Pre-Meal Classification: Alpha-adrenergic agonist	phenylpropanolamine HCl
Dexchlor Classification: Antihistamine	dexchlorpheniramine maleate
Dexchlorpheniramine Maleate Classification: Antihistamine	dexchlorpheniramine maleate

*Available in Canada only

BRAND NAME	GENERIC NAME

Dexedrine
Classification:
CNS stimulant

dextroamphetamine sulfate

Dexedrine Spansules
Classification:
CNS stimulant

dextroamphetamine sulfate

DexFerrum
Classification:
Iron preparation

iron dextran

Dexitac
Classification:
Analeptic

caffeine

Dexone
Classification:
Glucocorticoid

dexamethasone sodium phosphate

Dexone LA
Classification:
Glucocorticoid

dexamethasone acetate

Dexpanthenol
Classification:
Gastrointestinal stimulant

dexpanthenol

Dextran 40
Classification:
Plasma volume expander

dextran 40

Dextran 70
Classification:
Plasma volume expander

dextran 70/75

Dextran 75
Classification:
Plasma volume expander

dextran 70/75

Dextroamphetamine sulfate
Classification:
CNS stimulant

dextroamphetamine sulfate

Dextromethorphan
Classification:
Non-narcotic antitussive

dextromethorphan

BRAND NAME	GENERIC NAME
Dextrose (d-Glucose) Classification: Caloric agent	dextrose (d-Glucose)
Dextrostat Classification: CNS stimulant	destroamphetamine
Dey-Pak Sodium Chloride 3% and 10% Classification: Hyperosmolar preparation	sodium chloride, hypertonic
DHEA (EL 10) Classification: Biologic response modifier (Investigational)	DHEA (EL 10)
DHS Tar Classification: Keratolytic	coal tar
DHS Zinc Classification: Antiseborrheic	pyrithione zinc
DHT Classification: Vitamin, fat soluble	dihydrotachysterol (DHT)
DHT Intensol Solution Classification: Vitamin, fat soluble	dihydrotachysterol (DHT)
Di-Spaz Classification: Antispasmodic	dicyclomine HCl
DiaBeta Classification: Antidiabetic; sulfonylurea	glyburide
Diabetic Tussin EX Classification: Expectorant	guaifenesin

BRAND NAME	GENERIC NAME

Diabinese
Classification:
Antidiabetic; sulfonylurea

chlorpropamide

Dialose
Classification:
Laxative, softener

docusate sodium

Dialume
Classification:
Antacid

aluminum hydroxide gel

Diamine T.D.
Classification:
Antihistamine

brompheniramine maleate

Diamox
Classification:
Diuretic; carbonic anhydrase inhibitor

acetazolamide

Diamox Parenteral
Classification:
Diuretic; carbonic anhydrase inhibitor

acetazolamide sodium

Diamox Sequels
Classification:
Diuretic; carbonic anhydrase inhibitor

acetazolamide

Diapid
Classification:
Posterior pituitary hormone

lypressin (8-Lysine Vasopressin)

Diastat
Classification:
Anticonvulsant; benzodiazepine

diazepam rectal gel

Diatrizoate Meglumine 76%
Classification:
Radiopaque agent

diatrizoate meglumine 76%

Diazemuls*
Classification:
Antianxiety; benzodiazepine

diazepam

Diazepam
Classification:
Antianxiety; benzodiazepine

diazepam

*Available in Canada Only

BRAND NAME	GENERIC NAME
Diazepam Intensol Classification: Antianxiety; benzodiazepine	diazepam
Dibent Classification: Antispasmodic	dicyclomine HCl
Dibenzyline Classification: Antihypertensive; alpha-adrenergic blocker	phenoxybenzamine HCl
Dibromodulcitol Classification: Antineoplastic (Orphan)	dibromodulcitol
Dibucaine Classification: Local anesthetic	dibucaine HCl, topical
Dicarbosil Classification: Antacid; calcium supplement	calcium carbonate
Diclofenac Sodium Classification: Nonsteroidal anti-inflammatory	diclofenac sodium
Dicloxacillin Sodium Classification: Antibiotic; penicillinase-resistant penicillin	dicloxacillin sodium
Dicyclomine HCl Classification: Antispasmodic	dicyclomine HCl
Didrex Classification: CNS stimulant; anorexiant	benzphetamine HCl
Didronel Classification: Bone resorption inhibitor	etidronate disodium, oral

BRAND NAME	GENERIC NAME

Didronel IV
Classification:
Bone resorption inhibitor

etidronate disodium, parenteral

Diet Aid Maximum Strength
Classification:
Alpha-adrenergic agonist

phenylpropanolamine HCl

Diet AYDS
Classification:
Local anesthetic

benzocaine

Diethylpropion HCl
Classification:
CNS stimulant; anorexiant

diethylpropion HCl

Differin
Classification:
Anti-acne product

adapalene

Diflucan
Classification:
Antifungal; bis-triazole

fluconazole

Diflunisal
Classification:
Salicylate analgesic

diflunisal

Digibind
Classification:
Antidigoxin antibody

digoxin immune fab (ovine)

Digitaline*
Classification:
Cardiac glycoside

digitoxin

Digitoxin
Classification:
Cardiac glycoside

digitoxin

Digoxin
Classification:
Cardiac glycoside

digoxin

Dilacor XR
Classification:
Calcium channel blocker

diltiazem HCl

BRAND NAME	GENERIC NAME
Dilantin-125 Classification: Anticonvulsant; hydantoin	phenytoin
Dilantin Classification: Anticonvulsant; hydantoin	phenytoin sodium, parenteral
Dilantin Infatab Classification: Anticonvulsant; hydantoin	phenytoin
Dilantin Kapseals Classification: Anticonvulsant; hydantoin	phenytoin sodium, extended
Dilatrate-SR Classification: Antianginal	isosorbide dinitrate, oral
Dilaudid-5 Classification: Opicid analgesic	hydromorphone HCl
Dilaudid Classification: Opioid analgesic	hydromorphone HCl
Dilaudid-HP Classification: Opioid analgesic	hydromorphone HCl
Dilocaine Classification: Local anesthetic	lidocaine HCl, local
Dilor Classification: Bronchodilator; xanthine	dyphylline (dihydroxypropyl theophylline)
Dimelor* Classification: Antidiabetic; sulfonylurea	acetohexamide
Dimenhydrinate Classification: Antiemetic; anticholinergic	dimenhydrinate

BRAND NAME	GENERIC NAME

Dimetane Extentabs
Classification:
Antihistamine

brompheniramine maleate

Dinate
Classification:
Antiemetic; anticholinergic

dimenhydrinate

Diocto
Classification:
Laxative, softener

docusate sodium

Diocto-K
Classification:
Laxative, softener

docusate potassium

Diodoquin*
Classification:
Amebicide

iodoquinol (diiodohydroxyquin)

Dioeze
Classification:
Laxative, softener

docusate sodium

Dionosil Oily
Classification:
Radiopaque agent

propyliodone 60%

Dioval 40
Classification:
Estrogen

estradiol valerate

Dioval XX
Classification:
Estrogen

estradiol valerate

Diovan
Classification:
Antihypertensive; angiotensin II
antagonist

valsartan

Dipentum
Classification:
GI anti-inflammatory

olsalazine sodium

Dipivefrin HCl
Classification:
Adrenergic agonist

dipivefrin HCl

BRAND NAME	GENERIC NAME
Diphen Cough Classification: Antihistamine	diphenhydramine HCl
Diphenhist Classification: Antihistamine	diphenhydramine HCl
Diphenhydramine HCl Classification: Antihistamine	diphenhydramine HCl
Diphtheria and Tetanus Toxoids, Adsorbed (for adult use) Classification: Toxoid	diphtheria and tetanus toxoids, combined (Td)
Diphtheria and Tetanus Toxoids, Adsorbed (for pediatric use) Classification: Toxoid	diphtheria and tetanus toxoids, combined (Td)
Diphtheria Antitoxin Classification: Antitoxin	diphtheria antitoxin
Diprivan Classification: General anesthetic	propofol
Diprolene Classification: Glucocorticoid	betamethasone dipropionate, augmented
Diprolene AF Classification: Glucocorticoid	betamethasone dipropionate, augmented
Diprosone Classification: Glucocorticoid	betamethasone dipropionate
Dipyridamole Classification: Antiplatelet	dipyridamole

BRAND NAME	GENERIC NAME

Dirame
Classification:
Opiod analgesic (Investigational)

propiram

Disalcid
Classification:
Salicylate analgesic

salsalate

Disodium Clodronate
Classification:
Bone resorption inhibitor (Orphan)

disodium clodronate

Disodium Clodronate Tetrahydrate
Classification:
Bone resorption inhibitor (Orphan)

disodium clodronate tetrahydrate

Disonate
Classification:
Laxative, softener

docusate sodium

Disopyramide Phosphate
Classification:
Antiarrhythmic

disopyramide

Disotate
Classification:
Chelating agent

edetate disodium (EDTA)

Disulfiram
Classification:
Antialcoholic

disulfiram

Dital
Classification:
CNS stimulant; anorexiant

phendimetrazine tartrate

Ditropan
Classification:
Urinary antispasmodic

oxybutynin chloride

Diucardin
Classification:
Thiazide diuretic

hydroflumethiazide

Diuchlor H*
Classification:
Thiazide diuretic

hydrochlorothiazide

*Available in Canada Only

BRAND NAME	GENERIC NAME
Diuril Classification: Thiazide diuretic	chlorothiazide
Diuril Sodium Classification: Thiazide diuretic	chlorothiazide
Diurese Classification: Thiazide diuretic	trichlormethiazide
Dixarit* Classification: Antihypertensive, centrally acting	clonidine HCl
Dizac Classification: Antianxiety; benzodiazepine	diazepam
Dizmiss Classification: Antiemetic; anticholinergic	meclizine
DMP-450 Classification: Antiviral (Investigational)	DMP-450
Doan's Pills Classification: Salicylate analgesic	magnesium salicylate
Dobutamine HCl Classification: Adrenergic agonist	dobutamine HCl
Dobutrex Classification: Adrenergic agonist	dobutamine HCl
Doctar Classification: Keratolytic	coal tar
Docusate Calcium Classification: Laxative, softener	docusate calcium

*Available in Canada only

BRAND NAME	GENERIC NAME
Docusate Sodium Classification: Laxative, softener	docusate sodium
DOK Classification: Laxative, softener	docusate sodium
Dolene Classification: Opioid analgesic	propoxyphene HCl
Dolobid Classification: Salicylate analgesic	diflunisal
Dolophine HCl Classification: Opioid analgesic	methadone HCl
Dolorac Classification: Analgesic	capsaicin
Domeboro Classification: Astringent	aluminum acetate solution
Donnamar Classification: GI anticholinergic	hyoscyamine sulfate
Donnazyme Classification: Digestive enzyme	pancreatin
Dopamet* Classification: Antihypertensive, centrally acting	methyldopa/methyldopate HCl
Dopamine HCl Classification: Adrenergic agonist	dopamine HCl
Dopar Classification: Antiparkinson agent	levodopa

BRAND NAME	GENERIC NAME
Dopram Classification: Analeptic	doxapram HCl
Doral Classification: Sedative-hypnotic; benzodiazepine	quazepam
Dorcol Children's Decongestant Classification: Nasal decongestant	pseudoephedrine HCl
Dormarex Classification: Antihistamine	pyrilamine maleate
Dormin Classification: Antihistamine	diphenhydramine HCl
Doryx Classification: Antibiotic; tetracycline	doxycycline hyclate
Dosalax Classification: Laxative, irritant	senna
DOS Softgel Classification: Laxative, softener	docusate sodium
Doxtinex Classification: Dopamine receptor agonist	cabergoline
Dovonex Classification: Antipsoriatic	calcipotriene
Doxepin HCl Classification: Antianxiety; antidepressant	doxepin HCl
Doxorubicin HCl Classification: Antineoplastic; antibiotic	doxorubicin HCl (ADR)

BRAND NAME	GENERIC NAME

Doxy 100
Classification:
Antibiotic; tetracycline

doxycycline hyclate

Doxy 200
Classification:
Antibiotic; tetracycline

doxycycline hyclate

Doxy Caps
Classification:
Antibiotic; tetracycline

doxycycline hyclate

Doxychel Hyclate
Classification:
Antibiotic; tetracycline

doxycycline hyclate

Doxycin*
Classification:
Antibiotic; tetracycline

doxycycline hyclate

Doxycycline
Classification:
Antibiotic; tetracycline

doxycycline hyclate

Dr. Caldwell Senna Laxative
Classification:
Laxative, irritant

senna

Dr. Scholl's Athlete's Foot
Classification:
Antifungal

tolnaftate

Dr. Scholl's Corn/Callus Remover
Classification:
Keratolytic

salicylic acid, topical

Dr. Scholl's Maximum Strength Tritin
Classification:
Antifungal

tolnaftate

Dr. Scholl's Wart Removal Kit
Classification:
Keratolytic

salicylic acid, topical

*Available in Canada Only

BRAND NAME	GENERIC NAME
Dramamine Classification: Antiemetic; anticholinergic	dimenhydrinate
Dramamine II Classification: Antiemetic; anticholinergic	meclizine
Dramanate Classification: Antiemetic; anticholinergic	dimenhydrinate
Drenison ¼ Classification: Glucocorticoid	flurandrenolide
Drenison Tape* Classification: Glucocorticoid	flurandrenolide
Drepanol Classification: Blood Modifier (Orphan)	OM 401
Drisdol Classification: Vitamin, fat soluble	ergocalciferol D_2
Drisdol Drops Classification: Vitamin, fat soluble	ergocalciferol D_2
Dristan 12-Hr Nasal Classification: Nasal decongestant	oxymetazoline HCl, nasal
Dristan Saline Spray Classification: Nasal decongestant	sodium chloride, nasal
Dristan Long Lasting Classification: Nasal decongestant	oxymetazoline HCl, nasal
Drithocreme Classification: Antipsoriatic	anthralin (dithranol)

*Available in Canada only

BRAND NAME	GENERIC NAME

Drithocreme HP 1%
Classification:
Antipsoriatic

anthralin (dithranol)

Dritho-Scalp
Classification:
Antipsoriatic

anthralin (dithranol)

Drixoral Cough Liquid Caps
Classification:
Non-narcotic antitussive

dextromethorphan

Droperidol
Classification:
General anesthetic

droperidol

Droxia
Classification:
Antineoplastic, miscellaneous

hydroxyurea

Dryox 2.5
Classification:
Anti-acne product

benzoyl peroxide

Dryox 5
Classification:
Anti-acne product

benzoyl peroxide

Dryox 10
Classification:
Anti-acne product

benzoyl peroxide

Dryox 20
Classification:
Anti-acne product

benzoyl peroxide

Dryox Wash 5
Classification:
Anti-acne product

benzoyl peroxide

Drysol
Classification:
Antihyperhydrosis agent

aluminum chloride hexahydrate

DTIC-Dome
Classification:
Antineoplastic, miscellaneous

dacarbazine (DTIC, imidazole carboxamide)

BRAND NAME	GENERIC NAME
Dulcagen Classification: Laxative, irritant	bisacodyl
Dulcolax Classification: Laxative, irritant	bisacodyl
Dull-C Classification: Vitamin, water soluble	ascorbic acid (vitamin C)
Duo-Trach Kit Classification: Local anesthetic	lidocaine HCl, local
Duoderm Classification: Debriding agent	flexible hydroactive dressings and granules
Duofilm Classification: Keratolytic	salicylic acid, topical
DuoPlant Classification: Keratolytic	salicylic acid, topical
Duphalac Classification: Laxative	lactulose
Duplex T Classification: Keratolytic	coal tar
Durabolin Classification: Anabolic steroid	nandrolone phenpropionate
Duraclon Classification: Analgesic	clonidine HCl
Duract Classification: Nonsteroidal anti-inflammatory	bromfenac sodium

BRAND NAME	GENERIC NAME
Duracton* Classification: Anterior pituitary hormone	corticotropin injection, repository
Duragesic-25 Classification: Opioid analgesic	fentanyl transdermal
Duragesic-50 Classification: Opioid analgesic	fentanyl transdermal
Duragesic-75 Classification: Opioid analgesic	fentanyl transdermal
Duragesic-100 Classification: Opioid analgesic	fentanyl transdermal
Duralone-40 Classification: Glucocorticoid	methylprednisolone acetate
Duralone-80 Classification: Glucocorticoid	methylprednisolone acetate
Duramist Plus Classification: Nasal decongestant	oxymetazoline HCl, nasal
Duramorph Classification: Opioid analgesic	morphine sulfate
Duranest Classification: Local anesthetic	etidocaine HCl
Duranest MPF Classification: Local anesthetic	etidocaine HCl
Duratears Naturale Classification: Ophthalmic lubricant	ocular lubricants

BRAND NAME	GENERIC NAME
Duratest-100 Classification: Androgen	testosterone cypionate (in oil)
Duratest-200 Classification: Androgen	testosterone cypionate (in oil)
Durathate-200 Classification: Androgen	testosterone enanthate (in oil)
Duration Classification: Nasal decongestant	oxymetazoline HCl, nasal
Duratuss-G Classification: Expectorant	guaifenesin
Duricef Classification: Antibiotic; cephalosporin	cefadroxil
Duvoid Classification: Cholinergic stimulant	bethanechol chloride
Dwelle Classification: Ophthalmic lubricant	artificial tears solutions
Dycill Classification: Antibiotic; penicillinase-resistant penicillin	dicloxacillin sodium
Dyclone Classification: Local anesthetic	dyclonine HCl
Dymelor Classification: Antidiabetic; sulfonylurea	acetohexamide
Dymenate Classification: Antiemetic; anticholinergic	dimenhydrinate

BRAND NAME	GENERIC NAME

Dynabac
Classification:
Antibiotic; macrolide

dirithromycin

Dynacin
Classification:
Antibiotic; tetracycline

minocycline HCl

DynaCirc
Classification:
Calcium channel blocker

isradipine

Dynafed IB
Classification:
Nonsteroidal anti-inflammatory

ibuprofen

Dynafed Pseudo
Classification:
Nasal decongestant

pseudoephedrine HCl

Dynamine
Classification:
Anti-myasthenia agent (Orphan)

dynamine

Dynapen
Classification:
Antibiotic; penicillinase-resistant
penicillin

dicloxacillin sodium

Dyna-Hex Skin Cleanser
Classification:
Germicidal

chlorhexidine gluconate, topical

Dyna-Hex 2 Skin Cleanser
Classification:
Germicidal

chlorhexidine gluconate, topical

Dyox Wash 10
Classification:
Anti-acne product

benzoyl peroxide

Dyphylline
Classification:
Bronchodilator; xanthine

dyphylline (dihydroxypropyl
theophylline)

Dyrenium
Classification:
Potassium-sparing diuretic

triamterene

*Available in Canada Only

BRAND NAME	GENERIC NAME
Dyrexan-OD Classification: CNS stimulant; anorexiant	phendimetrazine tartrate
Dysport Classification: Paralytic (Orphan)	botulinum toxin type A

E

E-R-O Ear Classification: Emulsifier	carbamide peroxide (urea peroxide)
E-Base Classification: Antibiotic; macrolide	erythromycin base
E-Complex-600 Classification: Vitamin, fat soluble	vitamin E
E-Mycin Classification: Antibiotic; macrolide	erythromycin base
E-Pam* Classification: Antianxiety; benzodiazepine	diazepam
E-Vista Classification: Antianxiety	hydroxyzine
E-200 I.U. Softgells Classification: Vitamin, fat soluble	vitamin E
E-Vitamin Succinate Classification: Vitamin, fat soluble	vitamin E
E.E.S. 200 Classification: Antibiotic; macrolide	erythromycin ethylsuccinate

*Available in Canada only

BRAND NAME	GENERIC NAME
E.E.S. 400 Classification: Antibiotic; macrolide	erythromycin ethylsuccinate
Easprin Classification: Salicylate analgesic; antipyretic	aspirin
EC-Naprosyn Classification: Nonsteroidal anti-inflammatory	naproxen
Econopred Classification: Glucocorticoid	prednisolone acetate ophthalmic, suspension
Ecotrin Classification: Salicylate analgesic; antipyretic	aspirin
Ecotrin Adult Low Strength Classification: Salicylate analgesic; antipyretic	aspirin
Ecotrin Maximum Strength Classification: Salicylate analgesic; antipyretic	aspirin
Edecrin Classification: Loop diuretic	ethacrynate sodium/ethacrynic acid
Edecrin Sodium Classification: Loop diuretic	ethacrynate sodium/ethacrynic acid
Edetate Disodium Classification: Chelating agent	edetate disodium (EDTA)
Edex Classification: Prostaglandin	alprostadil (PGE_1)
ED-SPAZ Classification: GI anticholinergic	hyoscyamine sulfate

BRAND NAME	GENERIC NAME
Efed II Classification: Alpha-adrenergic agonist	phenylpropanolamine HCl
Efidac 24 Chlorpheniramine Classification: Antihistamine	chlorpheniramine maleate
Effer-K Classification: Electrolyte replacement; potassium	potassium bicarbonate/acetate/citrate
Effer-Syllium Classification: Laxative, bulk-producing	psyllium
Effexor Classification: Antidepressant	venlafaxine
Effexor-XR Classification: Antidepressant	venlafaxine
Efidac/24 Classification: Nasal decongestant	pseudoephedrine HCl
Efodine Classification: Antiseptic; germicidal	povidone-iodine
Efudex Classification: Antineoplastic; antimetabolite	fluorouracil, topical
Elavil Classification: Antidepressant	amitriptyline HCl
Eldepryl Classification: Antiparkinson agent	selegiline HCl (L-deprenyl)
Eldopaque Classification: Depigmentation agent	hydroquinone

BRAND NAME	GENERIC NAME
Eldopaque-Forte Classification: Depigmentation agent	hydroquinone
Eldoquin Classification: Depigmentation agent	hydroquinone
Elimite Classification: Scabicide; pediculicide	permethrin
Elixomin Classification: Bronchodilator; xanthine	theophylline
Elixophyllin Classification: Bronchodilator; xanthine	theophylline
Elmiron Classification: Urinary tract analgesic	pentosan polysulfate sodium
Elocon Classification: Glucocorticoid	mometasone furoate
Elspar Classification: Antineoplastic, miscellaneous	asparaginase
Eltor* Classification: Nasal decongestant	pseudoephedrine HCl
Eltroxin Classification: Thyroid hormone	levothyroxine sodium (T_4; L-thyroxine)
Emadine Classification: Antihistamine, ophthalmic	emedastine difumarate
Emcyt Classification: Antineoplastic; hormone	estramustine phosphate sodium

BRAND NAME	GENERIC NAME
Emecheck Classification: Antiemetic	phosphorated carbohydrate solution
Emersal Classification: Antipsoriatic	ammoniated mercury
Emetrol Classification: Antiemetic	phosphorated carbohydrate solution
Eminase Classification: Antithrombotic	anistreplase (APSAC)
Empirin Classification: Salicylate analgesic; antipyretic	aspirin
Emko Classification: Spermicide	nonoxynol
Emko Pre-Fil Classification: Spermicide	nonoxynol
Emulsoil Classification: Laxative, irritant	castor oil
Enable Classification: Anti-inflammatory (Investigational)	tenidap
Encare Classification: Spermicide	nonoxynol
Endrate Classification: Chelating agent	edetate disodium (EDTA)
Enduron Classification: Thiazide diuretic	methylclothiazide

BRAND NAME	GENERIC NAME
Enecat Classification: Radiopaque agent	barium sulfate
Ener-B Classification: Vitamin, water soluble	cyanocobalamin (vitamin B_{12})
Enflurane Classification: General anesthetic	enflurane
Engerix-B Classification: Vaccine	hepatitis B vaccine
Enisyl Classification: Amino acid	lysine
Enlon Classification: Anticholinesterase	edrophonium chloride
Entolase-HP Classification: Digestive enzyme	pancrelipase
Entrobar Classification: Radiopaque agent	barium sulfate
Entrophen* Classification: Salicylate analgesic; antipyretic	aspirin
Enuclene Classification: Artificial eye lubricant	tyloxapol
Enulose Classification: Laxative	lactulose
Ephedrine Classification: Adrenergic agonist	ephedrine

BRAND NAME	GENERIC NAME
Ephedrine Sulfate Classification: Adrenergic agonist	ephedrine
Epidermal Growth Factor (human) Classification: Growth hormone, ophthalmic (Orphan)	epidermal growth factor (human)
Epi-C Classification: Radiopaque agent	barium sulfate
Epifrin Classification: Adrenergic agonist	epinephrine HCl, ophthalmic
Epinal Classification: Adrenegic agonist	epinephryl borate
Epinephrine Classification: Adrenergic agonist	epinephrine
Epinephrine HCl Classification: Adrenergic agonist	epinephrine
Epinephrine HCl Classification: Adrenergic agonist	epinephrine HCl, ophthalmic
Epinephrine Pediatric Classification: Adrenergic agonist	epinephrine
Epipen Classification: Adrenergic agonist	epinephrine
Epipen Jr. Classification: Adrenergic agonist	epinephrine
Epitol Classification: Anticonvulsant	carbamazepine

BRAND NAME	GENERIC NAME

Epivir
Classification:
Antiviral; nucleoside

lamivudine (3TC)

Epogen
Classification:
Hormone; amino acid polypeptide

epoetin alfa (erythropoietin, EPO)

Eprex*
Classification:
Hormone; amino acid polypeptide

epoetin alfa (erythropoietin, EPO)

Epsom Salt
Classification:
Laxative, saline

magnesium sulfate

Epsom Salt
Classification:
Laxative, saline

saline laxatives

Equalactin
Classification:
Laxative, bulk-producing

polycarbophil

Equanil
Classification:
Antianxiety

meprobamate

Equilet
Classification:
Antacid; calcium supplement

calcium carbonate

Eramycin
Classification:
Antibiotic; macrolide

erythromycin stearate

Ergamisol
Classification:
Antineoplastic, miscellaneous

levamisole HCl

Ergoloid Mesylates
Classification:
Ergot alkaloid

ergoloid mesylates

Ergomar
Classification:
Antimigraine; ergot alkaloid

ergotamine tartrate

BRAND NAME	GENERIC NAME

Ergotrate Maleate
Classification:
Oxytocic

ergonovine maleate

Ery-Sol
Classification:
Anti-acne product

erythromycin, topical

Ery-Tab
Classification:
Antibiotic; macrolide

erythromycin base

Eryc
Classification:
Antibiotic; macrolide

erythromycin base

Erycette
Classification:
Anti-acne product

erythromycin, topical

Eryderm 2%
Classification:
Anti-acne product

erythromycin, topical

Erygel
Classification:
Anti-acne product

erythromycin, topical

Erymax
Classification:
Anti-acne product

erythromycin, topical

EryPed
Classification:
Antibiotic; macrolide

erythromycin ethylsuccinate

EryPed 200
Classification:
Antibiotic; macrolide

erythromycin ethylsuccinate

EryPed 400
Classification:
Antibiotic; macrolide

erythromycin ethylsuccinate

Erythra-Derm
Classification:
Anti-acne product

erythromycin, topical

BRAND NAME	GENERIC NAME
Erythrocin Stearate Classification: Antibiotic; macrolide	erythromycin stearate
Erythromid* Classification: Antibiotic; macrolide	erythromycin estolate
Erythromycin Classification: Antibiotic; macrolide	erythromycin, ophthalmic
Erythromycin Classification: Antibiotic; macrolide	erythromycin, topical
Erythromycin Base Classification: Antibiotic; macrolide	erythromycin base
Erythromycin Estolate Classification: Antibiotic; macrolide	erythromycin estolate
Erythromycin Ethylsuccinate Classification: Antibiotic; macrolide	erythromycin ethylsuccinate
Erythromycin Filmtabs Classification: Antibiotic; macrolide	erythromycin base
Erythromycin Lactobionate Classification: Antibiotic; macrolide	erythromycin I.V.
Erythromycin Stearate Classification: Antibiotic; macrolide	erythromycin stearate
Eserine Sulfate Classification: Miotic	physostigmine, ophthalmic
Esidrix Classification: Thiazide diuretic	hydrochlorothiazide

*Available in Canada Only

BRAND NAME	GENERIC NAME
Eskalith Classification: Antimanic	lithium carbonate
Eskalith CR Classification: Antimanic	lithium carbonate
Esoterica Facial Classification: Depigmentation agent	hydroquinone
Esoterica Fortified Classification: Depigmentation agent	hydroquinone
Esoterica Regular Classification: Depigmentation agent	hydroquinone
Espotabs Classification: Laxative, irritant	phenolphthalein
Estazolam Classification: Sedative-hypnotic; benzodiazepine	estazolam
Estinyl Classification: Estrogen	ethinyl estradiol
Estra-L 20 Classification: Estrogen	estradiol valerate
Estra-L 40 Classification: Estrogen	estradiol valerate
Estrace Classification: Estrogen	estradiol, oral
Estraderm Classification: Estrogen	estradiol transdermal system

BRAND NAME	GENERIC NAME

Estradiol Cypionate
Classification:
Estrogen

estradiol cypionate

Estradiol Valerate
Classification:
Estrogen

estradiol valerate

Estratab
Classification:
Estrogen

estrogens, esterified

Estring
Classification:
Estrogen

estradiol vaginal ring

Estro-Cyp
Classification:
Estrogen

estradiol cypionate

Estrogenic Substance Aqueous
Classification:
Estrogen

estrogenic substance or estrogens
aqueous suspension

Estrone-5
Classification:
Estrogen

estrone

Estrone Aqueous
Classification:
Estrogen

estrone

Estropipate
Classification:
Estrogen

estropipate

Ethamolin
Classification:
Sclerosing agent

ethanolamine oleate

Ethiodol
Classification:
Radiopaque agent

ethiodized oil

Ethmozine
Classification:
Antiarrhythmic

moricizine HCl

BRAND NAME	GENERIC NAME

Ethon
Classification:
Thiazide diuretic

methylclothiazide

Ethosuximide
Classification:
Anticonvulsant; succinimide

ethosuximide

Ethrane
Classification:
General anesthetic

enflurane

Ethyol
Classification:
Antineoplstic adjuvant; cytoprotective

amifostine

Etibi*
Classification:
Antitubercular

ethambutol HCl

Etiocholanedione
Classification:
Blood modifier (Orphan)

etiocholanedione

Etodolac
Classification:
Nonsteroidal anti-inflammatory

etodolac

Etopophos
Classification:
Antineoplastic; mitotic inhibitor

etoposide (VP-16-123)

Euflex*
Classification:
Antineoplastic; antiandrogen

flutamide

Eulexin
Classification:
Antineoplastic; antiandrogen

flutamide

Eurax
Classification:
Scabicide; pediculicide

crotamiton

Evac-U-Gen
Classification:
Laxative, irritant

phenolphthalein

*Available in Canada only

BRAND NAME	GENERIC NAME
Evalose Classification: Laxative	lactulose
Everone 200 Classification: Androgen	testosterone enanthate (in oil)
Evista Classification: Estrogen receptor modulator	raloxifene
Ex-Lax Gentle Nature Classification: Laxative, irritant	calcium slats of sennosides A&B
Exact Classification: Anti-acne product	benzoyl peroxide
Exegran Classification: Anticonvulsant (Investigational)	zonisamide
Exelderm Classification: Antifungal	sulconozole nitrate
Exemestane Classification: Antineoplastic (Orphan)	exemestane
Exidine-2 Scrub Classification: Germicidal	chlorhexidine gluconate, topical
Exidine-4 Scrub Classification: Germicidal	chlorhexidine gluconate, topical
Exidine Skin Cleanser Classification: Germicidal	chlorhexidine gluconate, topical
Exna Classification: Thiazide diuretic	benzthiazide

BRAND NAME	GENERIC NAME
Exocaine Medicated Classification: Counterirritant	methyl salicylate
Exocaine Plus Classification: Counterirritant	methyl salicylate
Exsel Classification: Antiseborrheic	selenium sulfide
Extra Strength Alkets Antacid Classification: Antacid; calcium supplement	calcium carbonate
Extra Strength Bayer Enteric 500 Aspirin Classification: Salicylate analgesic; antipyretic	aspirin
Extra Strength Denorex Classification: Keratolytic	coal tar
Extra Strength Dynafed E.X. Classification: Analgesic; antipyretic	acetaminophen
Extra Strength Gas-X Classification: Antiflatulent	simethicone
Eye-Sed Classification: Ophthalmic astringent	zinc sulfate solution
Eyesine Classification: Ophthalmic vasoconstrictor	tetrahydrozoline HCl, ophthalmic

F

Fabrase Classification: Enzyme replacement (Orphan)	alpha-galactosidase A

*Available in Canada only

BRAND NAME	GENERIC NAME

Factor VIIIa (recombinant, DNA origin)
Classification:
Hemostatic (Orphan)

factor VIIIa (recombinant, DNA origin)

Factrel
Classification:
Hormone

gonadorelin HCl

Famvir
Classification:
Antiviral

famciclovir

Fareston
Classification:
Antineoplastic; anti-estrogen

toremifene citrate

Fastin
Classification:
CNS stimulant

phentermine HCl

Fe50
Classification:
Iron preparation

ferrous sulfate

Feen-a-mint
Classification:
Laxative, irritant

phenolphthalein

Feen-a-mint Gum
Classification:
Laxative, irritant

phenolphthalein

Feiba VH Immuno
Classification:
Hemostatic

anti-inhibitor coagulant complex

Felbatol
Classification:
Anticonvulsant

felbamate

Feldene
Classification:
Nonsteroidal anti-inflammatory

piroxicam

Femara
Classification:
Antineoplastic; anti-estrogen

letrozole

BRAND NAME	GENERIC NAME
Femizol-M Classification: Antifungal	miconazole nitrate, vaginal
Femogen Forte* Classification: Estrogen	estrone
FemPatch Classification: Estrogen	estradiol, transdermal system
Femstat 3 Classification: Antifungal	butoconazole nitrate, vaginal
Fenesin Classification: Expectorant	guaifenesin
Fenicol* Classification: Antibacterial	chloramphenicol, ophthalmic
Fenoprofen Classification: Nonsteroidal anti-inflammatory	fenoprofen calcium
Fenretinide Classification: Retinoid (Investigational)	fenretinide
Fentanyl Classification: Opioid analgesic	fentanyl citrate
Fentanyl Oralet Classification: Opioid analgesic	fentanyl transmucosal system
Feosol Classification: Iron preparation	ferrous sulfate
Feostat Classification: Iron preparation	ferrous fumarate

*Available in Canada only

BRAND NAME	GENERIC NAME
Fer-Iron Classification: Iron preparation	ferrous sulfate
Fer-In-Sol Classification: Iron preparation	ferrous sulfate
Feratab Classification: Iron preparation	ferrous sulfate
Fergon Classification: Iron preparation	ferrous gluconate
Fero-Gradumet Classification: Iron preparation	ferrous sulfate
Ferospace Classification: Iron preparation	ferrous sulfate
Ferra-TD Classification: Iron preparation	ferrous sulfate
Ferralet Classification: Iron preparation	ferrous gluconate
Ferralet Slow Release Classification: Iron preparation	ferrous gluconate
Ferralyn Classification: Iron preparation	ferrous sulfate
Ferrets Classification: Iron preparation	ferrous fumarate
Ferrous Fumarate Classification: Iron preparation	ferrous fumarate

*Available in Canada Only

BRAND NAME	GENERIC NAME
Ferrous Gluconate Classification: Iron preparation	ferrous gluconate
Ferrous Sulfate Classification: Iron preparation	ferrous sulfate
Fertinex Classification: Ovulation stimulant	urofollitropin
Festal II Tablets Classification: Digestive enzyme	pancrelipase
Feverall Infants Classification: Analgesic; antipyretic	acetaminophen
Fiacitabine (FIAC) Classification: Antiviral (Investigational)	fiacitabine (FIAC)
Fialuridine (FIAU) Classification: Antiviral (Investigational)	Fialuridine (FIAU)
Fiberall Classification: Laxative, bulk-producing	psyllium
Fiberall, Chewable Classification: Laxative, bulk-producing	polycarbophil
Fiberall Natural Flavor and Orange Flavor Classification: Laxative, bulk-producing	psyllium
Fibercon Classification: Laxative, bulk-producing	polycarbophil
Fiber-Lax Classification: Laxative, bulk-producing	polycarbophil

*Available in Canada only

BRAND NAME	GENERIC NAME

FiberNorm
Classification:
Laxative, bulk-producing

polycarbophil

Fibrinogen (human)
Classification:
Hemostatic (Orphan)

fibrinogen (human)

Fibrogammin P
Classification:
Hemostatic (Orphan)

factor XIII (plasma-derived)

Fire Ant Venom, Allergenic Extract, Imported
Classification:
Biologic response modifier (Orphan)

fire ant venom, allergenic extract, imported

FK-565
Classification:
Biologic response modifier
(Investigational)

FK-565

Flagyl
Classification:
Antibacterial; amebicide

metronidazole

Flagyl ER
Classification:
Antibiotic; amebicide

metronidazole

Flagyl IV
Classification:
Antibacterial; amebicide

metronidazole

Flagyl IV RTU
Classification:
Antibacterial; amebicide

metronidazole

Flagyl 375
Classification:
Antibiotic; amebicide

metronidazole

Flarex
Classification:
Ophthalmic glucocorticoid

fluorometholone

BRAND NAME	GENERIC NAME
Flavorcee Classification: Vitamin, water soluble	ascorbic acid (vitamin C)
Fleet Babylax Classification: Hyperosmotic	glycerine (glycerol)
Fleet Bisacodyl Classification: Laxative, irritant	bisacodyl
Fleet Flavored Castor Oil Classification: Laxative, irritant	castor oil
Fleet Laxative Classification: Laxative, irritant	bisacodyl
Fleet Mineral Oil Enema Classification: Laxative, irritant	mineral oil
Fleet Phospho-soda Classification: Laxative, saline	saline laxatives
Fletcher's Castoria Classification: Laxative, irritant	senna
Flexeril Classification: Skeletal muscle relaxant, centrally acting	cyclobenzaprine HCl
Flexoject Classification: Skeletal muscle relaxant, centrally acting	orphenadrine citrate
Flexon Classification: Skeletal muscle relaxant, centrally acting	orphenadrine citrate
Flo-Coat Classification: Radiopaque agent	barium sulfate

*Available in Canada only

BRAND NAME	GENERIC NAME
Flolan Classification: Antihypertensive	epoprostenol sodium
Flomax Classification: Alpha-adrenergic blocker	tamsulosin HCl
Flonase Classification: Glucocorticoid	fluticasone propionate, nasal
Florinef Acetate Classification: Mineralocorticoid	fludrocortisone acetate
Florone Classification: Glucocorticoid	diflorasone diacetate
Florone E Classification: Glucocorticoid	diflorasone diacetate
Flovent Classification: Glucocorticoid	fluticasone propionate
Flovent Rotadisk Classification: Glucocorticoid	fluticasone propionate
Floxin Classification: Antibiotic; fluoroquinolone	ofloxacin
Floxin IV Classification: Antibiotic; fluoroquinolone	ofloxacin
Floxin Otic Classification: Antibiotic; fluoroquinolone	ofloxacin, otic
Floxuridine Classification: Antineoplastic; antimetabolite	floxuridine

*Available in Canada Only

BRAND NAME	GENERIC NAME
Flubriprofen Classification: Nonsteroidal anti-inflammatory	flubiprofen
Flubiprofen Sodium Ophthalmic Classification: Ophthalmic nonsteroidal anti-inflammatory	flubiprofen sodium
Fludara Classification: Antineoplastic; antimetabolite	fludarabine
Fluimucil Classification: Biologic response modifier (Investigational)	acetylcysteine
Flumadine Classification: Antiviral	rimantadine HCl
Fluocinolone Classification: Glucocorticoid	fluocinolone acetonide
Fluocinolone Acetonide Classification: Glucocorticoid	fluocinolone acetonide
Fluocinonide Classification: Glucocorticoid	fluocinonide
Fluogen Classification: Vaccine	influenza virus vaccine
Fluonid Classification: Glucocorticoid	fluocinolone acetonide
Fluor-A-Day* Classification: Electrolyte replacement; fluoride	sodium fluoride

*Available in Canada only

BRAND NAME	GENERIC NAME
Fluor-Op Classification: Ophthalmic glucocorticoid	fluorometholone
Fluor-I-Strip Classification: Ophthalmic diagnostic	fluorescein sodium
Fluor-I-Strip-A.T. Classification: Ophthalmic diagnostic	fluorescein sodium
Fluorescein Sodium Classification: Ophthalmic diagnostic	fluorescein sodium
Fluorescite Classification: Ophthalmic diagnostic	fluorescein sodium
Fluorets Classification: Ophthalmic diagnostic	fluorescein sodium
Fluoride Loz Classification: Electrolyte replacement; fluoride	sodium fluoride
Fluorigard Classification: Electrolyte replacement; fluoride	sodium fluoride
Fluorinse Classification: Electrolyte replacement; fluoride	sodium fluoride
Fluoritab Classification: Electrolyte replacement; fluoride	sodium fluoride
Fluoroplex Classification: Antineoplastic; antimetabolite	fluorouracil, topical
Fluorosoft Classification: Ophthalmic diagnostic	fluorexon

BRAND NAME	GENERIC NAME
Fluorothymidine (FLT) Classification: Antiviral (Investigational)	fluorothymidine (FLT)
Fluorouracil Classification: Antineoplastic; antimetabolite	fluorouracil (5-fluorouracil; 5-FU)
Fluosol Classification: Perfluorochemical emulsion	intravascular perfluorochemical emulsion
Fluothane Classification: General anesthetic	halothane
Fluotic* Classification: Electrolyte replacement; fluoride	sodium fluoride
Fluoxymesterone Classification: Androgen	fluoxymesterone
Fluphenazine Decanoate Classification: Antipsychotic	fluphenazine enanthate and decanoate
Fluphenazine HCl Classification: Antipsychotic	fluphenazine HCl
Flura Classification: Electrolyte replacement; fluoride	sodium fluoride
Flura-Drops Classification: Electrolyte replacement; fluoride	sodium fluoride
Flura-Loz Classification: Electrolyte replacement; fluoride	sodium fluoride
Flurandrenolide Classification: Glucocorticoid	flurandrenolide

*Available in Canada only

BRAND NAME	GENERIC NAME
Flurazepam Classification: Sedative-hypnotic; benzodiazepine	flurazepam HCl
Flurosyn Classification: Glucocorticoid	fluocinolone acetonide
FluShield Classification: Vaccine	influenza virus vaccine
Flutex Classification: Glucocorticoid	triamcinolone acetonide, topical
Fluviral* Classification: Vaccine	influenza virus vaccine
Fluvirin Classification: Vaccine	influenza virus vaccine
Fluzone Classification: Vaccine	influenza virus vaccine
FML Classification: Ophthalmic glucocorticoid	fluorometholone
FML Liquifilm Classification: Ophthalmic glucocorticoid	fluorometholone
Foille Classification: Local anesthetic	benzocaine, topical
Foille Medicated First Aid Classification: Local anesthetic	benzocaine, topical
Foille Plus Classification: Local anesthetic	benzocaine topical

*Available in Canada Only

BRAND NAME	GENERIC NAME
Folex PFS Classification: Antineoplastic; antimetabolite	methotrexate sodium (amethopterin, MTX)
Folic Acid Classification: Vitamin B complex group	folic acid, folacin, folate
Follistim Classification: Ovulation stimulant	follitropin beta
Folvite Classification: Vitamin B complex group	folic acid, folacin, folate
Forane Classification: General anesthetic	isoflurane
Formulex* Classification: Antispasmodic	dicyclomine HCl
Fortaz Classification: Antibiotic; cephalosporin	ceftazidime
Fortovase Classification: Antiviral; protease inhibitor	saquinavir mesylate
Fosamax Classification: Bone resorption inhibitor	alendronate sodium
Foscavir Classification: Antiviral	foscarnet sodium
Fostex Classification: Anti-acne product	benzoyl peroxide
Fostex 10% BPO Classification: Anti-acne product	benzoyl peroxide

*Available in Canada only

BRAND NAME	GENERIC NAME
Fostex BPO Wash Classification: Anti-acne product	benzoyl peroxide
Fourneau 309 Classification: CDC anti-infective	suramin
Fragmin Classification: Anticoagulant	dalteparin sodium
FreAmine HBC Classification: Nitrogen product	amino acid solution, stress
FreAmine III Classification: Nitrogen product	amino acid solution
Freezone Classification: Keratolytic	salicylic acid, topical
FS Shampoo Classification: Glucocorticoid	fluocinolone acetonide
FUDR Classification: Antineoplastic; antimetabolite	floxuridine
Ful-Glo Classification: Ophthalmic diagnostic	fluorescein sodium
Fulvicin-U/F Classification: Antifungal	griseofulvin microsize
Fulvicin P/G Classification: Antifungal	griseofulvin ultramicrosize
Fumasorb Classification: Iron preparation	ferrous fumarate

BRAND NAME	GENERIC NAME
Fumerin Classification: Iron preparation	ferrous fumarate
Funduscein-10 Classification: Ophthalmic diagnostic	fluorescein sodium
Funduscein-25 Classification: Ophthalmic diagnostic	fluorescein sodium
Fungizone Classification: Antifungal	amphotericin B, topical
Fungizone* Classification: Antifungal	amphotericin B
Fungizone Intravenous Classification: Antifungal	amphotericin B
Fungizone Oral Classification: Antifungal	amphotericin B
Fungoid AF Classification: Antifungal	undecylenic acid
Fungoid Creme Classification: Antifungal	miconazole nitrate, topical
Fungoid Solution Classification: Antifungal	clotrimazole, topical
Fungoid Tincture Classification: Antifungal	miconazole nitrate, topical
Furacin Classification: Antibacterial	nitrofurazone

*Available in Canada only

BRAND NAME	GENERIC NAME

Furadantin
Classification:
Urinary anti-infective

nitrofurantoin

Furamide
Classification:
CDC anti-infective

diloxanide furoate

Furosemide
Classification:
Loop diuretic

furosemide

Furoxone
Classification:
Antibiotic, broad-spectrum

furazolidone

G

G-myticin
Classification:
Aminoglycoside

gentamicin sulfate, topical

G-well
Classification:
Scabicide; pediculicide

lindane (gamma benzene hexachloride)

Gabbromicina
Classification:
Antitubercular (Orphan)

aminosidine

Gabitril
Classification:
Anticonvulsant

tiagabine

Galardin
Classification:
Ophthalmic (Orphan)

matrix metalloproteinase inhibitor

Gamimune N
Classification:
Immune globulin

immune globulin intravenous (IGIV)

Gammagard S/D
Classification:
Immune serum

immune globulin intravenous (IVIG)

BRAND NAME	GENERIC NAME
Gamma-hydroxybutyrate Classification: CNS stimulant (Orphan)	gamma-hydroxybutyrate
Gammalinolenic Acid Classification: Antirheumatic (Orphan)	gammalinolenic acid
Gammar-P I.V. Classification: Immune globulin	immune globulin intravenous (IGIV)
Gamulin Rh Classification: Immune serum	Rho (D) immune globulin
Ganaxolone Classification: Antispasmodic (Orphan)	ganaxolone
Ganite Classification: Bone resorption inhibitor	gallium nitrate
Gantanol Classification: Antibiotic; sulfonamide	sulfamethoxazole
Gantrisin Classification: Antibiotic; sulfonamide	sulfisoxazole
Garamycin Classification: Aminoglycoside	gentamicin sulfate
Garamycin Classification: Aminoglycoside	gentamicin sulfate, topical
Garamycin Intrathecal Classification: Aminoglycoside	gentamicin sulfate
Garamycin Ophthalmic Classification: Aminoglycoside	gentamicin sulfate, ophthalmic

*Available in Canada only

BRAND NAME	GENERIC NAME

Garamycin Pediatric
Classification:
Aminoglycoside

gentamicin sulfate

Gardrin
Classification:
Prostaglandin (Investigational)

enprostil

Gastrosed
Classification:
GI anticholinergic

hyoscyamine sulfate

Gas-X
Classification:
Antiflatulent

simethicone

Gastrocom
Classification:
Antiasthmatic

cromolyn sodium (disodium cromoglycate)

Gastrografin
Classification:
Radiopaque

diatrizoate meglumine 66% and diatrizoate sodium 10%

Gastrosed
Classification:
Anticholinergic

hyoscyamine sulfate

gBh*
Classification:
Scabicide; pediculicide

lindane (gamma benzene hexachloride)

Gee-Gee
Classification:
Expectorant

guaifenesin

Gelfilm
Classification:
Hemostatic

absorbable gelatin

Gelfilm Ophthalmic
Classification:
Hemostatic

absorbable gelatin

Gelfoam
Classification:
Hemostatic

absorbable gelatin

BRAND NAME	GENERIC NAME
Gel-Kam Classification: Electrolyte replacement; fluoride	sodium fluoride
Gelsolin, recombinant human Classification: Respiratory agent (Orphan)	gelsolin, recombinant human
Gel-Tin Classification: Electrolyte replacement; fluoride	sodium fluoride
Gemzar Classification: Antineoplastic, miscellaneous	gemicitabine HCl
Gen-xene Classification: Antianxiety; benzodiazepine	clorazepate dipotassium
Gen-K Classification: Electrolyte replacement; potassium	potassium chloride
Genahist Classification: Antihistamine	diphenhydramine HCl
Genapap Classification: Analgesic; antipyretic	acetaminophen
Genapap Extra Strength Classification: Analgesic; antipyretic	acetaminophen
Genapap Infant's Drops Classification: Analgesic; antipyretic	acetaminophen
Genaphed Classification: Nasal decongestant	pseudoephedrine HCl
Genasal Classification: Nasal decongestant	oxymetazoline HCl, nasal

BRAND NAME	GENERIC NAME

Genaspor
Classification:
Antifungal

tolnaftate

Genatuss
Classification:
Expectorant

guaifenesin

Gencalc 600
Classification:
Antacid; calcium supplement

calcium carbonate

Gendex 75
Classification:
Plasma volume expander

dextran 70/75

Genebs Extra Strength
Classification:
Analgesic; antipyretic

acetaminophen

GenESA
Classification:
In vivo diagnostic

arbutamine

Genevax
Classification:
Vaccine (Investigational)

HIV vaccine

Genevax-HIV-Px
Classification:
Vaccine (Investigational)

genevax-HIV-Px

Geneye
Classification:
Ophthalmic vasoconstrictor

tetrahydrozoline HCl, ophthalmic

Geneye Extra
Classification:
Ophthalmic vasoconstrictor

tetrahydrozoline HCl, ophthalmic

Genoptic Ophthalmic
Classification:
Aminoglycoside

gentamicin sulfate, ophthalmic

Genoptic S.O.P.
Classification:
Aminoglycoside

gentamicin sulfate, ophthalmic

BRAND NAME	GENERIC NAME
Genotropin Classification: Growth hormone	somatropin
Genpril Classification: Nonsteroidal anti-inflammatory	ibuprofen
Genprin Classification: Salicylate analgesic; antipyretic	aspirin
Gentacidin Classification: Aminoglycoside	gentamicin sulfate, ophthalmic
Gentak Classification: Aminoglycoside	gentamicin sulfate, ophthalmic
Gentamicin Classification: Aminoglycoside	gentamicin sulfate, ophthalmic
Gentamicin Ophthalmic Classification: Aminoglycoside	gentamicin sulfate, ophthalmic
Gentamicin Sulfate Classification: Aminoglycoside	gentamicin sulfate
Gentlax Classification: Laxative, irritant	senna
Gentran 40 Classification: Plasma volume expander	dextran 40
Gentran 75 Classification: Plasma volume expander	dextran 70/75
Geocillin Classification: Antibiotic; extended spectrum penicillin	carbenicillin indanyl sodium

BRAND NAME	GENERIC NAME

Gepirone HCl
Classification:
Antianxiety (Investigational)

gepirone HCl

Geref
Classification:
Polypeptide; in vivo diagnostic aid

sermorelin acetate

Geref
Classification:
Hormone (Orphan)

sermorelin acetate

Geridium
Classification:
Urinary analgesic

phenazopyridine HCl

Gerimal
Classification:
Ergot alkaloid

ergoloid mesylates

Germanin
Classification:
CDC anti-infective

suramin

GG-Cen
Classification:
Expectorant

guaifenesin

GlaucTabs
Classification:
Diuretic, carbonic anhydrase inhibitor

methazolamide

Glaucon
Classification:
Adrenergic agonist

epinephrine HCl, ophthalmic

Gliadel
Classification:
Antineoplastic; alkylating agent

carmustine (BCNU)

Glipizide
Classification:
Antidiabetic; sulfonylurea

glipizide

Glucagon
Classification:
Glucose elevating agent

glucagon

BRAND NAME	GENERIC NAME
Glucocerebrosidase, recombinant retroviral Classification: Enzyme (Orphan)	glucocerebrosidase, recombinant retroviral
Glucophage Classification: Antidiabetic; biguanides	metformin HCl
Glucose-40 Classification: Hyperosmolar preparation	glucose, ophthalmic
Glucotrol Classification: Antidiabetic; sulfonylurea	glipizide
Glucotrol XL Classification: Antidiabetic; sulfonylurea	glipizide
Glutamic Acid HCl Classification: Gastric acidifier	glutamic acid HCl
Glutethimide Classification: Sedative-hypnotic; nonbarbiturate	glutethimide
Glutose Classification: Glucose elevating agent	glucose
Gly-Oxide Liquid Classification: Antiseptic	carbamide peroxide (urea peroxide)
Glyate Classification: Expectorant	guaifenesin
Glyburide Classification: Antidiabetic; sulfonylurea	glyburide
Glycerin USP Classification: Hyperosmotic	glycerin (glycerol)

BRAND NAME	GENERIC NAME
Glycopyrrolate Classification: Anticholinergic	glycopyrrolate
Glycotuss Classification: Expectorant	guaifenesin
Glylorin Classification: Dermatological (Orphan)	terlipressin
Glynase Prestab Classification: Antidiabetic; sulfonylurea	glyburide
Glypressin Classification: Posterior pituitary hormone (Orphan)	terlipressin
Glyset Classification: Antidiabetic	miglitol
Glytuss Classification: Expectorant	guaifenesin
Go-Evac Classification: Bowel evacuant	polyethylene glycol-electrolyte solution
GoLYTELY Classification: Bowel evacuant	polyethylene glycol-electrolyte solution
Gonak Classification: Ophthalmic viscoelastic	hydroxypropyl methycellulose
Gonal-F Classification: Ovulation stimulant	follitropin alpha
Gonic Classification: Chorionic gonadotropin	chorionic gonadotropin, human (HCG)

BRAND NAME	GENERIC NAME
Gonioscope Classification: Gonioscopic aid	hydroxyethylcellulose
Goniosol Classification: Ophthalmic viscoelastic	hydroxypropyl methylcellulose
Gordofilm Classification: Keratolytic	salicylic acid, topical
Gordon's Urea Classification: Emollient	urea (carbamide), topical
Gormel Creme Classification: Emollient	urea (carbamide), topical
Gossypol Classification: Antineoplastic (Orphan)	gossypol
gp 160 Vaccine Classification: Vaccine (Investigational)	gp 160 vaccine
Gravol* Classification: Antiemetic; anticholinergic	dimenhydrinate
Grifulvin V Classification: Antifungal	griseofulvin microsize
Gris-PEG Classification: Antifungal	griseofulvin ultramicrosize
Grisactin 500 Classification: Antifungal	griseofulvin microsize
Grisactin Ultra Classification: Antifungal	griseofulvin ultramicrosize

*Available in Canada only

BRAND NAME	GENERIC NAME
Guaifenesin Classification: Expectorant	guaifenesin
Guaifenex LA Classification: Expectorant	guaifenesin
Guanabenz Acetate Classification: Antihypertensive, centrally acting	guanabenz acetate
Guanidine HCl Classification: Cholinergic muscle stimulant	guanidine HCl
Guiatuss Classification: Expectorant	guaifenesin
Gusperimus Classification: Immunosuppressive (Orphan)	gusperimus
Gyne-Lotrimin Classification: Antifungal	clotrimazole, vaginal
Gyne-Sulf Classification: Antibiotic; sulfonamide	triple sulfa
Gynecort 10 Classification: Glucocorticoid	hydrocortisone acetate
Gynecort Classification: Glucocorticoid	hydrocortisone acetate
Gynogen L.A. "20" Classification: Estrogen	estradiol valerate
Gynol II Classification: Spermicide	nonoxynol

BRAND NAME	GENERIC NAME

H

H-BIG
Classification:
Immune serum

hepatitis B immune globulin (HBIG)

H-BIGIV
Classification:
Immune serum (Orphan)

hepatitis B immune globulin, intravenous

H-F Gel
Classification:
Antidote (Orphan)

calcium gluconate gel 2.5%

H.P. Acthar Gel
Classification:
Anterior pituitary hormone

corticotropin injection, repository

Habitrol
Classification:
Smoking deterrent

nicotine transdermal system

Halcion
Classification:
Sedative-hypnotic; benzodiazepine

triazolam

Haldol
Classification:
Antipsychotic

haloperidol

Haldol Decanoate 50
Classification:
Antipsychotic

haloperidol decanoate

Haldol Decanoate 100
Classification:
Antipsychotic

haloperidol decanoate

Halenol Children's
Classification:
Analgesic; antipyretic

acetaminophen

Halfprin 81
Classification:
Salicylate analgesic; antipyretic

aspirin

BRAND NAME	GENERIC NAME
Halofantrine Classification: Antimalarial (Orphan)	halofantrine
Halofed Classification: Nasal decongestant	pseudoephedrine HCl
Halog Classification: Glucocorticoid	halcinonide
Halog-E Classification: Glucocorticoid	halcinonide
Haloperidol Classification: Antipsychotic	haloperidol
Halotestin Classification: Androgen	fluoxymesterone
Halotex Classification: Antifungal	haloprogin
Halothane Classification: General anesthetic	halothane
Halotussin Classification: Expectorant	guaifenesin
Haltran Classification: Nonsteroidal anti-inflammatory	ibuprofen
Havrix Classification: Vaccine	hepatitis A vaccine, inactivated
HD 85 Classification: Radiopaque agent	barium sulfate

BRAND NAME	GENERIC NAME
HD 200 Plus Classification: Radiopaque agent	barium sulfate
Head & Shoulders Classification: Antiseborrheic	pyrithione zinc
Head & Shoulders Intensive Treatment Classification: Antiseborrheic	selenium sulfide
Healon Classification: Ophthalmic viscoelastic	sodium hyaluronate
Healon GV Classification: Ophthalmic viscoelastic	sodium hyaluronate
Helixate Classification: Hemostatic	antihemophilic factor (AHF, Factor VIII)
Heartline Classification: Salicylate analgesic; antipyretic	aspirin
Hemocyte Classification: Iron preparation	ferrous fumarate
Hemofil M Classification: Hemostatic	antihemophilic factor (AHF, Factor VIII)
Hemonyne Classification: Hemostatic	factor IX complex (human)
Hemopad Classification: Hemostatic	microfibrillar collagen hemostat
Hemotene Classification: Hemostatic	microfibrillar collagen hemostat

BRAND NAME	GENERIC NAME
Hep-B-Gammagee Classification: Immune serum	hepatitis B immune globulin (HBIG)
Hep-Lock Classification: Anticoagulant	heparin sodium injection, USP
Hepalean* Classification: Anticoagulant	heparin calcium
Heparin Lock Flush Classification: Anticoagulant	heparin sodium injection, USP
Heparin Sodium Classification: Anticoagulant	heparin sodium injection, USP
Heparin Sodium and 0.45% **Sodium Chloride** Classification: Anticoagulant	heparin sodium and sodium chloride
Heparin Sodium and 0.9% **Sodium Chloride** Classification: Anticoagulant	heparin sodium and sodium chloride
HepatAmine Classification: Nitrogen product	amino acid solution, hepatic
Heptalac Classification: Laxative	lactulose
Hespan Classification: Plasma volume expander	hetastarch
Hetrazan Classification: Anthelmintics	diethylcarbamazine citrate

BRAND NAME	GENERIC NAME
Hexabrix Classification: Radiopaque agent	ioxaglate meglumine 39.3% and ioxaglate sodium 19.6%
Hexadrol Phosphate Classification: Glucocorticoid	dexamethasone sodium phosphate
Hexalen Classification: Antineoplastic, miscellaneous	altretamine (hexamethylmelamine)
Hi-Cor 2.5 Classification: Glucocorticoid	hydrocortisone, topical
Hibiclens Classification: Germicidal	chlorhexidine gluconate, topical
Hibiclens Antiseptic/Antimicrobial Skin Cleanser Classification: Germicidal	chlorhexidine gluconate, topical
Hibistat Germicidal Hand Rinse Classification: Germicidal	chlorhexidine gluconate, topical
HibTITER Classification: Vaccine	hemophilus b conjugate vaccine
High Potency Tar Classification: Keratolytic	coal tar
Hip-Rex* Classification: Urinary anti-infective	methenamine hippurate
Hiprex Classification: Urinary anti-infective	methenamine hippurate
Hismanal Classification: Antihistamine	astemizole

*Available in Canada only

BRAND NAME	GENERIC NAME
Histerone-100 Classification: Androgen	testosterone aqueous suspension
Histolyn-CYL Classification: In vivo diagnostic	histoplasmin
Histoplasmin, Diluted Classification: In vivo diagnostic	histoplasmin
Hi-Vegi-Lip Classification: Digestive enzyme	pancreatin
HIV Vaccine Classification: Vaccine (Investigational)	HIV vaccine
Hivid Classification: Antiviral	zalcitabine (ddC; dideoxycytidine)
Hivig Classification: Immune serum (Orphan)	human immunodeficiency virus immune globulin
HMS Classification: Ophthalmic glucocorticoid	medrysone
Hold DM Classification: Non-narcotic antitussive	dextromethorphan
Homatropine HBr Ophthalmic Classification: Mydriatic	homatropine hydrobromide, ophthalmic
Honvol* Classification: Estrogen	diethylstilbestrol
Humalog Classification: Antidiabetic	insulin lispro

*Available in Canada Only

BRAND NAME	GENERIC NAME
Humate-P Classification: Hemostatic	antihemophilic factor (AHF; Factor VIII)
Humatin Classification: Aminoglycoside	paromomycin sulfate
Humatrope Classification: Growth hormone	somatotropin (human growth hormone)
Humegon Classification: Gonadotropin	menotropins
Humibid Classification: Expectorant	guaifenesin
Humibid LA Classification: Expectorant	guaifenesin
HuMist Saline Nasal Mist Classification: Nasal decongestant	sodium chloride, nasal
Humorsol Classification: Miotic	demecarium bromide
Humulin 30/70* Classification: Antidiabetic	insulin, isophane suspension and insulin injection
Humulin 50/50 Classification: Antidiabetic	insulin, isophane suspension and insulin injection
Humulin 70/30 Classification: Antidiabetic	insulin, isophane suspension and insulin injection
Humulin L Classification: Antidiabetic	insulin, zinc suspension (lente)

*Available in Canada only

BRAND NAME	GENERIC NAME

Humulin N
Classification:
Antidiabetic

insulin, isophane suspension (NPH)

Humulin-R*
Classification:
Antidiabetic

insulin injection

Humulin R
Classification:
Antidiabetic

insulin injection

Humulin-U*
Classification:
Antidiabetic

insulin, zinc suspension extended (ultralente)

Humulin U Ultralente
Classification:
Antidiabetic

insulin, zinc suspension extended (ultralente)

Hurricaine
Classification:
Local anesthetic

benzocaine, topical

Hyalagan
Classification:
Viscoelastic

sodium hyaluronate

Hybolin Decanoate-50
Classification:
Anabolic steroid

nandrolone decanoate

Hybolin Decanoate-100
Classification:
Anabolic steroid

nandrolone decanoate

Hybolin Improved
Classification:
Anabolic steroid

nandrolone phenpropionate

Hycamtin
Classification:
Antineoplastic; hormone

topotecan HCl

Hycort
Classification:
Glucocorticoid

hydrocortisone, topical

BRAND NAME	GENERIC NAME
Hydeltrasol Classification: Glucocorticoid	prednisolone sodium phosphate
Hydergine Classification: Ergot alkaloid	ergoloid mesylates
Hydergine LC Classification: Ergot alkaloid	ergoloid mesylates
Hydralazine HCl Classification: Antihypertensive; vasodilator	hydralazine HCl
Hydrate Classification: Antiemetic; anticholinergic	dimenhydrinate
Hydrazol Classification: Diuretic; carbonic anhydrase inhibitor	acetazolamide
Hydrea Classification: Antineoplastic	hydroxyurea
Hydrex Classification: Thiazide diuretic	benzthiazide
Hydro-Chlor Classification: Thiazide diuretic	hydrochlorothiazide
Hydro-Crysti 12 Classification: Vitamin, water soluble	hydroxocobalamin (vitamin B_{12})
Hydrochlorothiazide Classification: Thiazide diuretic	hydrochlorothiazide
Hydrocil Instant Powder Classification: Laxative, bulk-producing	psyllium

BRAND NAME	GENERIC NAME
Hydrocortisone Classification: Glucocorticoid	hydrocortisone
Hydrocortisone Acetate Classification: Glucocorticoid	hydrocortisone acetate
Hydrocortone Classification: Glucocorticoid	hydrocortisone
Hydrocortone Acetate Classification: Glucocorticoid	hydrocortisone acetate
Hydrocortone Phosphate Classification: Glucocorticoid	hydrocortisone sodium phosphate
HyroDiuril Classification: Thiazide diuretic	hydrochlorothiazide
Hydroflumethiazide Classification: Thiazide diuretic	hydroflumethiazide
Hydromorphone HCl Classification: Opioid analgesic	hydromorphone HCl
Hydromox Classification: Thiazide diuretic	quinethazone
HydroStat IR Classification: Opioid analgesic	hydromorphone HCl
HydroTex Classification: Glucocorticoid	hydrocortisone, topical
Hydroxychloroquine Sulfate Classification: Antimalarial	hydroxychloroquine sulfate

BRAND NAME	GENERIC NAME

Hydroxycobalamin
Classification:
Vitamin, water soluble

hydroxocobalamin (vitamin B_{12})

Hydroxyzine HCl
Classification:
Antianxiety

hydroxyzine

Hydroxyzine Pamoate
Classification:
Antianxiety

hydroxyzine

Hydrozide*
Classification:
Thiazide diuretic

hydrochlorothiazide

Hygroton
Classification:
Thiazide-like diuretic

chlorthalidone

Hylorel
Classification:
Antihypertensive

guanadrel sulfate

Hylutin
Classification:
Progestin

hydroxyprogesterone caproate

Hyoscyamine Sulfate
Classification:
GI anticholinergic

hyoscyamine sulfate

Hypaque-76
Classification:
Radiopaque agent

diatrizoate meglumine 60% and
diatrizoate sodium 10%

Hypaque-M 75%
Classification:
Radiopaque agent

diatrizoate meglumine 50% and
diatrizoate sodium 30%

Hypaque Meglumine 30%
Classification:
Radiopaque agent

diatrizoate meglumine 30%

Hypaque Meglumine 60%
Classification:
Radiopaque agent

diatrizoate meglumine 60%

*Available in Canada only

BRAND NAME	GENERIC NAME
Hypaque Sodium 20% Classification: Radiopaque agent	diatrizoate sodium 20%
Hypaque Sodium 25% Classification: Radiopaque agent	diatrizoate sodium 25%
Hypaque Sodium 50% Classification: Radiopaque agent	diatrizoate sodium
Hypaque Sodium Classification: Radiopaque agent	diatrizoate sodium
Hypaque Sodium Classification: Radiopaque agent	diatrizoate sodium 41.66%
Hyper-Tet Classification: Immune serum	tetanus immune globulin
Hyperab Classification: Rabies prophylaxis	rabies immune globulin human (RIG)
HyperHep Classification: Immune serum	hepatitis B immune globulin (HBIG)
Hyperstat IV Classification: Antihypertensive; vasodilator	diazoxide, parenteral
Hypo Tears Classification: Ophthalmic solutions	artificial tears solutions
Hypo Tears Classification: Ophthalmic lubricant	ocular lubricants
Hypotears PF Classification: Ophthalmic solutions	artificial tears solutions

BRAND NAME	GENERIC NAME
HypRho-D Classification: Immune serum	Rho (D) immune globulin
HypRho-D Mini-Dose Classification: Immune serum	Rho (D) immune globulin Micro-Dose
Hyrexine-50 Classification: Antihistamine	diphenhydramine HCl
Hyskon Classification: In vivo diagnostic	hysteroscopy fluid
Hytakerol Classification: Vitamin, fat soluble	dihydrotachysterol (DHT)
Hytinic Classification: Iron preparation	polysaccharide iron complex
Hytone Classification: Glucocorticoid	hydrocortisone, topical
Hytrin Classification: Antihypertensive; alpha-adrenergic blocker	terazosin
Hytuss Classification: Expectorant	guaifenesin
Hytuss 2X Classification: Expectorant	guaifenesin
Hyzine-50 Classification: Antianxiety	hydroxyzine

BRAND NAME	GENERIC NAME

I

I-123 murine monoclonal antibody to alpha-fetoprotein
Classification:
In vivo diagnostic (Orphan)

I-123 murine monoclonal antibody to alpha-fetoprotein

I-123 murine monoclonal antibody to hCG
Classification:
In vivo diagnostic (Orphan)

I-123 murine monoclonal antibody to hCG

I-131 6B-iodomethyl-19-norcholesterol
Classification:
In vivo diagnostic (Orphan)

I-131 6B-iodomethyl-19-norcholesterol

I-131 murine monoclonal antibody to IgG2a to B cell
Classification:
In vivo diagnostic (Orphan)

I-131 murine monoclonal antibody to IgG2a to B cell

I-131 murine monoclonal antibody to alpha-fetoprotein
Classification:
In vivo diagnostic (Orphan)

I-131 murine monoclonal antibody to alpha-fetoprotein

I-131 murine monoclonal antibody to hCG
Classification:
In vivo diagnostic (Orphan)

I-131 murine monoclonal antibody to hCG

I-131 radiolabeled B1 monoclonal antibody
Classification:
Antineoplastic (Orphan)

I-131 radiolabeled B1 monoclonal antibody

IBU
Classification:
Nonsteroidal anti-inflammatory

ibuprofen

Ibuprin
Classification:
Nonsteroidal anti-inflammatory

ibuprofen

BRAND NAME	GENERIC NAME
Ibuprohm Classification: Nonsteroidal anti-inflammatory	ibuprofen
Idamycin Classification: Antineoplastic; antibiotic	idarubicin HCl
Idamycin PFS Classification: Antineoplastic; antibiotic	idarubicin HCl
Idoxuridine Classification: Antineoplastic (Orphan)	idoxuridine
Ifex Classification: Antineoplastic; alkylating agent	ifosfamide
IGF-I Classification: Growth hormone (Orphan)	insulin-like growth factor-I (recombinant human)
IgG monoclonal anti-CD4 (M-T412) Classification: Biologic response modifier (Orphan)	IgG monoclonal anti-CD4 (M-T412)
IgG monoclonal anti-TNF antibody (cA2) Classification: Biologic response modifier (Orphan)	IgG monoclonal anti-TNF antibody (cA2)
Iletin* Classification: Antidiabetic	insulin injection
Iletin II L* Classification: Antidiabetic	insulin, zinc suspension (lente)
Iletin II NPH* Classification: Antidiabetic	insulin, isophane suspension (NPH)

*Available in Canada only

BRAND NAME	GENERIC NAME

Iletin II*
Classification:
Antidiabetic

insulin injection

**Iletin II U-500 Regular
(Concentrated)**
Classification:
Antidiabetic

insulin injection concentrated

Iletin L*
Classification:
Antidiabetic

insulin, zinc suspension (lente)

Iletin NPH*
Classification:
Antidiabetic

insulin, isophane suspension (NPH)

Iletin PZI*
Classification:
Antidiabetic

insulin, protamine zinc suspension (PZI)

Iletin Ultralente*
Classification:
Antidiabetic

insulin zinc suspension extended
(ultralente)

Ilopan
Classification:
Gastrointestinal stimulant

dexpanthenol

Ilopan-Choline
Classification:
Gastrointestinal stimulant

dexpanthenol with choline bitartrate

Ilosone
Classification:
Antibiotic; macrolide

erythromycin estolate

Ilosone Pulvules
Classification:
Antibiotic; macrolide

erythromycin estolate

Ilotycin
Classification:
Antibiotic; macrolide

erythromycin, ophthalmic

Ilotycin Gluceptate
Classification:
Antibiotic; macrolide

erythromycin IV

BRAND NAME	GENERIC NAME
Ilozyme Tablets Classification: Digestive enzyme	pancrelipase
Imdur Classification: Antianginal	isosorbide mononitrate
Imipramine HCl Classification: Antidepressant	imipramine HCl
Imitrex Classification: Serotonin antagonist	sumatriptan succinate
Imitrex Nasal Classification: Antimigraine	sumatriptan, nasal
Immther Classification: Antineoplastic (Orphan)	disaccharide tripeptide glycerol dipalmitoyl
ImmuCyst* Classification: Antineoplastic, miscellaneous	BCG, intravesical
Immuraid, AFP-Tc-99m Classification: In vivo diagnostic (Orphan)	technetium Tc-99m monoclonal antibody to AFP
Immuraid, hCG-Tc-99m Classification: In vivo diagnostic (Orphan)	technetium Tc-99m monoclonal antibody to hCG
Imodium Classification: Antidiarrheal	loperamide
Imodium A-D Classification: Antidiarrheal	loperamide
Imodium A-D Caplet Classification: Antidiarrheal	loperamide

*Available in Canada only

BRAND NAME	GENERIC NAME

Imogam
Classification:
Rabies prophylaxis

rabies immune globulin human (RIG)

Imogam Rabies-HT
Classification:
Immune globulin

rabies immune globulin

Imovax Rabies I.D. Vaccine
Classification:
Rabies prophylaxis

rabies vaccine, human diploid cell cultures (HDCV)

Imovax Rabies Vaccine
Classification:
Rabies prophylaxis

rabies vaccine, human diploid cell cultures (HDCV)

Impril*
Classification:
Antidepressant

imipramine HCl

Imreg-1
Classification:
Biologic response modifier
(Investigational)

imreg-1

Imuran
Classification:
Immunosuppressive

azathioprine

Imuthiol
Classification:
Biologic response modifier
(Investigational)

diethyldithiocarbamate

Imuvert
Classification:
Antineoplastic (Orphan)

serretia marcescenes extract (polyribosomes)

Inapsine
Classification:
General anesthetic

droperidol

Indapamide
Classification:
Thiazide diuretic

indapamide

BRAND NAME	GENERIC NAME
Inderal Classification: Beta-adrenergic blocker	propranolol HCl
Inderal L.A. Classification: Beta-adrenergic blocker	propranolol HCl
Inderal 10 Classification: Beta-adrenergic blocker	propranolol HCl
Inderal 20 Classification: Beta-adrenergic blocker	propranolol HCl
Inderal 40 Classification: Beta-adrenergic blocker	propranolol HCl
Inderal 60 Classification: Beta-adrenergic blocker	propranolol HCl
Inderal 80 Classification: Beta-adrenergic blocker	propranolol HCl
Indigo Carmine Solution Classification: In vivo diagnostic	indigotindisulfonate sodium injection
Indocin Classification: Nonsteroidal anti-inflammatory	indomethacin
Indocin I.V. Classification: Nonsteroidal anti-inflammatory	indomethacin sodium trihydrate
Indocin SR Classification: Nonsteroidal anti-inflammatory	indomethacin
Indomethacin Classification: Nonsteroidal anti-inflammatory	indomethacin

BRAND NAME	GENERIC NAME
Infasurf Classification: Lung surfactant (Orphan)	surface active extract of saline lavage of bovine lungs
Infergen Classification: Biologic response modifier	interferon alfacon-1
InFeD Classification: Iron preparation	iron dextran
Inflamase Forte Classification: Glucocorticoid	prednisolone sodium phosphate ophthalmic, solution
Inflamase Mild Classification: Glucocorticoid	prednisolone sodium phosphate ophthalmic, solution
Infumorph 200 Classification: Opioid analgesic	morphine sulfate
Infumorph 500 Classification: Opioid analgesic	morphine sulfate
Inocor Classification: Cardiac inotrope	amrinone lactate
Insta-Glucose Classification: Glucose elevating element	glucose
Insulin Reaction Classification: Glucose elevating element	glucose
Intal Classification: Anti-inflammatory, antiasthmatic	cromolyn sodium (disodium cromoglycate)
Integrilin Classification: Antiplatelet	eptifibatide

BRAND NAME	GENERIC NAME
Interferon beta (recombinant human) Classification: Antineoplastic; biologic resonse modifier (Orphan)	interferon beta (recombinant human)
Interleukin-2 PEG Classification: Biologic response modifier (Investigational)	interleukin-2 PEG
Interleukin-2, recombinant liposome encapsulated Classification: Antineoplastic; biologic response modifier (Orphan)	interleukin-2, recombinant liposome encapsulated
Interleukin-3, recombinant human Classification: Biologic response modifier (Investigational)	interleukin-3, recombinant human
Intralipid 10% Classification: Caloric, fat	fat emulsions
Intralipid 20% Classification: Caloric, fat	fat emulsions
Intron A Classification: Antineoplastic; biologic response modifier	interferon alfa-2b (IFN-alpha 2; rIFN- 2; 2-interferon)
Intropin Classification: Adrenergic agonist	dopamine HCl
Inulin Classification: In vivo diagnostic	inulin iodine
Inversine Classification: Antihypertensive; ganglionic blocker	mecamylamine HCl

*Available in Canada only

BRAND NAME	GENERIC NAME

Invirase
Classification:
Antiviral; protease inhibitor

saquinavir mesylate

Iobenguane sulfate I-131
Classification:
In vivo diagnostic (Orphan)

iobenguane sulfate I-131

Iocon
Classification:
Keratolytic

coal tar

Iodex regular
Classification:
Antiseptic; germicidal

povidone-iodine

Iodine Tincture
Classification:
Antiseptic

iodine products

Iodine Topical Solution
Classification:
Antiseptic

iodine products

Iodotope
Classification:
Antithyroid

iodine products

Iodotope
Classification:
Antithyroid agent

sodium iodide I 131

Ionamin
Classification:
CNS stimulant; anorexiant

phenteramine HCl

Ionax Scrub*
Classification:
Germicidal

benzalkonium chloride

Ionil T Plus
Classification:
Keratolytic

coal tar

Iophen
Classification:
Expectorant

iodinated glycerol

BRAND NAME	GENERIC NAME

Iopidine
Classification:
Adrenergic agonist

apraclonidine HCl

Ipecac Syrup
Classification:
Emetic

ipecac syrup

IPOL
Classification:
Vaccine

poliovirus vaccine, inactivated
(IPV:SALK)

Ipratopium Bromide
Classification:
Anticholinergic

ipratropium bromide

Ircon
Classification:
Iron preparation

ferrous fumarate

Iscador
Classification:
Antiviral (Investigational)

iscador

Ismelin
Classification:
Antihypertensive

guanethidine monosulfate

ISMO
Classification:
Antianginal

isosorbide mononitrate

Ismotic
Classification:
Antianginal

isosorbide

Isobutyramide
Classification:
Blood modifier (Orphan)

isobutyramide

Isocaine HCl
Classification:
Local anesthetic

mepivacaine HCl

Isoetharine HCl
Classification:
Bronchodilator; beta-adrenergic agonist

isoetharine HCl

BRAND NAME	GENERIC NAME

Isoniazid
Classification:
Antitubercular

isoniazid (INH)

Isoprinosine
Classification:
Biologic response modifier (Orphan)

inosine pranobex

Isoproterenol HCl
Classification:
Adrenergic agonist

isoproterenol

Isopto Homatropine
Classification:
Mydriatic

homatropine hydrobromide, ophthalmic

Isoptin
Classification:
Calcium channel blocker

verapamil HCl

Isoptin SR
Classification:
Calcium channel blocker

verapamil HCl

Isopto Alkaline
Classification:
Ophthalmic lubricants

artificial tears solution

Isopto Atropine
Classification:
Mydriatic

atropine sulfate, ophthalmic

Isopto Carbachol
Classification:
Miotic

carbachol, topical

Isopto Carpine
Classification:
Miotic

pilocarpine HCl

Isopto Cetamide
Classification:
Antibiotic; sulfonamide

sulfacetamide sodium, ophthalmic

Isopto Fenical*
Classification:
Antibacterial

chloramphenicol, ophthalmic

*Available in Canada Only

BRAND NAME	GENERIC NAME
Isopto Hyoscine Classification: Mydriatic	scopolamine hydrobromide, otic
Isopto Plain Classification: Ophthalmic lubricants	artificial tears solution
Isopto Tears Classification: Ophthalmic lubricants	artificial tears solution
Isordil Classification: Antianginal	isosorbide dinitrate sublingual and chewable
Isordil Tembids Classification: Antianginal	isosorbide dinitrate, oral
Isordil Titradose Classification: Antianginal	isosorbide dinitrate, oral
Isosorbide Dinitrate Classification: Antianginal	isosorbide dinitrate, oral
Isosorbide Dinitrate Classification: Antianginal	isosorbide dinitrate sublingual and chewable
Isotamine* Classification: Antitubercular	isoniazid (INH)
Isovorin Classification: Folic acid antagonist (Orphan)	L-leucovorin
Isovue-128 Classification: Radiopaque agent	iopamidol 26%
Isovue-200, Isovue-M 200 Classification: Radiopaque agent	iopamidol 41%

*Available in Canada only

BRAND NAME	GENERIC NAME
Isovue-300, Isovue-M 300 Classification: Radiopaque agent	iopamidol 61%
Isovue-370 Classification: Radiopaque agent	iopamidol 76%
Isoxsuprine HCl Classification: Peripheral vasodilator	isoxsuprine HCl
Isuprel Classification: Adrenergic agonist	isoproterenol
Isuprel Mistometer Classification: Adrenergic agonist	isoproterenol
Itch-X Classification: Local anesthetic	pramoxine HCl, topical
Iveegam Classification: Immune serum	immune globulin intravenous (IVIG)

J

Jenamicin Classification: Aminoglycoside	gentamicin sulfate
JE-VAX Classification: Vaccine	Japanese encephalitis virus vaccine
Junior Strength Feverall Classification: Analgesic; antipyretic	acetaminophen
Just Tears Classification: Ophthalmic, lubricants	artificial tears solution

*Available in Canada Only

BRAND NAME	GENERIC NAME

K

K-Dur
Classification:
Electrolyte replacement; potassium

potassium chloride

K-G Elixir
Classification:
Electrolyte replacement; potassium

potassium gluconate

K-Lease
Classification:
Electrolyte replacement; potassium

potassium chloride

K-Lyte
Classification:
Electrolyte replacement; potassium

potassium bicarbonate/acetate/citrate

K-Lyte*
Classification:
Urinary alkalinizer

potassium citrate

K-Lyte/Cl
Classification:
Electrolyte replacement; potassium

potassium chloride

K-Lyte DS
Classification:
Electrolyte replacement; potassium

potassium bicarbonate/acetate/citrate

K-Norm
Classification:
Electrolyte replacement; potassium

potassium chloride

K-Phos No. 2
Classification:
Urinary acidifier

potassium acid phosphate and sodium acid phosphate

K-Phos Original
Classification:
Urinary acidifier

potassium acid phosphate

K-Phos-Neutral
Classification:
Electrolyte replacement

phosphorous (replacement products)

BRAND NAME	GENERIC NAME
K-Tab Classification: Electrolyte replacement; potassium	potassium chloride
K-Y Plus Classification: Spermicide	nonoxynol
K+ Care Classification: Electrolyte replacement; potassium	potassium chloride
Kabikinase Classification: Antithrombotic	streptokinase
Kadian Classification: Opioid analgesic	morphine sulfate
Kala Classification: Antidiarrheal	lactobacillus
Kanamycin Sulfate Classification: Aminoglycoside	kanamycin sulfate
Kantrex Classification: Aminoglycoside	kanamycin sulfate
Kaochlor Classification: Electrolyte replacement; potassium	potassium chloride
Kaochlor S-F Classification: Electrolyte replacement; potassium	potassium chloride
Kaon-Cl Classification: Electrolyte replacement; potassium	potassium chloride
Kaon-Cl-10 Classification: Electrolyte replacement; potassium	potassium chloride

BRAND NAME	GENERIC NAME
Kaopectate Advanced Formula Classification: Antidiarrheal	lactobacillus
Karidium Classification: Electrolyte replacement; fluoride	sodium fluoride
Karigel Classification: Electrolyte replacement; fluoride	sodium fluoride
Karigel-N Classification: Electrolyte replacement; fluoride	sodium fluoride
Kasof Classification: Laxative, softener	docusate potassium
Kay Ciel Classification: Electrolyte replacement; potassium	potassium chloride
Kayexalate Classification: Potassium-removing resin	sodium polystyrene sulfonate
Keflex Classification: Antibiotic; cephalosporin	cephalexin monohydrate
Keftab Classification: Antibiotic; cephalosporin	cephalexin HCl monohydrate
Kefurox Classification: Antibiotic; cephalosporin	cefuroxime sodium
Kefzol Classification: Antibiotic; cephalosporin	cefazolin sodium
Kemadrin Classification: Anticholinergic	procyclidine HCl

BRAND NAME	GENERIC NAME

Kemsol*
Classification:
Anti-inflammatory

dimethyl sulfoxide (DMSO)

Kenacort
Classification:
Glucocorticoid

triamcinolone

Kenaject-40
Classification:
Glucocorticoid

triamcinolone acetonide

Kenalog-10
Classification:
Glucocorticoid

triamcinolone acetonide

Kenalog-40
Classification:
Glucocorticoid

triamcinolone acetonide

Kenalog
Classification:
Glucocorticoid

triamcinolone acetonide

Kenalog
Classification:
Glucocorticoid

triamcinolone acetonide, topical

Kenalog-H
Classification:
Glucocorticoid

triamcinolone acetonide, topical

Kenalog in Orabase
Classification:
Glucocorticoid

triamcinolone acetonide (topical-oral)

Kerlone
Classification:
Beta-adrenergic blocker

betaxolol HCl

Kestrone-5
Classification:
Estrogen

estrone

Ketalar
Classification:
General anesthetic

ketamine HCl

BRAND NAME	GENERIC NAME

Ketorolac Tromethamine
Classification:
Nonsteroidal anti-inflammatory

ketorolac tromethamine

Key-Pred 25
Classification:
Glucocorticoid

prednisolone acetate

Key-Pred 50
Classification:
Glucocorticoid

prednisolone acetate

Key-Pred SP
Classification:
Glucocorticoid

prednisolone sodium phosphate

Kinevac
Classification:
Gastrointestinal function test

sincalide

KL4-surfactant
Classification:
Lung surfactant (Orphan)

KL4-surfactant

Klaron
Classification:
Antisebborheic

sulfacetamide sodium, topical

Klonopin
Classification:
Anticonvulsant; benzodiazepine

clonazepam

Klor-Con 10
Classification:
Electrolyte replacement; potassium

potassium chloride

Klor-Con 25
Classification:
Electrolyte replacement; potassium

potassium chloride

Klor-Con
Classification:
Electrolyte replacement; potassium

potassium chloride

Klorvess
Classification:
Electrolyte replacement; potassium

potassium bicarbonate/acetate/citrate

BRAND NAME	GENERIC NAME

Klorvess Liquid
Classification:
Electrolyte replacement; potassium

potassium chloride

Klotrix
Classification:
Electrolyte replacement; potassium

potassium chloride

Koāte-H.P.
Classification:
Hemostatic

antihemophilic factor (AHF, Factor VIII)

Kogenate
Classification:
Hemostatic

antihemophilic factor (AHF, Factor VIII)

Konakion
Classification:
Vitamin K

phytonadione (vitamin K_1)

Kondremul Plain
Classification:
Laxative, emollient

mineral oil

Konsyl
Classification:
Laxative, bulk-producing

psyllium

Konsyl-D
Classification:
Laxative, bulk-producing

psyllium

Konsyl Fiber
Classification:
Laxative, bulk-producing

polycarbophil

Konsyl-Orange
Classification:
Laxative, bulk-producing

psyllium

Konyne 80
Classification:
Hemostatic

factor IX complex (human)

Koromex
Classification:
Spermicide

nonoxynol

BRAND NAME	GENERIC NAME
Kryobulin VH* Classification: Hemostatic	antihemophilic factor (AHF, Factor VIII)
Ku-Zyme HP Capsules Classification: Digestive enzyme	pancrelipase
Kutapressin Classification: Anti-inflammatory	liver derivative complex
Kwellada* Classification: Scabicide; pediculicide	lindane (gamma benzene hexachloride)
Kybernin Classification: Antithrombin (Orphan)	antithrombin III concentrate, intravenous

L

L-5 hydroxytryptophan Classification: Muscle stimulant (Orphan)	L-5 hydroxytryptophan
L-Carnitine Classification: Amino acid	levocarnitine
L-cycloserine Classification: Amino acid (Orphan)	L-cycloserine
L-cysteine Classification: Amino acid (Orphan)	L-cysteine
L-Lysine Classification: Amino acid	lysine
LA-12 Classification: Vitamin, water soluble	hydroxocobalamin (vitamin B_{12})

*Available in Canada only

BRAND NAME	GENERIC NAME
Lacipil Classification: Calcium channel blocker (Investigational)	lacidipine
Lacri-Lube NP Classification: Ophthalmic lubricant	ocular lubricants
Lacri-Lube S.O.P. Classification: Ophthalmic lubricant	ocular lubricants
Lacril Classification: Ophthalmic lubricants	artificial tears solution
Lacrisert Classification: Ophthalmic lubricants	artificial tear insert
Lactaid Classification: Food modifier	lactase enzyme
Lacticare-HC Classification: Glucocorticoid	hydrocortisone, topical
Lactinex Classification: Dietary supplement	lactobacillus
Lamictal Classification: Anticonvulsant	lamotrigine
Lamisil Classification: Antifungal	terbinafine HCl
Lampit Classification: CDC anti-infective	nifurtimox
Lamprene Classification: Leprostatic	clofazimine

*Available in Canada Only

BRAND NAME	GENERIC NAME
Lanacane Classification: Local anesthetic	benzocaine, topical
Lanacort 5 Classification: Glucocorticoid	hydrocortisone acetate
Lanacort 10 Classification: Glucocorticoid	hydrocortisone acetate
Lanaphilic Classification: Emollient	urea (carbamide), topical
Laniazid Classification: Antitubercular	isoniazid (INH)
Laniazid CT Classification: Antitubercular	isoniazid (INH)
Lanophyllin Classification: Bronchodilator; xanthine	theophylline
Lanoxicaps Classification: Cardiac glycoside	digoxin
Lanoxin Classification: Cardiac glycoside	digoxin
Lanvis* Classification: Antineoplastic; antimetabolite	thioguanine (TG; 6-thioguanine)
Largon Classification: Sedative-hypnotic, nonbarbiturate	propiomazine HCl
Lariam Classification: Antimalarial	mefloquine HCl

*Available in Canada only

BRAND NAME	GENERIC NAME

Larodopa
Classification:
Antiparkinson agent

levodopa

Lasix
Classification:
Loop diuretic

furosemide

Lax-Pills
Classification:
Laxative, irritant

phenolphthalein

Legatrin PM
Classification:
Antimalarial

quinine sulfate

Lentard Monotard*
Classification:
Antidiabetic

insulin, zinc suspension (lente)

Lente Iletin I
Classification:
Antidiabetic

insulin, zinc suspension (lente)

Lente Iletin II
Classification:
Antidiabetic

insulin zinc suspension (lente)

Lente Insulin
Classification:
Antidiabetic

insulin, zinc suspension (lente)

Lente L
Classification:
Antidiabetic

insulin, zinc suspension (lente)

Lentinan
Classification:
Biologic response modifier
(Investigational)

lentinan

Lescol
Classification:
Antilipemic

fluvastatin

BRAND NAME	GENERIC NAME

Leucomax
Classification:
Biologic response modifier
(Investigational)

molgramostim

Leucovorin Calcium
Classification:
Folic acid antagonist

leucovorin calcium (citrovorum factor, folic acid)

Leukeran
Classification:
Antineoplastic; alkylating agent

chlorambucil

Leukine
Classification:
Biologic response modifier

sargramostim (granulocyte macrophage colony stimulating factor, GM-CSF)

Leustatin
Classification:
Antineoplastic; miscellaneous

cladribine

Levaquin
Classification:
Antibiotic; fluoroquinolone

levofloxacin

Levate*
Classification:
Antidepressant

amitriptyline HCl

Levatol
Classification:
Antihypertensive; beta-adrenergic blocker

penbutolol

Levbid
Classification:
GI anticholinergic

hyoscyamine sulfate

Levobunolol HCl
Classification:
Beta-adrenergic blocker

levobunolol HCl

Levo-Dromoran
Classification:
Opioid analgesic

levorphanol tartrate

Levodopa & Carbidopa
Classification:
Antiparkinson agent

levodopa/carbidopa

*Available in Canada only

BRAND NAME	GENERIC NAME
Levophed Classification: Adrenergic agonist	norepinephrine injection (levarterenol)
Levoprome Classification: Analgesic	methotrimeprazine HCl
Levo-T Classification: Thyroid hormone	levothyroxine sodium (T_4; L-thyroxine)
Levothroid Classification: Thyroid hormone	levothyroxine sodium (T_4; L-thyroxine)
Levothyroxine Sodium Classification: Thyroid hormone	levothyroxine sodium (T_4; L-thyroxine)
Levoxine Classification: Thyroid hormone	levothyroxine sodium (T_4; L-thyroxine)
Levoxyl Classification: thyroid hormone	levothyroxine sodium (T_4; L-thyroxine)
Levsin Classification: GI anticholinergic	hyoscyamine sulfate
Levsin Drops Classification: GI anticholinergic	hyoscyamine sulfate
Levsin/SL Classification: GI anticholinergic	hyoscyamine sulfate
Levsinex Timecaps Classification: GI anticholinergic	hyoscyamine sulfate
Libritabs Classification: Antianxiety; benzodiazepine	chlordiazepoxide HCl

BRAND NAME	GENERIC NAME

Librium
Classification:
Antianxiety; benzodiazepine

chlordiazepoxide HCl

Lidemol*
Classification:
Glucocorticoid

fluocinonide

Lidex
Classification:
Glucocorticoid

fluocinonide

Lidocaine HCl
Classification:
Local anesthetic

lidocaine HCl, local

Lidocaine HCl IV for Cardiac Arrhythmias
Classification:
Antiarrhythmic

lidocaine HCl, IV

Lidocaine HCl, Topical
Classification:
Local anesthetic

lidocaine HCl, topical

Lidocaine Viscous
Classification:
Local anesthetic

lidocaine HCl, topical

Lidoderm Patch
Classification:
Local anesthetic (Orphan)

liposomal prostaglandin E_1

Lidoject-1
Classification:
Local anesthetic

lidocaine HCl, local

Lidoject-2
Classification:
Local anesthetic

lidocaine HCl, local

Lidopen Auto-Injector
Classification:
Local anesthetic

lidocaine HCl

Lifocort-100
Classification:
Glucocorticoid

hydrocortisone sodium succinate

BRAND NAME	GENERIC NAME

Lincocin
Classification:
Antibiotic; lincosamide

lincomycin HCl

Lincorex
Classification:
Antibiotic; lincosamide

lincomycin HCl

Lindane
Classification:
Scabicide; pediculicide

lindane (gamma benzene hexachloride)

Linomide
Classification:
Biologic response modifier
(Investigational)

roquinimex

Lioresal
Classification:
Skeletal muscle relaxant, direct acting

baclofen

Liothyronine Sodium
Classification:
Thyroid hormone

liothyronine sodium (T_3)

Lipitor
Classification:
Antilipemic

atorvastatin calcium

Lipomul
Classification:
Modular supplement

corn oil

Liposomal prostaglandin E$_1$
Classification:
Prostaglandin (Orphan)

liposomal prostaglandin E$_1$

Liposyn II 10%
Classification:
Caloric, fat

fat emulsions

Liposyn II 20%
Classification:
Caloric, fat

fat emulsions

Liposyn III 10%
Classification:
Caloric, fat

fat emulsions

BRAND NAME	GENERIC NAME

Liposyn III 20%
Classification:
Caloric fat

fat emulsions

Liqui-Char
Classification:
Adsorbent

charcoal, activated

Liquibid
Classification:
Expectorant

guaifenesin

Liquid Barosperse
Classification:
Radiopaque agent

barium sulfate

Liquid Pred
Classification:
Glucocorticoid

prednisone

Liquifilm Forte
Classification:
Ophthalmic lubricants

artificial tears solutions

Liquimat
Classification:
Anti-acne product

sulfur

Liquipake
Classification:
Radiopaque agent

barium sulfate

Liquiprin Drops for Children
Classification:
Analgesic; antipyretic

acetaminophen

Lithane
Classification:
Antimanic

lithium carbonate

Lithium Carbonate
Classification:
Antimanic

lithium carbonate

Lithium Citrate
Classification:
Antimanic

lithium citrate

BRAND NAME	GENERIC NAME
Lithonate Classification: Antimanic	lithium carbonate
Lithostat Classification: Urinary urease inhibitor	acetohydroxamic acid (AHA)
Lithotabs Classification: Antimanic	lithium carbonate
Livostin Classification: Ophthalmic antihistamine	levocabastine HCl
LMD 10% Classification: Plasma volume expander	dextran 40
Locoid Classification: Glucocorticoid	hydrocortisone butyrate
Lodine Classification: Nonsteroidal anti-inflammatory	etodolac
Lodine XL Classification: Nonsteroidal anti-inflammatory	etodolac
Lodosyn Classification: Antiparkinson agent	carbidopa
Loniten Classification: Antihypertensive; vasodilator	minoxidil
Loperamide Classification: Antidiarrheal	loperamide
Lopid Classification: Antilipemic	gemfibrozil

BRAND NAME	GENERIC NAME
Lopresor* Classification: Antihypertensive; beta-adrenergic blocker	metoprolol
Lopressor Classification: Antihypertensive; beta-adrenergic blocker	metoprolol
Loprox Classification: Antifungal	ciclopirox olamine
Lopurin Classification: Uricosuric	allopurinol
Lorabid Classification: Antibiotic; cephalosporin	loracarbef
Lorazepam Classification: Antianxiety; benzodiazepine	lorazepam
Lorazepam Intensol Classification: Antianxiety; benzodiazepine	lorazepam
Lorelco Classification: Antilipemic	probucol
Lorothidol Classification: CDC anti-infective	bithionol
Lotema Classification: Ophthalmic corticosteroid	loteprednol
Lotensin Classification: Antihypertensive; angiotensin converting enzyme inhibitor	benazepril HCl
Lotrimin AF Classification: Antifungal	miconazole nitrate, topical

*Available in Canada only

BRAND NAME	GENERIC NAME

Lotrimin AF Lotion
Classification:
Antifungal

clotrimazole, topical

Lovenox
Classification:
Anticoagulant

enoxapirin sodium

Lowsium
Classification:
Antacid

magaldrate (hydroxymagnesium aluminate)

Loxapax*
Classification:
Antipsychotic

loxapine succinate/loxapine HCl

Loxapine Succinate
Classification:
Antipsychotic

loxapine succinate/loxapine HCl

Loxitane/Loxitane-C
Classification:
Antipsychotic

loxapine succinate/loxapine HCl

Loxitane
Classification:
Antipsychotic

loxapine succinate/loxapine HCl

Loxitane IM
Classification:
Antipsychotic

loxapine succinate/loxapine HCl

Lozide*
Classification:
Thiazide diuretic

indapamide

Lozol
Classification:
Thiazide diuretic

indapamide

Ludiomil
Classification:
Antidepressant, tetracyclic

maprotiline HCl

Lufyllin-400
Classification:
Bronchodilator; xanthine

dyphylline (dihydroxypropyl theophylline)

BRAND NAME	GENERIC NAME
Lufyllin Classification: Bronchodilator; xanthine	dyphylline (dihydroxypropyl theophylline)
Luminal Sodium Classification: Sedative-hypnotic; barbiturate	phenobarbital/phenobarbital sodium
Luoxide Classification: Anti-acne product	benzoyl peroxide
Lupron Classification: Antineoplastic; hormone	leuprolide acetate
Lupron Depot Classification: Antineoplastic; hormone	leuprolide acetate
Lupron Depot 3 Month Classification: Antineoplastic; hormone	leuprilide acetate
Lupron Depot 4 Month Classification: Antineoplastic; hormone	leuprolide acetate
Lupron Depot-Ped Classification: Antineoplastic; hormone	leuprolide acetate
Luride Classification: Electrolyte replacement; fluoride	sodium fluoride
Luride 0.25 Lozi-Tabs Classification: Electrolyte replacement; fluoride	sodium fluoride
Luride 0.5 Lozi-Tabs Classification: Electrolyte replacement; fluoride	sodium fluoride
Luride Lozi-Tabs Classification: Electrolyte replacement; fluoride	sodium fluoride

BRAND NAME	GENERIC NAME

Luride-SF
Classification:
Electrolyte replacement; fluoride

sodium fluoride

**Lutenizing Hormone
(recombinant human)**
Classification:
Hormone (Orphan)

lutenizing hormone (recombinant human)

Lutrepulse
Classification:
Gonadotropin-releasing hormone

gonadorelin acetate

Luvox
Classification:
Antidepressant

fluvoxamine maleate

Lyme Borreliosis Vaccine
Classification:
Vaccine (Investigational)

lyme borreliosis vaccine

Lymphazurin 1%
Classification:
Radiopaque agent

isosulfan blue

LymphoScan
Classification:
In vivo diagnostic (Orphan)

technetiujm Tc-99m monoclonal
antibody to B cell

Lyphocin
Classification:
Antibiotic; tricyclic glycopeptide

vancomycin HCl

Lysodase
Classification:
Enzyme (Orphan)

PEG-glucocerebrosidase

Lysodren
Classification:
Antineoplastic miscellaneous

mitotane (O, p-DDD)

M

M-M-R II
Classification:
Vaccine

measles, mumps, and rubella virus
vaccine, live

BRAND NAME	GENERIC NAME
M-R-Vax II Classification: Vaccine	measles, (Rubeola) and rubella virus vaccine, live
M-CAPS Classification: Amino acid	methionine
M-Prednisol-40 Classification: Glucocorticoid	methylprednisolone acetate
M-Prednisol-80 Classification: Glucocorticoid	methylprednisolone acetate
M-Zole 7 Dual Pak Classification: Antifungal	miconazole nitrate, vaginal
M.O.M. Classification: Laxative, saline	saline laxatives
Maalox Antacid Classification: Antacid; calcium supplement	calcium carbonate
Maalox Anti-Gas Classification: Antiflatulent	simethicone
Maalox Daily Fiber Therapy Classification: Laxative, bulk-producing	psyllium
Macil* Classification: Skeletal muscle relaxant, centrally acting	chlorphenesin carbamate
Macrobid Classification: Urinary anti-infective	nitrofurantoin macrocrystals
Macrodantin Classification: Urinary anti-infective	nitrofurantoin macrocrystals

*Available in Canada only

BRAND NAME	GENERIC NAME

Macrodex
Classification:
Plasma volume expander

dextran 70/75

Mag-Ox 400
Classification:
Electrolyte replacement

magnesium oxide

Mag-Tab SR
Classification:
Electrolyte replacement

magnesium lactate

Magan
Classification:
Salicylate analgesic

magnesium salicylate

Magnaprin
Classification:
Salicylate analgesic; antipyretic

aspirin

Magnaprin Arthritis Strength Aspirin
Classification:
Salicylate analgesic; antipyretic

aspirin

Magnesium Sulfate
Classification:
Electrolyte replacement

magnesium sulfate

Magnesium Sulfate Concentrated
Classification:
Electrolyte replacement

magnesium sulfate

Magnevist
Classification:
Radiopaque agent

gadopentetate dimeglumine 46.9%

Magonate
Classification:
Electrolyte replacement

magnesium gluconate

Maltec
Classification:
Antibiotic; aminoglycoside (Orphan)

gentamicin liposome

BRAND NAME	GENERIC NAME

Mallamint
Classification:
Antacid; calcium supplement

calcium carbonate

Mallisol
Classification:
Antiseptic; germicidal

povidone-iodine

Mandol
Classification:
Antibiotic; cephalosporin

cefamandole naftate

Manganese
Classification:
Trace element

manganese

Manganese Sulfate
Classification:
Trace element

manganese

Mannitol
Classification:
Osmotic diuretic

mannitol

Maolate
Classification:
Skeletal muscle relaxant, centrally acting

chlorphenesin carbamate

Maox 420
Classification:
Electrolyte replacement

magnesium oxide

Mapap Children's
Classification:
Analgesic; antipyretic

acetaminophen

Mapap Extra Strength
Classification:
Analgesic; antipyretic

acetaminophen

Mapap Infant Drops
Classification:
Analgesic; antipyretic

acetaminophen

Mapap Regular Strength
Classification:
Analgesic; antipyretic

acetaminophen

BRAND NAME	GENERIC NAME
Maprotiline HCl Classification: Antidepressant, tetracyclic	maprotiline HCl
Maranox Classification: Analgesic; antipyretic	acetaminophen
Marcaine HCl Classification: Local anesthetic	bupivacaine HCl
Marcaine Spinal Classification: Local anesthetic	bupivacaine HCl
Marcaine with Epinephrine Classification: Local anesthetic	bupivacaine HCl
Marcillin Classification: Antibiotic; aminopenicillin	ampicillin, oral
Marezine Classification: Antiemetic; anticholinergic	cyclizine
Marimastat Classification: Antineoplastic (Investigational)	marimastat
Marinol Classification: Antiemetic	dronabinol
Marmine Classification: Antiemetic; anticholinergic	dimenhydrinate
Marogen Classification: Hormone; amino acid polypeptide (Orphan)	epoetin beta
Marthritic Classification: Salicylate analgesic	salsalate

*Available in Canada Only

BRAND NAME	GENERIC NAME
Matulane Classification: Antineoplastic miscellaneous	procarbazine HCl (N-methyl hydrazine, MIH)
Mavik Classification: Antihypertensive; angiotensin converting enzyme inhibitor	trandolapril
Max-Card Classification: Vitamin, fat soluble	beta-carotene
Maxair Classification: Bronchodilator; beta-adrenergic agonist	pirbuterol acetate
Maxaquin Classification: Antibiotic; fluoroquinolone	lomefloxacin HCl
Maxeran* Classification: Antidopaminergic	metoclopramide
Maxidex Classification: Ophthalmic glucocorticoid	dexamethasone, ophthalmic
Maxiflor Classification: Glucocorticoid	diflorasone diacetate
Maximum Bayer Classification: Salicylate analgesic; antipyretic	aspirin
Maximum Strength Anbesol Classification: Local anesthetic	benzocaine, oral
Maximum Strength Corticaine Classification: Glucocorticoid	hydrocortisone, topical
Maxipime Classification: Antibiotic; cephalosporin	cefepime HCl

*Available in Canada only

BRAND NAME	GENERIC NAME
Maxivate Classification: Glucocorticoid	betamethasone dipropionate
Maxolon Classification: Antidopaminergic	metoclopramide
Mazanar Classification: CNS stimulant; anorexiant	mazindol
Mazepine* Classification: Anticonvulsant	carbamazepine
MCT Oil Classification: Modular supplement	medium chain triglycerides
MD-Gastroview Classification: Radiopaque agent	diatrizoate meglumine 66% and diatrizoate sodium 10%
MD-60 Classification: Radiopaque agent	diatrizoate meglumine 52% and diatrizoate sodium 8%
MD-76 Classification: Radiopaque agent	diatrizoate meglumine 66% and diatrizoate sodium 10%
Mebadin Classification: CDC anti-infective	dehydroemetine
Mebaral Classification: Sedative-hypnotic; barbiturate	mephobarbital
Mecasermin Classification: Biologic response modifier (Orphan)	mecasermin
Meclan Classification: Anti-acne product	meclocycline sulfosalicylate

*Available in Canada Only

BRAND NAME	GENERIC NAME
Meclizine HCl Classification: Antiemetic; anticholinergic	meclizine
Meclofenamate Classification: Nonsteroidal anti-inflammatory	meclofenamate sodium
Meda Cap Classification: Analgesic; antipyretic	acetaminophen
Meda Tab Classification: Analgesic; antipyretic	acetaminophen
Medicone Classification: Local anesthetic	benzocaine, topical
Medicycline* Classification: Antibiotic; tetracycline	tetracycline HCl
Medihaler-Iso Classification: Adrenergic agonist	isoproterenol
Medilium* Classification: Antianxiety; benzodiazepine	chlordiazepoxide HCl
Medimet* Classification: Antihypertensive, centrally acting	methyldopa/methyldopate HCl
MeDiplast Classification: Keratolytic	salicylic acid, topical
Meditran* Classification: Antianxiety	meprobamate
Medralone 40 Classification: Glucocorticoid	methylprednisolone acetate

*Available in Canada only

BRAND NAME	GENERIC NAME
Medralone 80 Classification: Glucocorticoid	methylprednisolone acetate
Medrol Classification: Glucocorticoid	methylprednisolone
Medroxyprogesterone Acetate Classification: Progestin	medroxyprogesterone acetate
Mefoxin Classification: Antibiotic; cephalosporin	cefoxitin sodium
Megace Classification: Progestin	megestrol acetate
Megacillin* Classification: Antibiotic; penicillin	penicillin G benzathine, parenteral
Megestrol Acetate Classification: Progestin	megestrol acetate
Melacine Classification: Vaccine (Orphan)	melanoma vaccine
Melanex Classification: Depigmentation agent	hydroquinone
Melanoma Cell Vaccine Classification: Vaccine (Orphan)	melanoma cell vaccine
Melfiat-105 Unicelles Classification: CNS stimulant; anorexiant	phendimetrazine tartrate
Melimmune Classification: Biologic response modifier (Orphan)	monoclonal antidiotype melanoma-associate antigen

*Available in Canada Only

BRAND NAME	GENERIC NAME
Mellaril-5 Classification: Antipsychotic	thioridazine HCl
Mellaril Classification: Antipsychotic	thioridazine HCl
Mellaril Concentrate Classification: Antipsychotic	thioridazine HCl
Menadol Classification: Nonsteroidal anti-inflammatory	ibuprofen
Menest Classification: Estrogen	estrogens, esterified
Meni-D Classification: Antiemetic; anticholinergic	meclizine
Menomune-A/C/Y/W-135 Classification: Vaccine	meningococcal polysaccharide vaccine
Mentax Classification: Antifungal	butenafine HCl
Meperidine HCl Classification: Opioid analgesic	meperidine HCl
Mephyton Classification: Vitamin K	phytonadione (vitamin K_1)
MEPIG Classification: Immune serum (Orphan)	pseudomanas hyperimmune globulin
Mepivicane HCl Classification: Local anesthetic	mepivicaine HCl

BRAND NAME	GENERIC NAME
Meprobamate Classification: Antianxiety	meprobamate
Mepron Classification: Antiprotozoal	atovaquone
Meravil* Classification: Antidepressant	amitriptyline HCl
Mercurochrome Classification: Antiseptic	merbromin
Meridia Classification: CNS stimulant; anorexiant	sibutramine HCl monohydrate
Merrem IV Classification: Antibiotic; carbapenem	meropenem
Mersol Classification: Antiseptic	thimerosal
Meruvax II Classification: Vaccine	rubella virus vaccine, live
Mesantoin Classification: Anticonvulsant; hydantoin	mephenytoin
Mesnex Classification: Antineoplastic adjuvant; cytoprotective	mesna
Mestinon Classification: Anticholinesterase	pyridostigmine bromide
Metamucil Classification: Laxative, bulk-producing	psyllium

BRAND NAME	GENERIC NAME
Metamucil Instant Mix Lemon-Lime Classification: Laxative, bulk-producing	psyllium
Metamucil Instant Mix Orange Classification: Laxative, bulk-producing	psyllium
Metamucil Orange Flavor Classification: Laxative, bulk-producing	psyllium
Metamucil Sugar Free Classification: Laxative, bulk-producing	psyllium
Metamucil Sugar Free Orange Flavor Classification: Laxative, bulk-producing	psyllium
Metaprel Classification: Bronchodilator; beta-adrenergic agonist	metaproterenol sulfate
Metastron Classification: Antineoplastic; radiopharmaceutical	strontium-89 chloride
Metaraminol Bitartrate Classification: Adrenergic agonist	metaraminol
Methadone HCl Classification: Opioid analgesic	methadone HCl
Methadone HCl diskets Classification: Opioid analgesic	methadone HCl
Methadone HCl Intensol Classification: Opioid analgesic	methadone HCl

*Available in Canada only

BRAND NAME	GENERIC NAME
Methadose Classification: Opioid analgesic	methdone HCl
Methazolamide Classification: Diuretic; carbonic anhydrase inhibitor	methazolamide
Methblue 65 Classification: Urinary anti-infective	methylene blue
Methenamine Mandelate Classification: Urinary anti-infective	methenamine mandelate
Methergine Classification: Oxytocic	methylergonovine maleate
Methionine Classification: Amino acid	methionine
Methionyl Neutrotrophic Factor (brain-derived) Classification: Anti-amyotrophic lateral sclerosis agent (Orphan)	methionyl neutrotrophic factor (brain-derived)
Methocarbamol Classification: Skeletal muscle relaxant, centrally acting	methocarbamol
Methotrexate Classification: Antineoplastic; antimetabolite	methotrexate sodium (amethopterin, MTX)
Methotrexate LPF Classification: Antineoplastic; antimetabolite	methotrexate sodium (amethopterin, MTX)
Methychlothiazide Classification: Thiazide diuretic	methyclothiazide

BRAND NAME	GENERIC NAME
Methyldopa/Methyldopate HCl Classification: Antihypertensive, centrally acting	methyldopa/methyldopate HCl
Methylene Blue Classification: Urinary anti-infective	methylene blue
Methylergobasine* Classification: Oxytocic	methylergonovine maleate
Methylnaltrexone Classification: Narcotic antagonist (Orphan)	methylnaltroxone
Methylphenidate HCl Classification: CNS stimulant	methylphenidate HCl
Methylprednisolone Classification: Glucocorticoid	methylprednisolone
Methylprednisolone Acetate Classification: Glucocorticoid	methylprednisolone acetate
Methylprednisolone Sodium Classification: Glucocorticoid	methylprednisolone sodium succinate
Methyltestosterone Classification: Androgen	methyltestosterone
Meticorten Classification: Glucocorticoid	prednisone
Metoclopramide Classification: Antidopaminergic	metoclopramide
Metoclopramide HCl Classification: Antidopaminergic	metoclopramide

*Available in Canada only

BRAND NAME	GENERIC NAME

Metopirone
Classification:
In vivo diagnostic

metyrapone

Metoprolol Tartrate
Classification:
Antihypertensive; beta-adrenergic blocker

metoprolol

Metreton Ophthalmic
Classification:
Glucocorticoid

prednisolone sodium phosphate
ophthalmic, solution

Metro I.V.
Classification:
Antibacterial, amebicide

metronidazole

Metrodin
Classification:
Ovulation stimulant

urofollitropin

MetroGel
Classification:
Anti-acne product

metronidazole, topical

MetroGel-Vaginal
Classification:
Antibacterial, amebicide

metronidazole, vaginal

Metubine Iodide
Classification:
Nondepolarizing neuromuscular blocker

metocurine iodide

Mevacor
Classification:
Antilipemic

lovastatin

Meval*
Classification:
Antianxiety; benzodiazepine

diazepam

Mexiletine HCl
Classification:
Antiarrhythmic

mexiletine HCl

Mexitil
Classification:
Antiarrhythmic

mexiletine HCl

BRAND NAME	GENERIC NAME
Mezlin Classification: Antibiotic; extended spectrum penicillin	mezlocillin sodium
MG 217 Medicated Classification: Keratolytic	coal tar
Miacalcin Classification: Parathyroid agent	calcitonin (salmon)
Micanol Classification: Antipsoriatic	anthralin (dithranol)
Micatin Classification: Antifungal; imidazole	miconazole nitrate, topical
Micatin Liquid Classification: Antifungal; imidazole	miconazole nitrate, topical
Miconazole Nitrate Classification: Antifungal; imidazole	miconazole nitrate, topical
MICRhoGAM Classification: Immune serum	Rho (D) immune globulin micro-dose
Micro-K Classification: Electrolyte replacement; potassium	potassium chloride
Microlipid Classification: Modular supplement	safflower
Micronase Classification: Antidiabetic	glyburide
MicroNefrin Classification: Adrenergic agonist	epinephrine

*Available in Canada only

BRAND NAME	GENERIC NAME
Micronized Glyburide Classification: Antidiabetic; sulfonylurea	glyburide
Micronor Classification: Progestin	norethindrone
Microx Classification: Thiazide-like diuretic	metolazone
Microzide Classification: Thiazide diuretic	hydrochlorothiazide
Midamor Classification: Potassium-sparing diuretic	amiloride HCl
Midol IB Classification: Nonsteroidal anti-inflammatory	ibuprofen
Migranol Classification: Antimigraine; ergot alkaloid	dihydroergotamine, nasal
Milkinol Classification: Laxative, emollient	mineral oil
Milk of Magnesia Classification: Laxative, saline	saline laxatives
Milk of Magnesia Concentrated Classification: Antacid; laxative	magnesia (magnesium hydroxide)
Milontin Kapseals Classification: Anticonvulsant; succinimide	phensuximide
Miltown 600 Classification: Antianxiety	meprobamate

BRAND NAME	GENERIC NAME
Mineral Oil Classification: Laxative, emollient	mineral oil
Mini-Gamulin Rh Classification: Immune serum	Rho (D) immune globulin micro-dose
Minipress Classification: Antihypertensive; alpha-adrenergic blocker	prazosin
Mini Thin Pseudo Classification: Nasal decongestant	pseudoephedrine HCl
Minitran Classification: Antianginal	nitroglycerin transdermal systems
Minocin Classification: Antibiotic; tetracycline	minocycline HCl
Minocin IV Classification: Antibiotic; tetracycline	minocycline HCl
Minocycline HCl Classification: Antibiotic; tetracycline	minocycline HCl
Minoxidil Classification: Antihypertensive; vasodilator	minoxidil
Minoxidil for Men Classification: Antihypertensive; vasodilator	minoxidil, topical
Mintezol Classification: Anthelmintic	thiabendazole
Minute-Gel Classification: Electrolyte replacement; fluoride	sodium fluoride

*Available in Canada only

BRAND NAME	GENERIC NAME
Miocarpine* Classification: Miotic	pilocarpine HCl
Miochol-E Classification: Miotic	acetylcholine chloride, intraocular
Miostat Classification: Miotic	carbachol, intraocular
Miradon Classification: Anticoagulant	anisindione
Mirapex Classification: Antiparkinson agent	pramipexole dihydrochloride
Mithracin Classification: Antineoplastic; antibiotic	plicamycin (mithramycin)
Mitoguazone Classification: Antineoplastic (Orphan)	mitoguazone
Mitran Classification: Antianxiety; benzodiazepine	chlordiazepoxide HCl
Mitrol Classification: Osmotic diuretic	mannitol
Mitrolan Classification: Laxative, bulk-producing	polycarbophil
Mivacron Classification: Nondepolarizing neuromuscular blocker	mivacurium chloride
Moban Classification: Antipsychotic	molindone HCl

*Available in Canada Only

BRAND NAME	GENERIC NAME
Mobenol* Classification: Antidiabetic; sulfonylurea	tolbutamide
Mobidin Classification: Salicylate analgesic	magnesium salicylate
Mobisyl Classification: Analgesic	trolamine salicylate
Moctanin Classification: Antilithic	monoctanoin
Modane Classification: Laxative, irritant	phenolphthalein
Modane Bulk Classification: Laxative, bulk-producing	psyllium
Modane Soft Classification: Laxative, softener	docusate sodium
Modified Burow's Solution Classification: Astringent	aluminum acetate solution
Moi-Stir 10 Classification: Oral lubricants	saliva substitutes
Moi-Stir Classification: Oral lubricants	saliva substitutes
Moi-Stir Swabsticks Classification: Oral lubricants	saliva substitutes
Moisture Drops Classification: Ophthalmic	artificial tears solution

*Available in Canada only

BRAND NAME	GENERIC NAME
Mol-Iron Classification: Iron preparation	ferrous sulfate
Mollifene Classification: Emulsifier	carbamide peroxide (urea peroxide)
Molypen Classification: Trace element	molybdenum
Monafed Classification: Expectorant	guaifenesin
Monistat 3 Classification: Antifungal	miconazole nitrate, vaginal
Monistat 7 Classification: Antifungal	miconazole nitrate, vaginal
Monistat-Derm Classification: Antifungal	miconazole nitrate, topical
Monistat Dual-Pak Classification: Antifungal	miconazole nitrate, vaginal
Monistat i.v. Classification: Antifungal; imidazole	miconazole
Monitan* Classification: Beta-adrenergic blocker	acebutolol
Mono-Chlor Classification: Cauterizing agent	monochloroacetic acid
Monocid Classification: Antibiotic; cephalosporin	cefonicid sodium

BRAND NAME	GENERIC NAME

Monoclate-P
Classification:
Hemostatic

antihemophilic factor (AHF, factor VIII)

Monoclonal Antibody (human), Hepatitis B Virus
Classification:
Biologic response modifier (Orphan)

monoclonal antibody (human), hepatitis B virus

Monoclonal Antibody 17-1A
Classification:
Biologic response modifier (Orphan)

monoclonal antibody 17-1A

Monoclonal Antibody PM-81
Classification:
Biologic response modifier (Orphan)

monoclonal antibody PM-81

Monoclonal Antibody to CD4,5a8
Classification:
Biologic response modifier (Orphan)

monoclonal antibody to CD4,5a8

Monoclonal Antibody, Lupus Nephritis
Classification:
Biologic response modifier (Orphan)

monoclonal antibody, lupus nephritis

Monodox
Classification:
Antibiotic; tetracycline

doxycycline hyclate

Mono-Gesic
Classification:
Salicylate analgesic

salsalate

Monoket
Classification:
Antianginal

isosorbide mononitrate

Mononine
Classification:
Hemostatic

monoclonal factor IX

Mono-Press
Classification:
Thiazide diuretic

trichlormethiazide

*Available in Canada only

BRAND NAME	GENERIC NAME

Mono Vacc Test (O.T.)
Classification:
In vivo diagnostic

tuberculin (Old), multiple puncture
devices

Monopril
Classification:
Antihypertensive; angiotensin converting
enzyme inhibitor

fosinopril sodium

Monurol
Classification:
Urinary anti-infective

fosfomycin tromethamine

Moranyl
Classification:
CDC anti-infective

suramin

MoreDophilus
Classification:
Dietary supplement

lactobacillus

Morphine Sulfate
Classification:
Opioid analgesic

morphine sulfate

Morrhuate Sodium
Classification:
Sclerosing agent

morrhuate sodium

Mosco
Classification:
Keratolytic

salicylic acid, topical

Motrin
Classification:
Nonsteroidal anti-inflammatory

ibuprofen

Motrin IB
Classification:
Nonsteroidal anti-inflammatory

ibuprofen

Motrin Junior Strength
Classification:
Nonsteroidal anti-inflammatory

ibuprofen

MouthKote F/R
Classification:
Electrolyte replacement; fluoride

sodium flouride

BRAND NAME	GENERIC NAME

MRV
Classification:
Vaccine

mixed respiratory vaccine

MS Contin
Classification:
Opioid analgesic

morphine sulfate

MS/L
Classification:
Opioid analgesic

morphine sulfate

MS/L-Concentrate
Classification:
Opioid analgesic

morphine sulfate

MS/S
Classification:
Opioid analgesic

morphine sulfate

MSIR
Classification:
Opioid analgesic

morphine sulfate

MSTA
Classification:
In vivo diagnostic

mumps skin test antigen

Muco-Fen-LA
Classification:
Expectorant

guaifenesin

Mucomyst
Classification:
Mucolytic

acetylcysteine (N-acetylcysteine)

Mucomyst 10 IV
Classification:
Mucolytic (Orphan)

acetylcysteine, intravenous

Mucosil-10
Classification:
Mucolytic

acetylcysteine (N-acetylcysteine)

Mucosil-20
Classification:
Mucolytic

acetylcysteine (N-acetylcysteine)

BRAND NAME	GENERIC NAME
Multitest CMI Classification: In vivo diagnostic	skin test antigens, multiple
Mumpsvax Classification: Vaccine	mumps virus vaccine, live
Murine Ear Classification: Emulsifier	carbamide peroxide, otic
Murine Plus Eye Drops Classification: Ophthalmic vasoconstrictor	tetrahydrozoline HCl, ophthalmic
Muro 128 Classification: Hyperosmolar preparation	sodium chloride, hypertonic
Murocel Classification: Ophthalmic lubricants	artificial tears solution
Mustargen Classification: Antineoplastic; alkylating agent	mechlorethamine HCl (nitrogen mustard; HN_2)
Mutamycin Classification: Antineoplastic	mitomycin (mitomycin-C; MTC)
Myambutol Classification: Antitubercular	ethambutol HCl
Mycelex Classification: Antifungal	clotrimazole, topical
Mycelex-7 Classification: Antifungal	clotrimazole, vaginal
Mycelex-7 Combination Pack Classification: Antifungal	clotrimazole, vaginal

BRAND NAME	GENERIC NAME
Mycelex-G Classification: Antifungal	clotrimazole, topical
Mycelex OTC Classification: Antifungal	clotrimazole, topical
Mycelex Troches Classification: Antifungal	clotrimazole, oral
Mycelex Twin Pack Classification: Antifungal	clotrimazole, vaginal
Mycifradin Sulfate Classification: Aminoglycoside	neomycin sulfate
Myciguent Classification: Aminoglycoside	neomycin sulfate, topical
Mycinettes Classification: Local anesthetic	benzocaine, oral
Mycobutin Classification: Antitubercular	rifabutin
Mycocide NS Classification: Germicidal	benzalkonium chloride
Mycostatin Classification: Antifungal	nystatin, oral
Mycostatin Classification: Antifungal	nystatin, vaginal
Mycostatin Pastilles Classification: Antifungal	nystatin, oral

BRAND NAME	GENERIC NAME

Mydriacyl Ophthalmic
Classification:
Mydriatic

tropicamide, ophthalmic

Myelin
Classification:
Anti-multiple sclerosis agent (Orphan)

myelin

Mykrox
Classification:
Thiazide-like diuretic

zaroxolyn

**Mylanta Natural Fiber
Supplement**
Classification:
Laxative, bulk-producing

psyllium

Myleran
Classification:
Antineoplastic; alkylating agent

busulfan

Mylicon
Classification:
Antiflatulent

simethicone

Myoflex
Classification:
Analgesic

trolamine salicylate

Myolin
Classification:
Skeletal muscle relaxant, centrally acting

orphenadrine citrate

Myoscint
Classification:
In vivo diagnostic (Orphan)

imiciromab penetrate

Myotrophin
Classification:
Growth hormone (Orphan)

insulin-like growth factor-I

Mysoline
Classification:
Anticonvulsant

primidone

Mytelase
Classification:
Anticholinesterase

ambenonium chloride

BRAND NAME	GENERIC NAME

Mytonachol
Classification:
Cholinergic stimulant

bethanechol chloride

Mytussin
Classification:
Expectorant

guaifenesin

N

Nadolol HCl
Classification:
Beta-adrenergic blocker

nadolol HCl

Nadostine*
Classification:
Antifungal

nystatin, oral

Nafazair
Classification:
Ophthalmic vasoconstrictor

naphazoline HCl ophthalmic

Nafcil
Classification:
Antibiotic; penicillinase-resistant
penicillin

nafcillin sodium

Nafcillin Sodium
Classification:
Antibiotic; penicillinase-resistant
penicillin

nafcillin sodium

Nafrine*
Classification:
Nasal decongestant

oxymetazoline HCl, nasal

Naftin
Classification:
Antifungal

naftifine HCl

Naganol
Classification:
CDC anti-infective

suramin

Nalbuphine HCl
Classification:
Opioid agonist-antagonist analgesic

nalbuphine HCl

*Available in Canada only

BRAND NAME	GENERIC NAME

Naldecon Senior EX
Classification:
Expectorant

guaifenesin

Nalfon
Classification:
Nonsteroidal anti-inflammatory

fenoprofen calcium

Nallpen
Classification:
Antibiotic; penicillinase-resistant
penicillin

nafcillin sodium

Naloxone HCl
Classification:
Narcotic antagonist

naloxone HCl

Nandrolone Decanoate
Classification:
Anabolic steroid

nandrolone phenpropionate

Naphazoline HCl
Classification:
Ophthalmic vasoconstrictor

naphazoline HCl, ophthalmic

Naphcon Forte
Classification:
Ophthalmic vasoconstrictor

naphazoline HCl, ophthalmic

Naphuride
Classification:
CDC anti-infective

suramin

Naprelan
Classification:
Nonsteroidal anti-inflammatory

naproxen

Napron X
Classification:
Nonsteroidal anti-inflammatory

naproxen

Naprosyn
Classification:
Nonsteroidal anti-inflammatory

naproxen

Naqua
Classification:
Thiazide diuretic

trichlormethiazide

BRAND NAME	GENERIC NAME
Narcan Classification: Narcotic antagonist	naloxone HCl
Nardil Classification: Monoamine oxidase inhibitor	phenelzine sulfate
Naropin Classification: Local anesthetic	ropivacaine HCl
Nasacort Classification: Glucocorticoid	triamcinolone acetonide, nasal
Nasacort AQ Classification: Glucocorticoid	triamcinolone acetonide, nasal
Nasahist-B Classification: Antihistamine	brompheniramine maleate
NāSal Classification: Nasal decongestant	sodium chloride, nasal
Nasalcrom Classification: Antiasthmatic	cromolyn sodium (disodium cromoglycate)
Nasalide Nasal Solution Classification: Glucocorticoid	flunisolide, nasal
Nasal Moist Classification: Nasal decongestant	sodium chloride, nasal
Nasarel Classification: Glucocorticoid	flunisolide, nasal
Nascobal Classification: Vitamin, water soluble	cyanocobalamin (vitamin B_{12})

BRAND NAME	GENERIC NAME
Nasonex Classification: Nasal corticosteroid	mometasone furoate monohydrate
Natacyn Classification: Ophthalmic antifungal	natamycin
Natulan* Classification: Antineoplastic, miscellaneous	procarbazine HCl (N-methylhydrazine, MIH)
Natural Vegetable Reguloid Classification: Laxative, bulk-producing	psyllium
Naturetin Classification: Thiazide diuretic	bendroflumethiazide
Nauseal* Classification: Antiemetic; anticholinergic	dimenhydrinate
Nausea Relief Classification: Antiemetic	phosphorated carbohydrate solution
Nauseatol* Classification: Antiemetic, anticholinergic	dimenhydrinate
Nausetrol Classification: Antiemetic	phosphorated carbohydrate solution
Navelbine Classification: Antineoplastic; mitotic inhibitor	vinorelbine tartrate
Navane Classification: Antipsychotic	thiothixene
ND Stat Classification: Antihistamine	brompheniramine maleate

*Available in Canada Only

BRAND NAME	GENERIC NAME
Nebcin Classification: Aminoglycoside	tobramycin sulfate
NebuPent Classification: Antiprotozoal	pentamidine isethionate
NegGram Classification: Urinary anti-infective	nalidixic acid
NegGram Caplets Classification: Urinary anti-infective	nalidixic acid
Nembutal Classification: Sedative-hypnotic; barbiturate	pentobarbital sodium
Nembutal Sodium Classification: Sedative-hypnotic; barbiturate	pentobarbital sodium
Nembutal Sodium Solution Classification: Sedative-hypnotic; barbiturate	pentobarbital sodium
Neo-Calglucon Classification: Electrolyte replacement; calcium	calcium glubionate
Neo-Codema* Classification: Thiazide diuretic	hydrochlorothiazide
Neo-Cultol Classification: Laxative, emollient	mineral oil
Neo-Diaral Classification: Antidiarrheal	loperamide
Neo-Durabolic Classification: Anabolic steroid	nandrolone decanoate

BRAND NAME	GENERIC NAME
Neo-Estrone* Classification: Estrogen	estrogens, esterified
Neo-fradin Classification: Aminoglycoside	neomycin sulfate
Neo-Synephrine Classification: Adrenergic agonist	phenylephrine HCl
Neo-Synephrine Classification: Nasal decongestant	phenylephrine HCl, nasal
Neo-Synephrine 12 Hour Classification: Nasal decongestant	oxymetazoline HCl, nasal
Neo-Synephrine 2.5% Classification: Adrenergic	phenylephrine HCl
Neo-Synephrine 10% Plain Classification: Ophthalmic vasoconstrictor	phenylephrine HCl, ophthalmic
Neo-Synephrine Viscous Classification: Ophthalmic vasoconstrictor	phenylephrine HCl, ophthalmic
Neo-Tabs Classification: Aminoglycoside	neomycin sulfate
Neo-Tetrine* Classification: Antibiotic; tetracycline	tetracycline HCl
Neo-Tran* Classification: Antianxiety	meprobamate
Neo-Tric* Classification: Antibacterial; amebicide	metronidazole

*Available in Canada Only

BRAND NAME	GENERIC NAME
Neoloid Classification: Laxative, irritant	castor oil
Neomycin Classification: Aminoglycoside	neomycin sulfate
Neomycin Sulfate Classification: Aminoglycoside	neomycin sulfate
Neoral Classification: Immunosuppressive	cyclosporine (cyclosporin A)
Neosar Classification: Antineoplastic; alkylating agent	cyclophosphamide
Neostigmine Classification: Anticholinesterase	neostigmine
Neostigmine Methylsulfate Classification: Anticholinesterase	neostigmine
NephrAmine Classification: Nitrogen product	amino acid solution, renal
Nephro-Calci Classification: Antacid; calcium supplement	calcium carbonate
Nephro-Fer Classification: Iron preparation	ferrous fumarate
Nephron Inhalant Classification: Adrenergic agonist	epinephrine
Nephronex* Classification: Urinary anti-infective	nitrofurantoin

*Available in Canada only

BRAND NAME	GENERIC NAME

Neptazane
Classification:
Diuretic; carbonic anhydrase inhibitor

methazolamide

Nervocaine 1%
Classification:
Local anesthetic

lidocaine HCl, local

Nesacaine
Classification:
Local anesthetic

chloroprocaine HCl

Nesacaine-MPF
Classification:
Local anesthetic

chloroprocaine HCl

Nestrex
Classification:
Vitamin, water soluble

pyridoxine HCl (vitamin B_6)

Netromycin
Classification:
Aminoglycoside

netilmicin sulfate

Neumega
Classification:
Biologic response modifier

oprelvekin

Neupogen
Classification:
Biologic response modifier

filgrastim (granulocyte colony stimulating factor, G-CSF)

Neuralgon
Classification:
Skeletal muscle relaxant (Orphan)

L-baclofen

Neurelan
Classification:
Antimultiple sclerosis agent (Orphan)

fampridine

Neurontin
Classification:
Anticonvulsant

gabapentin

Neurotrophin-1
Classification:
Anti-amyotrophic lateral sclerosis agent
(Orphan)

neurotrophin-1

BRAND NAME	GENERIC NAME
Neut Classification: Systemic alkalinizer	sodium bicarbonate
Neutra-Phos Classification: Electrolyte replacement	phosphorous (replacement products)
Neutra-Phos-K Classification: Electrolyte replacement	phosphorous (replacement products)
Neutrexin Classification: Anti-infective; folate antagonist	trimetrexate glucuronate
NGD 91-2 Classification: Antianxiety (Investigational)	NGD 91-2
Nia-Bid Classification: Vitamin, water soluble	niacin (vitamin B_3, nicotinic acid)
Niacinamide Classification: Vitamin, water soluble	nicotinamide (niacinamide)
Niacor Classification: Vitamin, water soluble	niacin (vitamin B_3, nicotinic acid)
Niaspan Classification: Antilipemic	niacin, sustained release
Nicardipine HCl Classification: Calcium channel blocker	nicardipine HCl
N'ice Vitamin C Drops Classification: Vitamin, water soluble	ascorbic acid (vitamin C)
Niclocide Classification: Anthelmintic	niclosamide

BRAND NAME	GENERIC NAME

Nico-400
Classification:
Vitamin, water soluble

niacin (vitamin B_3, nicotinic acid)

Nicobid
Classification:
Vitamin, water soluble

niacin (vitamin B_3, nicotinic acid)

Nicoderm
Classification:
Smoking deterrent

nicotine transdermal system

Nicolar
Classification:
Vitamin, water soluble

niacin (vitamin B_3, nicotinic acid)

Nicorette
Classification:
Smoking deterrent

nicotine polacrilex

Nicorette DS
Classification:
Smoking deterrent

nicotine polacrilex

Nicotinamide
Classification:
Vitamin, water soluble

nicotinamide (niacinamide)

Nicotinex
Classification:
Vitamin, water soluble

niacin (vitamin B_3, nicotinic acid)

Nicotinic acid
Classification:
Vitamin, water soluble

niacin (vitamin B_3, nicotinic acid)

Nicotrol
Classification:
Smoking deterrent

nicotine transdermal system

Nicotrol NS
Classification:
Smoking deterrent

nicotine nasal

Nico-Vert
Classification:
Antiemetic; anticholinergic

dimenhydrinate

*Available in Canada Only

BRAND NAME	GENERIC NAME
Nifedipine Classification: Calcium channel blocker	nifedipine
Niferex-150 Classification: Iron preparation	polysaccharide iron complex
Niferex Classification: Iron preparation	polysaccharide iron complex
Nilandron Classification: Antineoplastic; antiandrogen	nilutamide
Nilstat Classification: Antifungal	nystatin, topical
Nilstat Classification: Antifungal	nystatin, oral
Nimbex Classification: Nondepolarizing neuromuscular blocker	cisatracurium besylate
Nimotrop Classification: Calcium channel blocker	nimodipine
Nipent Classification: Antineoplastic; antibiotic	pentostatin (DCF; 2-Deoxycoformycin)
Nitazoxanide Classification: Antiprotazoal (Orphan)	nitazoxanide
Nitrek Classification: Antianginal	nitroglycerin, transdermal system
Nitro-Bid Classification: Antianginal	nitroglycerin, topical

BRAND NAME	GENERIC NAME
Nitro-Bid IV Classification: Antianginal	nitroglycerin, intravenous
Nitro-Dur Classification: Antianginal	nitroglycerin, transdermal systems
Nitro-Time Classification: Antianginal	nitroglycerin, sustained release
Nitrodisc Classification: Antianginal	nitroglycerin, transdermal systems
Nitrofurazone Classification: Antibacterial	nitrofurazone
Nitrogard Classification: Antianginal	nitroglycerin, transmucosal
Nitroglycerin Classification: Antianginal	nitroglycerin, topical
Nitroglycerin Classification: Antianginal	nitroglycerin, intravenous
Nitroglycerin Classification: Antianginal	nitroglycerin, sustained release
Nitroglycerin Transdermal Classification: Antianginal	nitroglycerin, transdermal systems
Nitroglyn Classification: Antianginal	nitroglycerin, sustained release
Nitrolingual Classification: Antianginal	nitroglycerin, translingual

BRAND NAME	GENERIC NAME
Nitrol Classification: Antianginal	nitroglycerin, topical
Nitrong Classification: Antianginal	nitroglycerin, sustained release
Nitropress Classification: Antihypertensive; vasodilator	nitroprusside sodium
Nitrostat Classification: Antianginal	nitroglycerin, sublingual
Nix Classification: Scabicide; pediculicide	permethrin
Nizoral Classification: Antifungal; imidazole	ketoconazole
Nizoral Classification: Antifungal; imidazole	ketoconazole, topical
Nō-Dōz Classification: Analeptic	caffeine
Nolahist Classification: Antihistamine	phenindamine tartrate
Nolvadex Classification: Antineoplastic; hormone	tamoxifen citrate
No Pain-HP Classification: Analgesic	capsaicin
Nootropil Classification: Muscle stimulant (Orphan)	piracetam

*Available in Canada only

BRAND NAME	GENERIC NAME
Nor-Q.D. Classification: Progestin	norethindrone
Nor-Tet Classification: Antibiotic; tetracycline	tetracycline HCl
Norastemizole Classification: Antihistamine (Investigational)	norastemizole
Norcuron Classification: Non-depolarizing neuromuscular blocker	vecuronium bromide
Norditropin Classification: Growth hormone	somatropin
Nordryl Classification: Antihistamine	diphenhydramine HCl
Nordryl Cough Classification: Antihistamine	diphenhydramine HCl
Norflex Classification: Skeletal muscle relaxant, centrally acting	orphenadrine citrate
Normiflo Classification: Anticoagulant	ardeparin sodium
Normodyne Classification: Antihypertensive	labetalol
Normosang Classification: Blood modifier (Orphan)	heme arginate
Noroxin Classification: Antibiotic; fluoroquinolone	norfloxacin

*Available in Canada Only

BRAND NAME	GENERIC NAME
Norpace Classification: Antiarrhythmic	disopyramide
Norpace CR Classification: Antiarrhythmic	disopyramide
Norplant System Classification: Progestin, synthetic	levonorgestrel implant
Norpramin Classification: Antidepressant, tricyclic	desipramine HCl
Nortriptyline HCl Classification: Antidepressant	nortriptyline HCl
Norvasc Classification: Calcium channel blocker	amlodipine
Norvir Classification: Antiviral; protease inhibitor	ritonavir
Norwich Extra-Strength Classification: Salicylate analgesic; antipyretic	aspirin
Nōstril Classification: Nasal decongestant	phenylephrine HCl, nasal
Nōstrilla Classification: Nasal decongestant	oxymetazoline HCl, nasal
Nova-Rectal* Classification: Sedative-hypnotic; barbiturate	pentobarbital sodium
Novamine Classification: Nitrogen product	amino acid solution

*Available in Canada only

BRAND NAME	GENERIC NAME

Novamoxin*
Classification:
Antibiotic; aminopenicillin

amoxicillin trihydrate

Novantrone
Classification:
Antineoplastic; antibiotic

mitoxantrone

Novapren
Classification:
Antiviral (Investigational)

novapren

Novapurol*
Classification:
Uricosuric

allopurinol

Novasen*
Classification:
Salicylate analgesic; antipyretic

aspirin

Novo-Gemfibrozil*
Classification:
Antilipemic

gemfibrozil

Novobutamide*
Classification:
Antidiabetic; sulfonylurea

tolbutamide

Novocain
Classification:
Local anesthetic

procaine HCl

Novochlorhydrate*
Classification:
Sedative-hypnotic; nonbarbiturate

chloral hydrate

Novochlorocap*
Classification:
Antibacterial; antirickettsial

chloramphenicol sodium succinate

Novochloroquine*
Classification:
Antimalarial

chloroquine phosphate

Novocloxin*
Classification:
Antibiotic; penicillinase-resistant
penicillin

cloxacillin sodium

*Available in Canada Only

BRAND NAME	GENERIC NAME
Novodimenate* Classification: Antiemetic; anticholinergic	dimenhydrinate
Novodipam* Classification: Antianxiety; benzodiazepine	diazepam
Novoflurazine* Classification: Antipsychotic	trifluoperazine HCl
Novofolacid* Classification: Vitamin B complex group	folic acid, folacin, folate
Novofuran Classification: Urinary anti-infective	nitrofurantoin
Novohexidyl* Classification: Anticholinergic	trihexyphenidyl HCl
Novohydrazide* Classification: Thiazide diuretic	hydrochlorothiazide
Novolexin* Classification: Antibiotic; cephalosporin	cephalexin monohydrate
Novolin 70/30 Classification: Antidiabetic	insulin, isophane suspension and injection
Novolin 70/30 PenFill Classification: Antidiabetic	insulin, isophane suspension and insulin injection
Novolin ge 30/70* Classification: Antidiabetic	insulin, isophane suspension and insulin injection
Novolin ge 50/50* Classification: Antidiabetic	insulin, isophane suspension and insulin injection

*Available in Canada only

BRAND NAME	GENERIC NAME
Novolin ge Lente* Classification: Antidiabetic	insulin, zinc suspension (lente)
Novolin ge NPH* Classification: Antidiabetic	insulin, isophane injection (NPH)
Novolin ge Toronto* Classification: Antidiabetic	insulin injection
Novolin ge Ultralente* Classification: Antidiabetic	insulin, zinc suspension extended (Ultralente)
Novolin L Classification: Antidiabetic	insulin, zinc suspension (lente)
Novolin N Classification: Antidiabetic	insulin, isophane suspension (NPH)
Novolin N PenFill Classification: Antidiabetic	insulin, isophane suspension (NPH)
Novolin R Classification: Antidiabetic	insulin injection
Novolin R PenFill Classification: Antidiabetic	insulin injection
Novolorazem* Classification: Antianxiety; benzodiazepine	lorazepam
Novomedopa* Classification: Antihypertensive, centrally acting	methyldopa/methyldopate HCl
Novomepro* Classification: Antianxiety	meprobamate

*Available in Canada Only

BRAND NAME	GENERIC NAME
Novoniacin* Classification: Vitamin, water soluble	niacin (vitamin B_3, nicotinic acid)
Novonidazole* Classification: Antibacterial; amebicide	metronidazole
Novopen-VK* Classification: Antibiotic; penicillin	penicillin V potassium
Novopoxide* Classification: Antianxiety; benzodiazepine	chlordiazepoxide HCl
Novopramine* Classification: Antidepressant	imipramine HCl
Novopropamide* Classification: Antidiabetic; sulfonylurea	chlorpropamide
Novoquine* Classification: Antimalarial	quinine sulfate
Novoridazine* Classification: Antipsychotic	thioridazine HCl
Novorythro* Classification: Antibiotic; macrolide	erythromycin base
Novosemide* Classification: Loop diuretic	furosemide
Novosoxazole* Classification: Antibiotic; sulfonamide	sulfisoxazole
Novosudac* Classification: Nonsteroidal anti-inflammatory	sulindac

*Available in Canada only

BRAND NAME	GENERIC NAME
Novotetra* Classification: Antibiotic; tetracycline	tetracycline HCl
Novothalidone* Classification: Thiazide-like diuretic	chlorthalidone
Novotriphyl* Classification: Bronchodilator; xanthine	oxtriphylline
Novotriptyn* Classification: Antidepressant	amitriptyline HCl
Novoxapam* Classification: Antianxiety; benzodiazepine	oxazepam
Nozinan* Classification: Analgesic	methotrimeprazine HCl
NP-27 Classification: Antifungal	tolnaftate
NPH Iletin I Classification: Antidiabetic	insulin, isophane suspension (NPH)
NPH insulin Classification: Antidiabetic	insulin, isophane suspension (NPH)
N-trifluoroacetyladriamycin-14-valerate Classification: Antineoplastic (Orphan)	N-trifluoroacetyladriamycin-14-valerate
NTZ Long-Acting Nasal Classification: Nasal decongestant	oxymetazoline HCl, nasal
Nu-Iron 150 Classification: Iron preparation	polysaccharide iron complex

*Available in Canada Only

BRAND NAME	GENERIC NAME
Nu-Iron Classification: Iron preparation	polysaccharide iron complex
Nubain Classification: Opioid agonist-antagonist analgesic	nalbuphine HCl
Nutropin AQ Classification: Growth hormone	somatropin
Numorphan Classification: Opioid analgesic	oxymorphone HCl
Numorphan HP Classification: Opioid analgesic	oxymorphone HCl
Nupercainal Classification: Local anesthetic	dibucaine HCl, topical
Nuprin Classification: Nonsteroidal anti-inflammatory	ibuprofen
Nuromax Classification: Nondepolarizing neuromuscular blocker	doxacurium chloride
Nutracort Classification: Glucocorticoid	hydrocortisone, topical
Nutraplus Classification: Osmotic diuretic	urea (carbamide), topical
Nydrazid Classification: Antitubercular	isoniazid (INH)
NyLytely Classification: Bowel evacuant	polyethylene glycol-electrolyte solution

*Available in Canada only

BRAND NAME	GENERIC NAME
Nystatin Classification: Antifungal	nystatin, oral
Nystatin Classification: Antifungal	nystatin, topical
Nystatin Classification: Antifungal	nystatin, vaginal
Nystatin-LF I.V. Classification: Antifungal (Investigational)	AR-121
Nystex Classification: Antifungal	nystatin, topical
Nytol Classification: Antihistamine	diphenhydramine HCl

O

Obe-Nix Classification: CNS stimulant; anorexiant	phentermine HCl
OBY-CAP Classification: CNS stimulant; anorexiant	phentermine HCl
Occlusal HP Classification: Keratolytic	salicylic acid, topical
Ocean Classification: Nasal decongestant	sodium chloride, nasal
Ocean Mist Classification: Nasal decongestant	sodium chloride, nasal

BRAND NAME	GENERIC NAME
OCL Classification: Bowel evacuant	polyethylene glycol-electrolyte solution
Octamide PFS Classification: Antidopaminergic	metoclopramide
Octocaine HCl Classification: Local anesthetic	lidocaine HCl, local
Ocuclear Classification: Nasal decongestant	oxymetazoline HCl, ophthalmic
Ocucoat Classification: Ophthalmic viscoelastic	hydroxypropyl methylcellulose
OcuCoat Classification: Ophthalmic lubricant	artificial tears solution
OcuCoat PF Classification: Ophthalmic lubricant	artificial tears solution
Ocufen Classification: Ophthalmic nonsteroidal anti- inflammatory	flurbiprofen sodium
Ocuflox Classification: Antibiotic; fluoroquinolone	ofloxacin, ophthalmic
Ocupress Classification: Beta-adrenergic blocker	carteolol HCl
Ocusert Pilo-20 Classification: Miotic	pilocarpine ocular therapeutic system
Ocusert Pilo-40 Classification: Miotic	pilocarpine ocular therapeutic system

*Available in Canada only

BRAND NAME	GENERIC NAME

Off-Ezy Wart Remover
Classification:
Keratolytic

salicylic acid, topical

Ogen
Classification:
Estrogen

estropipate

Omnicef
Classification:
Antibiotic; dephalosporin

cefdinir

OmniHIB
Classification:
Vaccine

hemophilus b conjugate vaccine

Omnipaque
Classification:
Radiopaque agent

iohexol

Omnipen
Classification:
Antibiotic; aminopenicillin

ampicillin, oral

Omnipen-N
Classification:
Antibiotic; aminopenicillin

ampicillin sodium, parenteral

OMS Concentrate
Classification:
Opioid analgesic

morphine sulfate

Oncaspar
Classification:
Antineoplastic miscellaneous

pegaspargase (PEG-L-asparaginase)

Onocorad Ov103
Classification:
Antineoplastic (Orphan)

onocorad Ov103

Oncoscint CR/OV
Classification:
In vivo diagnostic (Orphan)

satumomab pendetide

Oncotice*
Classification:
Antineoplastic, miscellaneous

BCG, intravesical

*Available in Canada Only

BRAND NAME	GENERIC NAME
Oncotrac Melanoma Imaging Kit Classification: In vivo diagnostic (Orphan)	technetium Tc-99m antimelanoma monoclonal antibody
Oncovin Classification: Antineoplastic; mitotic inhibitor	vincristine sulfate (VCR;LCR)
Ony-Clear Classification: Antifungal	miconazole nitrate, topical
Opcon Classification: Ophthalmic vasoconstrictor	naphazoline HCl, ophthalmic
Operand Classification: Antiseptic; germicidal	povidone-iodine
Ophthalgan Classification: Hyperosmolar preparation	glycerin, ophthalmic
Ophthetic Classification: Local anesthetic	proparacaine HCl
Opium Tincture Deodorized Classification: Opioid analgesic	opium
Opticrom 4% Classification: Anti-inflammatory	cromolyn sodium, ophthalmic
Opticyl Classification: Mydriatic	tropicamide, ophthalmic
Optigene 3 Eye Drops Classification: Ophthalmic vasoconstrictor	tetrahydrozoline HCl, ophthalmic
Optimine Classification: Antihistamine	azatadine maleate

*Available in Canada only

BRAND NAME	GENERIC NAME
Optimmune Classification: Immunosuppressive (Orphan)	cyclosporine, ophthalmic
Optimoist Classification: Oral lubricant	saliva substitute
Optipranolol Classification: Beta-adrenergic blocker	metipranolol HCl
Optiray 160 Classification: Radiopaque agent	ioversol 34%
Optiray 240 Classification: Radiopaque agent	ioversol 51%
Optiray 320 Classification: Radiopaque agent	ioversol 68%
Optiray 350 Classification: Radiopaque agent	ioversol 74%
Optison Classification: Radiopaque agent	octaflurorpropane and human albumin microspheres
OR-Tyl Classification: Antispasmodic	dicyclomine HCl
Orabase-B Classification: Local anesthetic	benzocaine, oral
Orabase Baby Classification: Local anesthetic	benzocaine, oral
Oracit Classification: Systemic alkalinizer	citrate and citric acid

BRAND NAME	GENERIC NAME
Oragrafin Calcium Classification: Radiopaque agent	ipodate calcium
Oragrafin Sodium Classification: Radiopaque agent	ipodate sodium
Orajel Classification: Local anesthetic	benzocaine, oral
Orajel Perioseptic Classification: Antiseptic	carbamide peroxide (urea peroxide)
Oralone Dental Classification: Glucocorticoid	triamcinolone acetonide (topical-oral)
Oramorph SR Classification: Opioid analgesic	morphine
Orap Classification: Antipsychotic	pimozide
Orasone Classification: Glucocorticoid	prednisone
Orazinc Classification: Electrolyte replacement; zinc	zinc sulfate
Orbenin* Classification: Antibiotic; penicillinase-resistant penicillin	cloxacillin sodium
Oretic Classification: Thiazide diuretic	hydrochlorothiazide
Oreton Methyl Classification: Androgen	methyltestosterone

*Available in Canada only

BRAND NAME	GENERIC NAME

Organidin
Classification:
Expectorant

iodinated glycerol

Organidin NR
Classification:
Expectorant

guaifenesin

Orgaran
Classification:
Anticoagulant

danaproid

Orgotein
Classification:
Anti-amyotrophic lateral sclerosis agent
(Orphan)

orgotein

Orimune
Classification:
Vaccine

poliovirus vaccine, live, oral, trivalent
(TOPV; SABINE)

Orinase
Classification:
Antidiabetic; sulfonylurea

tolbutamide

Orinase Diagnostic
Classification:
In vivo diagnostic; sulfonylurea

tolbutamide sodium

ORLAAM
Classification:
Opioid agonist

levomethadyl acetate HCl

Ormazine
Classification:
Antipsychotic

chlorpromazine HCl

Ornidyl
Classification:
Antiprotozoal

eflornithine HCl (DMFO)

Orphenadrine Citrate
Classification:
Skeletal muscle relaxant, centrally acting

orphenadrine citrate

Orthoclone OKT3
Classification:
Immunosuppressive

muromonab-CD3

*Available in Canada Only

BRAND NAME	GENERIC NAME
Ortho Dienestrol Classification: Estrogen	dienestrol
Ortho-Est Classification: Estrogen	estropipate
Orudis Classification: Nonsteroidal anti-inflammatory	ketoprofen
Orudis KT Classification: Nonsteroidal anti-inflammatory	ketoprofen
Os-Cal 500 Classification: Antacid; calcium supplement	calcium carbonate
Osmoglyn Classification: Hyperosmotic	glycerin (glycerol)
Osteo-D Classification: Vitamin, fat soluble (Orphan)	secalciferol
Osteocalcin Classification: Parathyroid agent	calcitonin (salmon)
Osytercal 500 Classification: Antacid; calcium supplement	calcium carbonate
Otrivin Classification: Nasal decongestant	xylometazoline HCl, nasal
Otrivin Pediatric Nasal Drops Classification: Nasal decongestant	xylometazoline HCl, nasal
Ovide Classification: Scabicide; pediculicide	malathion

*Available in Canada only

BRAND NAME	GENERIC NAME
Ovol* Classification: Antiflatulent	simethicone
Ovral* Classification: Progestin	norgestrel
Ovrette Classification: Progestin	norgestrel
Oxacillin Sodium Classification: Antibiotic; penicillinase-resistant penicillin	oxacillin sodium
Oxaliplatin Classification: Antineoplastic (Orphan)	oxaliplatin
Oxandrin Classification: Anabolic steroid	oxandrolone
Oxazepam Classification: Antianxiety; benzodiazepine	oxazepam
Oxistat Classification: Antifungal	oxiconazole nitrate
Oxsoralen Classification: Psoralen	methoxsalen, topical (8-methoxypsoralen, 8-MOP)
Oxsoralen-Ultra Classification: Psoralen	methoxsalen, oral (8-methoxypsoralen, 8-MOP)
Oxtriphylline Classification: Bronchodilator; xanthine	oxtriphylline
Oxy 5 Classification: Anti-acne product	benzoyl peroxide

*Available in Canada Only

BRAND NAME	GENERIC NAME
Oxy 10 Classification: Anti-acne product	benzoyl peroxide
Oxy 10 Wash Classification: Anti-acne product	benzoyl peroxide
Oxybutinin Chloride Classification: Urinary antispasmodic	oxybutynin chloride
Oxycel Classification: Hemostatic	oxidized cellulose
OxyContin Classification: Opioid analgesic	oxycodone HCl
Oxydess II Classification: CNS stimulant	dextroamphetamine sulfate
OxylR Classification: Opioid analgesic	oxycodone HCl
Oxymetazoline HCl Classification: Nasal decongestant	oxymetazoline HCl, nasal
Oxytetracycline HCl Classification: Antibiotic; tetracycline	oxytetracycline HCl
Oxytocin Classification: Oxytocic	oxytocin, parenteral
Oysco 500 Classification: Antacid; calcium supplement	calcium carbonate
Oyst-Cal 500 Classification: Antacid; calcium supplement	calcium carbonate

*Available in Canada only

BRAND NAME	GENERIC NAME

Oyster Shell Calcium 500
Classification:
Antacid; calcium supplement

calcium carbonate

P

Pacis*
Classification:
Antineoplastic, miscellaneous

BCG, intravesical

Packer's Pine Tar
Classification:
Keratolytic

coal tar

Palmitrate - A 5000
Classification:
Vitamin, fat soluble

vitamin A

PALS
Classification:
Systemic deodorizer

chlorophyl derivatives

Pamelor
Classification:
Antidepressant

nortriptyline HCl

Pamine
Classification:
Anticholinergic

methscopolamine bromide

Pamisyl
Classification:
Anti-inflammatory (Orphan)

4-aminosalicylic acid

Panadol
Classification:
Analgesic; antipyretic

acetaminophen

Panadol Infant's Drops
Classification:
Analgesic; antipyretic

acetaminophen

Panadol Junior Strength
Classification:
Analgesic; antipyretic

acetaminophen

BRAND NAME	GENERIC NAME
Panasol-S Classification: Glucocorticoid	prednisone
Panavir Classification: Antiviral (Investigational)	panavir
Pancrease Capsules Classification: Digestive enzyme	pancrelipase
Pancreas MT4 Classification: Digestive enzyme	pancrelipase
Pancrease MT10 Classification: Digestive enzyme	pancrelipase
Pancrease MT16 Classification: Digestive enzyme	pancrelipase
Pancrease MT 20 Classification: Digestive enzyme	pancrelipase
Pancrezyme 4X Classification: Digestive enzyme	pancreatin
Pancuronium Bromide Classification: Nondepolarizing neuromuscular blocker	pancuronium bromide
Pandel Classification: Glucocorticoid	hydrocortisone buteprate
Panectyl* Classification: Antihistamine	trimeprazine
Panhematin Classification: Antiporphyrial	hemin

BRAND NAME	GENERIC NAME

Panmycin
Classification:
Antibiotic; tetracycline

tetracycline HCl

PanOxyl 10
Classification:
Anti-acne product

benzoyl peroxide

PanOxyl 15
Classification:
Anti-acne product

benzoyl peroxide

PanOxyl AQ 2 ½
Classification:
Anti-acne product

benzoyl peroxide

PanOxyl AQ 5
Classification:
Anti-acne product

benzoyl peroxide

PanOxyl AQ 10
Classification:
Anti-acne product

benzoyl peroxide

Panretin Oral
Classification:
Biologic response modifier
(Investigational)

panretin oral

Panscol
Classification:
Keratolytic

salicylic acid, topical

Papaverine HCl
Classification:
Peripheral vasodilator

papaverine HCl

Paplex Ultra
Classification:
Keratolytic

salicylic acid, topical

Para-Aminobenzoic Acid
Classification:
Vitamin, water soluble

para-aminobenzoic acid (PABA)

Paraflex
Classification:
Skeletal muscle relaxant, centrally acting

chlorzoxazone

BRAND NAME	GENERIC NAME
Parafon Forte DSC Classification: Skeletal muscle relaxant, centrally acting	chlorzoxazone
Paral Classification: Anticonvulsant	paraldehyde
Paraldehyde Classification: Anticonvulsant	paraldehyde
Paraplatin Classification: Antineoplastic; alkylating agent	carboplatin
Parathar Classification: Hormone	teriparatide acetate
Paredrine 1% Ophthalmic Classification: Ophthalmic vasoconstrictor	hydroxyamphetamine HBr
Paregoric Classification: Opioid analgesic	opium
Paregorique* Classification: Opioid analgesic	opium
Par Glycerol Classification: Expectorant	iodinated glycerol
Parlodel Classification: Dopamine receptor agonist	bromocriptine mesylate
Parnate Classification: Monoamine oxidase inhibitor	tranylcypromine sulfate
Paromomycin Classification: Antitubercular (Orphan)	aminosidine

*Available in Canada only

BRAND NAME	GENERIC NAME
Paser Classification: Antitubercular	aminosalicylic acid
Patanol Classification: Antihistamine, ophthalmic	olopatidine
Pathilon Classification: Anticholinergic	tridihexethyl chloride
Pathocil Classification: Antibiotic; penicillinase-resistant penicillin	dicloxacillin sodium
Pavabid Plateau Caps Classification: Peripheral vasodilator	papaverine HCl
Pavagen TD Classification: Peripheral vasodilator	papaverine HCl
Pavatine Classification: Peripheral vasodilator	papaverine HCl
Pavulon Classification: Nondepolarizing neuromuscular blocker	pancuronium bromide
Paxarel Classification: Sedative-hypnotic; nonbarbiturate	acetylcarbromal
Paxil Classification: Antidepressant	paroxetine
Paxipam Classification: Antianxiety; benzodiazepine	halazepam
PBZ Classification: Antihistamine	tripelennamine HCl

*Available in Canada Only

BRAND NAME	GENERIC NAME
PBZ-SR Classification: Antihistamine	tripelennamine HCl
PCE Dispertab Classification: Antibiotic; macrolide	erythromycin base
Pedameth Classification: Amino acid	methionine
Pedi-Boro Soak Paks Classification: Astringent	aluminum acetate solution
Pedia Care Allergy Formula Classification: Antihistamine	chlorpheniramine meleate
Pedia Care Infant's Decongestant Classification: Nasal decongestant	pseudoephedrine HCl
Pediaflor Classification: Electrolyte replacement; fluoride	sodium fluoride
Pediapred Classification: Glucocorticoid	prednisolone sodium phosphate
Pediatric Gentamicin Sulfate Classification: Aminoglycoside	gentamicin sulfate
Pediatric Triban Classification: Antiemetic; anticholinergic	trimethobenzamide HCl
PedvaxHIB Classification: Vaccine	hemophilus b conjugate vaccine
Peganone Classification: Anticonvulsant	ethotoin

*Available in Canada only

BRAND NAME	GENERIC NAME
Pen-V Classification: Antibiotic; penicillin	penicillin V potassium
Pen-Vee K Classification: Antibiotic; penicillin	penicillin V potassium
Penecort Classification: Glucocorticoid	hydrocortisone, topical
Penetrex Classification: Antibiotic; fluoroquinolone	enoxacin
Penglobe* Classification: Antibiotic; aminopenicillin	bacampicillin HCl
Penicillin G Potassium Classification: Antibiotic; penicillin	penicillin G aqueous, parenteral
Penicillin G Sodium Classification: Antibiotic; penicillin	penicillin G aqueous, parenteral
Penicillin VK Classification: Antibiotic; penicillin	penicillin V potassium
Pentacarinat Classification: Antiprotozoal	pentamidine isethionate
Pentam 300 Classification: Antiprotozoal	pentamidine isethionate
Pentamidine Isethionate Classification: Antiprotazoal	pentamidine isethionate
Pentamycin* Classification: Antibacterial	chloramphenicol, ophthalmic

*Available in Canada Only

BRAND NAME	GENERIC NAME
Pentasa Classification: GI anti-inflammatory	mesalamine
Penthrane Classification: General anesthetic	methoxyflurane
Pentobarbital Sodium Classification: Sedative-hypnotic; barbiturate	pentobarbital sodium
Pentogen* Classification: Sedative-hypnotic; barbiturate	pentobarbital sodium
Pentostam Classification: CDC anti-infective	sodium antimony gluconate
Pentothal Classification: General anesthetic; barbiturate	thiopental sodium
Pentoxifylline Classification: Hemorheologic agent	pentoxifylline
Pentrax Classification: Keratolytic	coal tar
Pentrax Gold Classification: Keratolytic	coal tar
Penumomist Classification: Expectorant	guaifenesin
Pepcid Classification: Histamine H_2 receptor antagonist	famotidine
Pepcid AC Acid Controller Classification: Histamine H_2 receptor antagonist	famotidine

*Available in Canada only

BRAND NAME	GENERIC NAME
Pepcid IV Classification: Histamine H$_2$ receptor antagonist	famotidine
Peptavlon Classification: Antineoplastic; antibiotic	pentagastrin
Pepto-Bismol Classification: Antidiarrheal	bismuth subsalicylate
Pepto-Bismol Maximum Strength Classification: Antidiarrheal	bismuth subsalicylate
Perchloracap Classification: Radiopaque agent	potassium perchlorate
Perdiem Classification: Laxative, bulk-producing	psyllium
Pergonal Classification: Gonadotropin	menotropins
Periactne Classification: Antihistamine	cyproheptadine HCl
Peridex Classification: Antibacterial	chlorhexidine gluconate, oral
PerioGard Classification: Antibacterial	chlorhexidine gluconate, oral
Permapen Classification: Antibiotic; penicillin	penicillin G benzathine, parenteral
Permax Classification: Antiparkinson agent	pergolide mesylate

*Available in Canada Only

BRAND NAME	GENERIC NAME
Permitil Classification: Antipsychotic	fluphenazine HCl
Peroxin A5 Classification: Anti-acne product	benzoyl peroxide
Peroxin A10 Classification: Anti-acne product	benzoyl peroxide
Perphenazine Classification: Antipsychotic	perphenazine
Persa-Gel Classification: Anti-acne product	benzoyl peroxide
Pers-Gel W 5% Classification: Anti-acne product	benzoyl peroxide
Persa-Gel W 10% Classification: Anti-acne product	benzoyl peroxide
Persantine Classification: Antiplatelet	dipyridamole
Persantine IV Classification: Antiplatelet	dipyridamole
Pertussin Classification: Non-narcotic antitussive	dextromethorphan
Pertussin ES Classification: Non-narcotic antitussive	dextromethorphan
Petrogalar Plain Classification: Laxative, emollient	mineral oil

*Available in Canada only

BRAND NAME	GENERIC NAME

Pfeiffer's Allergy
Classification:
Antihistamine

chlorpheniramine maleate

Pfizerpen
Classification:
Antibiotic; penicillin

penicillin G (aqueous), parenteral

Pharmaflur
Classification:
Electrolyte replacement; fluoride

sodium fluoride

Pharmaflur df
Classification:
Electrolyte replacement; fluoride

sodium fluoride

Pharmaflur 1.1
Classification:
Electrolyte replacement; fluoride

sodium fluoride

Phazyme
Classification:
Antiflatulent

simethicone

Phazyme 95
Classification:
Antiflatulent

simethicone

Phazyme 125
Classification:
Antiflatulent

simethicone

Phenazo*
Classification:
Urinary analgesic

phenazopyridine HCl

Phenazopyridine HCl
Classification:
Urinary analgesic

phenazopyridine HCl

Phendimetrazine Tartrate
Classification:
CNS stimulant; anorexiant

phendimetrazine tartrate

Phenfomin
Classification:
Antidiabetic; biguanide (Investigational)

phenformin

BRAND NAME	GENERIC NAME

Phendry
Classification:
Antihistamine

diphenhydramine HCl

Phenergan
Classification:
Antihistamine

promethazine HCl

Phenergan Fortis
Classification:
Antihistamine

promethazine HCl

Phenergan Plain
Classification:
Antihistamine

promethazine HCl

Phenobarbital
Classification:
Sedative-hypnotic; barbiturate

phenobarbital sodium

Phenobarbital Sodium
Classification:
Sedative-hypnotic; barbiturate

phenobarbital sodium

Phenolax
Classification:
Laxative, irritant

phenolphthalein

Phenoxine
Classification:
Alpha-adrenergic agonist

phenylpropanolamine HCl

Phentermine HCl
Classification:
CNS stimulant; anorexiant

phentermine HCl

Phentermine Resin
Classification:
CNS stimulant; anorexiant

phentermine HCl

Phenylase
Classification:
Enzyme (Orphan)

phenylalanine ammonia-lyase

Phenylephrine HCl
Classification:
Adrenergic agonist

phenylephrine HCl

BRAND NAME	GENERIC NAME

Phenylephrine HCl
Classification:
Adrenergic agonist

phenylephrine HCl

Phenylephrine HCl
Classification:
Ophthalmic vasoconstrictor

phenylephrine HCl, ophthalmic

Phenylpropanolamine
Classification:
Alpha-adrenergic agonist

phenylpropanolamine HCl

Phenytoin Sodium
Classification:
Anticonvulsant; hydantoin

phenytoin sodium, parenteral

Phenytoin Sodium
Classification:
Anticonvulsant; hydantoin

phenytoin sodium, extended

Phenytoin Sodium
Classification:
Anticonvulsant; hydantoin

phenytoin sodium, prompt

Phillip's Milk of Magnesia
Classification:
Antacid; laxative

magnesia (magnesium hydroxide)

pHisoHex
Classification:
Germicidal

hexachlorophene

Phos-Flur
Classification:
Electrolyte replacement; fluoride

sodium fluoride

Phos-Lo
Classification:
Electrolyte replacement; calcium

calcium acetate

Phosphocol P32
Classification:
Antineoplastic; radiopharmaceutical

chromic phosphate P32

Phospholine Iodide
Classification:
Miotic

echothiophate iodide

BRAND NAME	GENERIC NAME
Photofrin Classification: Antineoplastic, miscellaneous	porfimer sodium
Phyllocontin Classification: Bronchodilator; xanthine	aminophylline (theophylline ethylenediamine)
Pilagan Classification: Miotic	pilocarpine nitrate
Pilocar Classification: Miotic	pilocarpine HCl
Pilocarpine HCl Classification: Miotic	pilocarpine HCl
Pilopine HS Classification: Miotic	pilocarpine HCl
Piloptic-1 Classification: Miotic	pilocarpine HCl
Piloptic-2 Classification: Miotic	pilocarpine HCl
Pima Classification: Expectorant	iodine products
Pin-Rid Classification: Anthelmintics	pyrantel pamoate
Pin-X Classification: Anthelmintics	pyrantel pamoate
Pindolol Classification: Antihypertensive; beta-adrenergic blocker	pindolol

*Available in Canada only

BRAND NAME	GENERIC NAME

Pipracil
Classification:
Antibiotic; extended spectrum penicillin

piperacillin sodium

Pitocin
Classification:
Oxytocic

oxytocin, parenteral

Pitressin Synthetic
Classification:
Posterior pituitary hormone

vasopressin

Placidyl
Classification:
Sedative-hypnotic; nonbarbiturate

ethchlorvynol

Plague Vaccine
Classification:
Vaccine

plague vaccine

Plaquase
Classification:
Enzyme (Orphan)

collagenase

Plaquenil Sulfate
Classification:
Antimalarial

hydroxychloroquine sulfate

Plasbumin-5
Classification:
Blood derivative

albumin human 5%

Plasbumin-25
Classification:
Blood derivative

albumin human 25%

Plasma-Plex
Classification:
Blood derivative

plasma protein fraction

Plasmanate
Classification:
Blood derivative

plasma protein fraction

Platinol-AQ
Classification:
Antineoplastic; alkylating agent

cisplatin (CDDP)

BRAND NAME	GENERIC NAME
Plavix Classification: Antiplatelet	clopidogrel
Plegine Classification: CNS stimulant; anorexiant	phendimetrazine tartrate
Plegisol Classification: Cardioplegic solution	cardioplegic solution
Plendil Classification: Calcium channel blocker	felodipine
PMEA Classification: Antiviral (Investigational)	PMEA
PMS-Bethanechol Chloride* Classification: Cholinergic stimulant	bethanechol chloride
PMS-Dicitrate* Classification: Urinary alkalinizer	sodium citrate/citric acid solution (Shohl's Solution)
PMS-Isoniazid* Classification: Antitubercular	isoniazid (INH)
PMS-Metronidazole* Classification: Antibacterial; amebicide	metronidazole
Pneumovax 23 Classification: Vaccine	pneumococcal vaccine, polyvalent
Pnu-Imune 23 Classification: Vaccine	pneumococcal vaccine, polyvalent
Pod-Ben-25 Classification: Keratolytic	podophyllum resin

*Available in Canada only

BRAND NAME	GENERIC NAME

Podocon-25
Classification:
Keratolytic

podophyllum resin

Podofilm*
Classification:
Keratolytic

podophyllum resin

Podofin
Classification:
Keratolytic

podophyllum resin

Point-Two
Classification:
Electrolyte replacement; fluoride

sodium fluoride

Polaramine
Classification:
Antihistamine

dexchlorpheniramine maleate

Polocaine
Classification:
Local anesthetic

mepivacaine HCl

Polocaine MPF
Classification:
Local anesthetic

mepivacaine HCl

Polycillin
Classification:
Antibiotic; aminopenicillin

ampicillin, oral

Polycillin-N
Classification:
Antibiotic; aminopenicillin

ampicillin sodium, parenteral

Polycillin Pediatric Drops
Classification:
Antibiotic; aminopenicillin

ampicillin, oral

Polycillin-PRB
Classification:
Antibiotic; aminopenicillin

ampicillin with probenecid

Polycitra
Classification:
System alkalinizer

citrate and citric acid

BRAND NAME	GENERIC NAME
Polycitra Classification: Urinary alkalinizer	potassium citrate and citric acid
Polycitra-K Classification: Urinary alkalinizer	potassium citrate and citric acid
Polycitra-LC Classification: Systemic alkalinizer	citrate and citric acid
Polycitra-LC Classification: Urinary alkalinizer	potassium citrate and citric acid
Polydine Classification: Antiseptic; germicidal	povidone and iodine
Polygam S/D Classification: Immune serum	immune globulin intravenous (IVIG)
Polymox Classification: Antibiotic; aminopenicillin	amoxicillin trihydrate
Polymox Drops Classification: Antibiotic; aminopenicillin	amoxicillin trihydrate
Polymyxin B Sulfate Classification: Antibiotic; polymyxin	polymyxin B sulfate, parenteral
Polymyxin B Sulfate, Ophthalmic Classification: Antibiotic; polymyxin	polymyxin B sulfate, sterile ophthalmic
Polytar Classification: Keratolytic	coal tar
Polytar Bath Classification: Keratolytic	coal tar

BRAND NAME	GENERIC NAME

Ponstel
Classification:
Nonsteroidal anti-inflammatory

mefenamic acid

Pontocaine Eye
Classification:
Local anesthetic

tetracaine HCl, ophthalmic

Pontocaine HCl
Classification:
Local anesthetic

tetracaine HCl, topical

Pontocaine HCl
Classification:
Local anesthetic

tetracaine HCl, ophthalmic

Pontocaine HCl
Classification:
Local anesthetic

tetracaine HCl

Porcelana
Classification:
Depigmentation

hydroquinone

Porcelana with Sunscreen
Classification:
Depigmentation

hydroquinone

Porfiromycin
Classification:
Antineoplastic (Orphan)

porfiromycin

Pork NPH Iletin II
Classification:
Antidiabetic

insulin, isophane suspension (NPH)

Pork Regular Iletin II
Classification:
Antidiabetic

insulin injection

Posicor
Classification:
Antihypertensive; calcium channel
blocker

mibefradil dihydrochloride

Posture
Classification:
Electrolyte replacement; calcium

tricalcium phosphate

BRAND NAME	GENERIC NAME
Potaba Classification: Vitamin, water soluble	para-aminobenzoic acid (PABA)
Potassium Chloride Classification: Electrolyte replacement; potassium	potassium chloride
Potassium Gluconate Classification: Electrolyte replacement; potassium	potassium gluconate
Potassium Iodide Classification: Expectorant	iodine products
Potassium Iodide Solution Classification: Antithyroid agent	potassium iodide
Povidine Classification: Antiseptic; germicidal	povidone-iodine
PPF Classification: Blood derivative	plasma protein fraction
Pralidoxime Chloride Classification: Cholinesterase reactivator	pralidoxime chloride (2-PAM)
Pramegel Classification: Local anesthetic	pramoxine HCl, topical
Prandase* Classification: Antidiabetic	acarbose
Prandin Classification: Antidiabetic; meglitinide	repaglinide
Pravachol Classification: Antilipemic	pravastatin sodium

*Available in Canada only

BRAND NAME	GENERIC NAME

Prax
Classification:
Local anesthetic

pramoxine HCl, topical

Prazepam
Classification:
Antianxiety; benzodiazepine

prazepam

Prazosin
Classification:
Antihypertensive; alpha-adrenergic
blocker

prazosin

Pre-Pen
Classification:
Skin test antigen

benzylpencilloyl-polylysine

Precose
Classification:
Antidiabetic

acarbose

Pred Forte
Classification:
Glucocorticoid

prednisolone acetate ophthalmic,
suspension

Pred Mild
Classification:
Glucocorticoid

prednisolone acetate ophthalmic,
suspension

Predalone 50
Classification:
Glucocorticoid

prednisolone acetate

Predcor-50
Classification:
Glucocorticoid

prednisolone acetate

Prednicen-M
Classification:
Glucocorticoid

prednisone

Prednisol TBA
Classification:
Glucocorticoid

prednisolone tebutate

Prednisolone
Classification:
Glucocorticoid

prednisolone

BRAND NAME	GENERIC NAME
Prednisolone Acetate Classification: Glucocorticoid	prednisolone acetate
Prednisolone Acetate Ophthalmic Classification: Ophthalmic glucocorticoid	prednisolone acetate ophthalmic, suspension
Prednisolone Tebutate Classification: Glucocorticoid	prednisolone tebutate
Prednisone Classification: Glucocorticoid	prednisone
Prednisone Intensol Concentrate Classification: Glucocorticoid	prednisone
Pregnyl Classification: Chorionic gonadotropin	chorionic gonadotropin, human (HCG)
Prelone Classification: Glucocorticoid	prednisolone
Prelu-2 Classification: CNS stimulant; anorexiant	phendimetrazine tartrate
Premarin Classification: Estrogen	estrogens, conjugated
Premarin Intravenous Classification: Estrogen	estrogens, conjugated
Prepcat Classification: Radiopaque agent	barium sulfate

BRAND NAME	GENERIC NAME

Prepidil Gel
Classification:
Oxytocic; prostaglandin

dinoprostone

Pretz
Classification:
Nasal decongestant

sodium chloride, nasal

Prevacid
Classification:
Antisecretory; benzimidazoles

lansoprazole

Prevalite
Classification:
Antilipemic

cholesyramine

Prevident
Classification:
Electrolyte replacement; fluoride

sodium fluoride

Prilosec
Classification:
Proton pump inhibitor

omeprazole

Primacor
Classification:
Cardiac inotrope

milrinone lactate

Primaquine Phosphate
Classification:
Antimalarial

primaquine phosphate

Primatene Mist
Classification:
Adrenergic agonist

epinephrine

Primaxin I.M.
Classification:
Antibiotic; carbapenem

imipenem-cilastatin

Primaxin I.V.
Classification:
Antibiotic; carbapenem

imipenem-cilastatin

Primidone
Classification:
Anticonvulsant

primidone

BRAND NAME	GENERIC NAME
Principen Classification: Antibiotic; aminopenicillin	ampicillin, oral
Prinivil Classification: Antihypertensive; angiotensin converting enzyme inhibitor	lisinopril
Priscoline Classification: Antihypertensive; vasodilator	tolazoline HCl
Privine Classification: Nasal decongestant	naphazoline HCl, nasal
Pro-Banthine Classification: Anticholinergic	propantheline bromide
Pro-Bionate Classification: Antidiarrheal	lactobacillus
Pro-Cal-Sof Classification: Laxative, softener	docusate calcium
Pro-Depo Classification: Progestin	hydroxyprogesterone caproate
ProAmatine Classification: Adrenergic agonist	midodrine HCl
Probampacin Classification: Antibiotic; aminopenicillin	ampicillin with probenecid
Probenecid Classification: Uricosuric	probenecid
Procainamide HCl Classification: Antiarrhythmic	procainamide sustained, release

BRAND NAME	GENERIC NAME
Procainamide HCl Classification: Antiarrhythmic	procainamide HCl
Procaine HCl Classification: Local anesthetic	procaine HCl
Procanabid Classification: Antiarrhythmic	procainamide, extended release
Procardia Classification: Calcium channel blocker	nifedipine
Procardia XL Classification: Calcium channel blocker	nifedipine
Prochlorperazine Classification: Antipsychotic	prochlorperazine
Procrit Classification: Hormone, amino acid polypeptide	epoetin alfa (erythropoietin, EPO)
Proctocort Classification: Glucocorticoid	hydrocortisone, topical
ProctoCream-HC Classification: Glucocorticoid	hydrocortisone, topical
Proctofoam NS Classification: Local anesthetic	pramoxine HCl, topical
Procyclid* Classification: Anticholinergic	procyclidine HCl
Procysteine Classification: Amino acid (Orphan)	L-2-oxothiazolidine-4-carboxylic acid

*Available in Canada Only

BRAND NAME	GENERIC NAME
Procytox* Classification: Antineoplastic; alkylating agent	cyclophosphamide
Prodiem Plain* Classification: Laxative, bulk-producing	psyllium
Prodium Classification: Urinary analgesic	phenazopyridine HCl
Profasi Classification: Chorionic gonadotropin	chorionic gonadotropin, human (HCG)
Profenal Classification: Ophthalmic nonsteroidal anti-inflammatory	suprofen
Profilnine SD Classification: Hemostatic	factor IX complex (human)
Progestasert Classification: Progestin	progesterone intrauterine system
Progesterone Classification: Progestin	progesterone powder
Progesterone In Oil Classification: Progestin	progesterone in oil
Proglycem Classification: Glucose elevating agent	diazoxide, oral
Prograf Classification: Immunosuppressive	tacrolimus (FK506)
ProHance Classification: Radiopaque agent	gadoteridol

*Available in Canada only

BRAND NAME	GENERIC NAME

ProHIBiT
Classification:
Vaccine

hemophilus b conjugate vaccine

Prolastin
Classification:
Enzyme replacement

alpha-1-proteinase inhibitor (human)

Proleukin
Classification:
Antineoplastic; biologic response
modifier

aldesleukin (interleukin-2; IL-2)

Prolixin
Classification:
Antipsychotic

fluphenazine HCl

Prolixin Decanoate
Classification:
Antipsychotic

fluphenazine enanthate and decanoate

Prolixin Enanthate
Classification:
Antipsychotic

fluphenazine enanthate and decanoate

Proloprim
Classification:
Antibiotic, folic acid antagonist

trimethoprim

Promanyl*
Classification:
Antipsychotic

promazine HCl

Promazine HCl
Classification:
Antipsychotic

promazine HCl

Promethazine HCl
Classification:
Antihistamine

promethazine HCl

Prometrium
Classification:
Progestin

progesterone

Promit
Classification:
Plasma volume expander

dextran 1

BRAND NAME	GENERIC NAME
Pronestyl Classification: Antiarrhythmic	procainamide HCl
Pronestyl-SR Classification: Antiarrhythmic	procainamide sustained release
Propagest Classification: Alpha-adrenergic agonist	phenylpropanolamine HCl
Propantheline Bromide Classification: Anticholinergic	propantheline bromide
Proparacaine HCl Classification: Local anesthetic	proparacaine HCl
Propecia Classification: Androgen inhibitor	finasteride
Propine Classification: Adrenergic agonist	dipivefrin HCl
Proplex T Classification: Hemostatic	factor IX complex (human)
Propoxyphene HCl Classification: Opioid analgesic	propoxyphene HCl
Propranolol HCl Classification: Beta-adrenergic blocker	propranolol HCl
Propranolol Intensol Classification: Beta-adrenergic blocker	propranolol HCl
Propulsid Classification: Gastrointestinal stimulant	cisapride

BRAND NAME	GENERIC NAME

Propyl-thyracil*
Classification:
Antithyroid agent
propylthiouracil (PTU)

Propylthiouracil
Classification:
Antithyroid agent
propylthiouracil (PTU)

Proscar
Classification:
Androgen inhibitor
finasteride

ProSom
Classification:
Sedative-hypnotic; benzodiazepine
estazolam

ProStep
Classification:
Smoking deterrent
nicotine transdermal system

Prostigmin
Classification:
Anticholinesterase
neostigmine

Prostin/15M
Classification:
Oxytocic; prostaglandin
carboprost tromethamine

Prostin VR Pediatric
Classification:
Prostaglandin
alprostadil (PGE$_1$)

Protamine Sulfate
Classification:
Heparin antagonist
protamine sulfate

Prostaphlin
Classification:
Antibiotic; penicillinase-resistant
penicillin
oxacillin sodium

Protar Protein
Classification:
Keratolytic
coal tar

Protectol
Classification:
Antifungal
undecylenic acid

BRAND NAME	GENERIC NAME
Protein C Concentrate Classification: Hemostatic (Orphan)	protein C concentrate
Protenate Classification: Blood derivative	plasma protein fraction
Prothazine Classification: Antihistamine	promethazine HCl
Prothazine Plain Classification: Antihistamine	promethazine HCl
Protopam Chloride Classification: Cholinesterase reactivator	pralidoxime chloride (2-PAM)
Protophylline* Classification: Bronchodilator, xanthine	dyphylline (dihydroxypropyl theophylline)
Protostat Classification: Antibacterial; amebicide	metronidazole
Protox Classification: Antimalarial (Orphan)	poloxamer 331
Protiptyline HCl Classification: Antidepressant, tricyclic	protriptyline HCl
Protropin Classification: Growth hormone	somatrem
Proventil Classification: Bronchodilator; beta-adrenergic agonist	albuterol
Proventil HFA Classification: Bronchodilator; beta-adrenergic agonist	albuterol sulfate

*Available in Canada only

BRAND NAME	GENERIC NAME
Proventil Repetabs Classification: Bronchodilator; beta-adrenergic agonist	albuterol
Provera Classification: Progestin	medroxyprogesterone acetate
Provigil Classification: Centrally acting alpha agonist	modafinil
Proviodine* Classification: Antiseptic; germicidal	povidone-iodine
Provocholine Classification: Cholinergic	methacholine chloride
Proxigel Classification: Antiseptic	carbamide peroxide (urea peroxide)
Prozac Classification: Antidepressant	fluoxetine
Prozine-50 Classification: Antipsychotic	promazine HCl
Prulet Classification: Laxative, irritant	phenolphthalein
Pseudoephedrine HCl Classification: Nasal decongestant	pseudoephedrine HCl
Pseudogest Decongestant Classification: Nasal decongestant	pseudoephedrine HCl
Psor-a-set Classification: Keratolytic	salicylic acid, topical

*Available in Canada Only

BRAND NAME	GENERIC NAME
Psorcon Classification: Glucocorticoid	diflorasone diacetate
Psorinail Classification: Keratolytic	coal tar
Pulmicort Turbuhaler Classification: Glucocorticoid	budesonide
Pulmozyme Classification: Mucolytic	dornase alfa
Puralube Tears Classification: Ophthalmic lubricant	artificial tears solution
Purge Classification: Laxative, irritant	castor oil
Purinol* Classification: Uricosuric	allopurinol
Purinethol Classification: Antineoplastic; antimetabolite	mercaptopurine (6-MP; 6-mercaptopurine)
PVFK* Classification: Antibiotic; penicillin	penicillin V potassium
Pyrazinamide Classification: Antitubercular	pyrazinamide
Pyridiate Classification: Urinary analgesic	phenazopyridine HCl
Pyridium Classification: Urinary analgesic	phenazopyridine HCl

BRAND NAME	GENERIC NAME

Pyridoxine HCl
Classification:
Vitamin, water soluble

pyridoxine HCl (vitamin B_6)

Q

Quadramet
Classification:
Radiopharmaceutical

samarium Sm 153 lexidronam

Quarzan
Classification:
Anticholinergic

clidinium bromide

Quelicin
Classification:
Depolarizing neuromuscular blocker

succinylcholine chloride

Questran
Classification:
Antilipemic

cholestyramine

Questran Light
Classification:
Antilipemic

cholestyramine

Quibron-T Dividose
Classification:
Bronchodilator; xanthine

theophylline

Quibron-T/SR Dividose
Classification:
Bronchodilator; xanthine

theophylline

Quick Pep
Classification:
Analeptic

caffeine

Quiess
Classification:
Antianxiety

hydroxyzine HCl

Quinaglute Dura-Tabs
Classification:
Antiarrhythmic

quinidine gluconate

BRAND NAME	GENERIC NAME
Quinalan Classification: Antiarrhythmic	quinidine gluconate
Quinidex Extentabs Classification: Antiarrhythmic	quinidine sulfate
Quinidine Gluconate Classification: Antiarrhythmic	quinidine gluconate
Quinidine Sulfate Classification: Antiarrhythmic	quinidine sulfate
Quinine Sulfate Classification: Antimalarial	quinine sulfate
Quinora Classification: Antiarrhythmic	quinidine sulfate
Quinsana Plus Classification: Antifungal	tolnaftate

R

R-Gel Classification: Analgesic	capsaicin
R-Gen Classification: Expectorant	iodinated glycerol
R-Gene 10 Classification: Pituitary function test	arginine HCl
RabAvert Classification: Vaccine	rabies vaccine

*Available in Canada only

BRAND NAME	GENERIC NAME

Ramses
Classification:
Spermicide

nonoxynol

Rantidine
Classification:
Histamine H_2 receptor antagonist

rantidine

Raxar
Classification:
Antibiotic; fluoroquinolone

grepafloxacin

Rebif
Classification:
Antimultiple sclerosis agent
(Investigational)

interferon beta-1a

Receptin
Classification:
Immune serum (Orphan)

CD4, recombinant soluble human (rCD4)

Reclomide
Classification:
Antidopaminergic

metoclopramide

Recombinate
Classification:
Hemostatic

antihemophilic factor (AHF, Factor VIII)

Recombivax HB
Classification:
Vaccine

hepatitis B vaccine

Redoxon*
Classification:
Vitamin, water soluble

ascorbic acid (vitamin C)

Redutemp
Classification:
Analgesic; antipyretic

acetaminophen

Reese's Pinworm
Classification:
Anthelmintics

pyrantel pamoate

REFACTO
Classification:
Hemostatic (Orphan)

R-VIII SQ

BRAND NAME	GENERIC NAME
Refludan Classification: Thrombin inhibitor	lepirudin
Refresh Classification: Ophthalmic lubricant	artificial tears solution
Refresh PM Classification: Ophthalmic lubricant	ocular lubricants
Regitine Classification: Antihypertensive; alpha-adrenergic blocker	phentolamine
Reglan Classification: Antidopaminergic	metoclopramide
Regonol Classification: Anticholinesterase	pyridostigmine bromide
Regranex Classification: Growth factor	becaplermin
Regular Insulin Classification: Antidiabetic	insulin injection
Regular Purified Pork Insulin Classification: Antidiabetic	insulin injection
Regular Strength Bayer Enteric Coated Caplets Classification: Salicylate analgesic; antipyretic	aspirin
Regulax SS Classification: Laxative, softener	docusate sodium

BRAND NAME	GENERIC NAME

Reguloid Natural
Classification:
Laxative, bulk-producing

psyllium

Reguloid Orange
Classification:
Laxative, bulk-producing

psyllium

Reguloid Sugar Free Regular
Classification:
Laxative, bulk-producing

psyllium

Relafen
Classification:
Nonsteroidal anti-inflammatory

nabumetone

Relaxin (recombinant, human)
Classification:
Anti-multiple sclerosis agent (Orphan)

relaxin (recombinant, human)

Remeron
Classification:
Antidepressant, tetracyclic

mirtazapine

Remular-S
Classification:
Skeletal muscle relaxant, centrally acting

chlorzoxazone

Remune
Classification:
Vaccine (Investigational)

gp 120 vaccine

Renamin
Classification:
Nitrogen product

amino acid solution, renal

Renese
Classification:
Thiazide diuretic

polythiazide

Reno-M-30
Classification:
Radiopaque agent

diatrizoate meglumine 30%

Reno-M-60
Classification:
Radiopaque agent

diatrizoate meglumine 60%

*Available in Canada Only

BRAND NAME	GENERIC NAME
Reno-M-Dip Classification: Radiopaque agent	diatrizoate meglumine 30%
Renografin-60 Classification: Radiopaque agent	diatrizoate meglumine 52% and diatrizoate sodium 8%
Renografin-76 Classification: Radiopaque agent	diatrizoate meglumine 66% and diatrizoate sodium 10%
Renova Classification: Anti-acne product	tretinoin
Renovist Classification: Radiopaque agent	diatrizoate meglumine 34.3% and diatrizoate sodium 35%
Renovist II Classification: Radiopaque agent	diatrizoate meglumine 28.5% and diatrizoate sodium 29.1%
Renovue-Dip Classification: Radiopaque agent	iodamide meglumine 24%
Renvue-65 Classification: Radiopaque agent	iodamide meglumine 65%
ReoPro Classification: Antiplatelet	ABCIXIMAB
Reposans-10 Classification: Antianxiety; benzodiazepine	chlordiazepoxide HCl
Requip Classification: Antiparkinson agent	ropinirole
Rescriptor Classification: Antiviral	delavirdine mesylate

BRAND NAME	GENERIC NAME

Resectisol
Classification:
Osmotic diuretic

mannitol

Reserfia*
Classification:
Antihypertensive

rauwolfia derivatives-reserpine

Reserpine
Classification:
Antihypertensive

rauwolfia derivatives-reserpine

Respa-GF
Classification:
Expectorant

guaifenesin

Respbid
Classification:
Bronchodilator; xanthine

theophylline

RespiGam
Classification:
Immune serum

respiratory syncytial virus immune
globulin IV (human) (RSV-IVIG)

Restore
Classification:
Laxative, bulk-producing

psyllium

Restoril
Classification:
Sedative-hypnotic; benzodiazepine

temazepam

Resyl*
Classification:
Expectorant

guaifenesin

Retavase
Classification:
Antithrombotic

retelpase, recombinant

Retin-A
Classification:
Anti-acne product

tretinoin (vitamin A acid, retinoic acid)

Retin-A Micro
Classification:
Anti-acne product

tretinoin (vitamin A acid, retinoic acid)

BRAND NAME	GENERIC NAME

Retinoin
Classification:
Antineoplastic (Orphan)

retinoin

Retrovir
Classification:
Antiviral

zidovudine, formerly azidothymidine or AZT

Rēv-Eyes
Classification:
Alpha-adrenergic blocker

dapiprazole HCl

Reversol
Classification:
Anticholinesterase

edrophonium chloride

Revex
Classification:
Narcotic antagonist

nalmefene HCl

ReVia
Classification:
Narcotic antagonist

naltrexone HCl

Revimine*
Classification:
Adrenergic

dopamine HCl

Rexolate
Classification:
Salicylate analgesic

sodium thiosalicylate

Rezipas
Classification:
Anti-inflammatory (Orphan)

4-aminosalicylic acid

Rezulin
Classification:
Antidiabetic

troglitazone

RGG0853,E1A lipid complex
Classification:
Antineoplastic (Orphan)

RGG0853,E1A lipid complex

Rheomacrodex
Classification:
Plasma volume expander

dextran 40

*Available in Canada only

BRAND NAME	GENERIC NAME

RheothRx copolymer
Classification:
Blood modifier (Orphan)

poloxamer 188

Rheumatrex Dose Pack
Classification:
Antineoplastic; antimetabolite

methotrexate sodium (amethopterin, MTX)

rhIL-12
Classification:
Biologic response modifier
(Investigational)

rhIL-12

Rhinalar*
Classification:
Glucocorticoid

flunisolide, nasal

Rhinall
Classification:
Nasal decongestant

phenylephrine HCl, nasal

Rhinocort
Classification:
Glucocorticoid

budesonide, nasal

Rhinocort Turbuhaler*
Classification:
Glucocorticoid

budesonide

RhoGAM
Classification:
Immune serum

Rho (D) immune globulin

Ricin (blocked) Conjugated Murine MCA (anti-b4)
Classification:
Antineoplastic (Orphan)

ricin (blocked) conjugated murine MCA (anti-b4)

Ricin (blocked) conjugated murine MCA (anti-my9)
Classification:
Antineoplastic (Orphan)

ricin (blocked) conjugated murine MCA (anti-my9)

Ricin (blocked) conjugated murine (MCA (n901)
Classification:
Antineoplastic (Orphan)

ricin (blocked) conjugated murine NCA (n901)

BRAND NAME	GENERIC NAME
Ridaura Classification: Gold compound	auranofin
Ridenol Classification: Analgesic; antipyretic	acetaminophen
R-IFN-beta Classification: Antineoplastic; biologic response modifier (Orphan)	interferon beta (reccombinant)
Rifadin Classification: Antitubercular	rifampin
Rifapentine Classification: Antitubercular (Orphan)	rifapentine
Rilutek Classification: Anti-amyotrophic lateral sclerosis agent	riluzole
RII Retinamide Classification: Anti-myelodysplastic agent (Orphan)	RII retinamide
Rimactine Classification: Antitubercular	rifampin
Rimso-50 Classification: Anti-inflammatory	dimethyl sulfoxide (DMSO)
Riopan Classification: Antacid	magaldrate (hydroxymagnesium aluminate)
Risperdal Classification: Antipsychotic	risperidone
Ritalin Classification: CNS stimulant	methylphenidate HCl

BRAND NAME	GENERIC NAME

Ritalin SR
Classification:
CNS stimulant

methylphenidate HCl

Ritanserin
Classification:
Serotonin S-2-antagonist (Investigational)

ritanserin

Ritodrine HCl
Classification:
Uterine relaxant

ritodrine HCl

Rituxan
Classification:
Antineoplastic

rituximab

RMS
Classification:
Opioid analgesic

morphine sulfate

Robaxin-750
Classification:
Skeletal muscle relaxant, centrally acting

methocarbamol

Robaxin
Classification:
Skeletal muscle relaxant, centrally acting

methocarbamol

Robicillin-VK
Classification:
Antibiotic; penicillin

penicillin V potassium

Robigesic*
Classification:
Analgesic; antipyretic

acetaminophen

Robimycin Robitabs
Classification:
Antibiotic; macrolide

erythromycin base

Robinul
Classification:
Anticholinergic

glycopyrrolate

Robinul Forte
Classification:
Anticholinergic

glycopyrrolate

*Available in Canada Only

BRAND NAME	GENERIC NAME
Robitussin Classification: Expectorant	guaifenesin
Robitussin Cough Calmers Classification: Non-narcotic antitussive	dextromethorphan
Robitussin Pediatric Classification: Non-narcotic antitussive	dextromethorphan
Rocaltrol Classification: Vitamin, fat soluble	calcitriol (1,25-dihydroxycholecalciferol)
Rocephin Classification: Antibiotic; cephalosporin	ceftriaxone sodium
Roferon-A Classification: Antineoplastic; biologic response modifier	interferon alfa-2a (rIFN-A; IFLrA)
Rogaine Classification: Antihypertensive; vasodilator	minoxidil
Rogitine* Classification: Antihypertensive; alpha-adrenergic blocker	phentolamine
Rolaids Calcium Rich Classification: Antacid; calcium supplement	calcium carbonate
Rolavil* Classification: Antidepressant	amitriptyline HCl
Romazicon Classification: Benzodiazepine antagonist	flumazenil

*Available in Canada only

BRAND NAME	GENERIC NAME
Rose Bengal Classification: Ophthalmic diagnostic	rose bengal
Rosets Classification: Ophthalmic diagnostic	rose bengal
RotaShield Classification: Vaccine	rotavirus vaccine
Rounax* Classification: Analgesic; antipyretic	acetaminophen
Rowasa Classification: GI anti-inflammatory	mesalamine
Roxanol 100 Classification: Opioid analgesic	morphine sulfate
Roxanol Classification: Opioid analgesic	morphine sulfate
Roxanol Rescudose Classification: Opioid analgesic	morphine sulfate
Roxanol SR Classification: Opioid analgesic	morphine sulfate
Roxicodone Classification: Opioid analgesic	oxycodone HCl
Roxicodone Intensol Classification: Opioid analgesic	oxycodone HCl
Roxin Classification: Histamine H_2 receptor antagonist (Investigational)	roxatidine acetate

BRAND NAME	GENERIC NAME
Ru-Vert-M Classification: Antiemetic; anticholinergic	meclizine
Rubex Classification: Antineoplastic; antibiotic	doxorubicin HCl (ADR)
Rubion* Classification: Vitamin, water soluble	cyanocobalamin (vitamin B_{12})
Run-K Classification: Electrolyte replacement; potassium	potassium chloride
Rynacrom* Classification: Antiasthmatic	cromolyn sodium (disodium cromoglycate)
Rythmol Classification: Antiarrhythmic	propafenone

S

BRAND NAME	GENERIC NAME
S-2 Inhalant Classification: Adrenergic agonist	epinephrine
S-T Cort Classification: Glucocorticoid	hydrocortisone, topical
Sabol Shampoo* Classification: Germicidal	benzalkonium chloride
Sabril Classification: Anticonvulsant (Investigational)	vigabatrin
Sacarasa Classification: Enzyme (Orphan)	sucrase

*Available in Canada only

BRAND NAME	GENERIC NAME

Sal-Acid
Classification:
Keratolytic

salicylic acid, topical

Sal-Adult*
Classification:
Salicylate analgesic; antipyretic

aspirin

Sal-Infant*
Classification:
Salicylate analgesic; antipyretic

aspirin

Sal Plant
Classification:
Keratolytic

salicylic acid, topical

Salactic Film
Classification:
Keratolytic

salicylic acid, topical

Salagen
Classification:
Cholinergic

pilocarpine, oral

Salazopyrin*
Classification:
Anti-inflammatory; sulfonamide

sulfasalazine

Salbutamol*
Classification:
Beta-adrenergic agonist

albuterol

Saleto-200
Classification:
Nonsteroidal anti-inflammatory

ibuprofen

Saleto-400
Classification:
Nonsteroidal anti-inflammatory

ibuprofen

Saleto-600
Classification:
Nonsteroidal anti-inflammatory

ibuprofen

Saleto-800
Classification:
Nonsteroidal anti-inflammatory

ibuprofen

BRAND NAME	GENERIC NAME
Salflex Classification: Salicylate analgesic	salsalate
SalineX Classification: Nasal decongestant	sodium chloride, nasal
Salivart Classification: Oral lubricant	saliva substitutes
Salix Classification: Oral lubricant	saliva substitute
Salmonine Classification: Parathyroid agent	calcitonin (salmon)
Salsalate Classification: Salicylate analgesic	salsalate
Salsitab Classification: Salicylate analgesic	salsalate
Sal-Tropine Classification: Anticholinergic	atropine sulfate
Saluron Classification: Thiazide diuretic	hydroflumethiazide
Sandimmune Classification: Immunosuppressive	cyclosporine
Sandoglobulin Classification: Immune serum	immune globulin intravenous (IGIV)
Sandostatin Classification: Somatostatin analog	octreotide acetate

BRAND NAME	GENERIC NAME
Sani-Supp Classification: Hyperosmotic	glycerin (glycerol)
Sanorex Classification: CNS stimulant; anorexiant	mazindol
Sansert Classification: Serotonin antagonist	methysergide maleate
Santyl Classification: Topical enzyme	collagenase
Sarisol No. 2 Classification: Sedative-hypnotic; barbiturate	butabarbital sodium
Scabene Classification: Scabicide; pediculicide	lindane (gamma benzene hexachloride)
Scaline* Classification: Depolarizing neuromuscular blocker	succinylcholine chloride
Scalpicin Classification: Glucocorticoid	hydrocortisone, topical
Scleromate Classification: Sclerosing agent	morrhuate sodium
Sclerosol Classification: Pleurodesis agent (Investigational)	talc, sterile aerosol
Scopace Classification: Anticholinergic	scopolamine hydrobromide
Scopolamine Hydrobromide Classification: Anticholinergic	scopolamine hydrobromide

*Available in Canada Only

BRAND NAME	GENERIC NAME
Scot-tussin Allergy Classification: Antihistamine	diphenhydramine HCl
Scot-tussin Expectorant Classification: Expectorant	guaifenesin
Scriptene Classification: Antiviral (Investigational)	AZT-P-ddI
SeaMist Classification: Nasal decongestant	sodium chloride, nasal
Sebizon Classification: Antiseborrheic	sulfacetamide sodium, topical
Secobarbital sodium Classification: Sedative-hypnotic; barbiturate	secobarbital sodium
Secogen Sodium* Classification: Sedative-hypnotic; barbiturate	secobarbital sodium
Seconal Sodium Classification: Sedative-hypnotic; barbiturate	secobarbital sodium
Secretin-Ferring Powder Classification: Gastrointestinal function test	secretin
Sectral Classification: Beta-adrenergic blocker	acebutolol
Sele-Pak Classification: Trace element	selenium
Selegiline HCl Classification: Antiparkinson agent	selegiline HCl (L-deprenyl)

BRAND NAME	GENERIC NAME
Selenium Classification: Trace element	selenium
Selenium Sulfide Classification: Antiseborrheic	selenium sulfide
Selepen Classification: Trace element	selenium
Selsun Classification: Antiseborrheic	selenium sulfide
Selsun Blue Classification: Antiseborrheic	selenium sulfide
Selsun Gold for Women Classification: Antiseborrheic	selinium sulfide
Semicid Classification: Spermicide	nonoxynol
Senna-Gen Classification: Laxative, irritant	senna
Senokot Classification: Laxative, irritant	senna
Senokotxtra Classification: Laxative, irritant	senna
Senolax Classification: Laxative, irritant	senna
Senoxen Classification: Laxative, irritant	senna

BRAND NAME	GENERIC NAME

SensoGARD
Classification:
Local anesthetic

benzocaine, oral

Sensorcaine
Classification:
Local anesthetic

bupivacaine HCl

Sensorcaine MPF
Classification:
Local anesthetic

bupivacaine HCl

Sensorcaine with Epinephrine
Classification:
Local anesthetic

bupivacaine HCl

Septisol
Classification:
Germicidal

hexachlorophene

Septisol Solution
Classification:
Germicidal

triclosan

Septopal
Classification:
Antibiotic, aminoglycoside (Orphan)

gentamicin impregnated PMMA beads

Septra
Classification:
Antibiotic; sulfonamide

trimethoprim and sulfamethoxazole
TMP-SMZ)

Septra DS
Classification:
Antibiotic; sulfonamide

trimethoprim and sulfamethoxazole
(TMP-SMZ)

Septra I.V.
Classification:
Antibiotic; sulfonamide

trimethoprim and sulfamethoxazole
(TMP-SMZ)

Seral*
Classification:
Sedative-hypnotic; barbiturate

secobarbital sodium

Serax
Classification:
Antianxiety; benzodiazepine

oxazepam

BRAND NAME	GENERIC NAME
Serazone Classification: Antidepressant	nefazadone HCl
Serentil Classification: Antipsychotic	mesoridazine besylate
Serevent Classification: Bronchodilator; beta-adrenergic agonist	salmeterol
Serevent Diskus Classification: Bronchodilator; beta adrenergic agonist	salmeterol
Serlect Classification: Antipsychotic (Investigational)	sertindole
Seromycin Pulvules Classification: Antitubercular	cycloserine
Serophene Classification: Ovulation stimulant	clomiphene citrate
Seroquel Classification: Antipsychotic	quetiapine
Serostim Classification: Growth hormone	somatropin
Serpalan Classification: Antihypertensive	rauwolfia derivatives-reserpine
Sertan* Classification: Anticonvulsant	primidone
Sertindole Classification: Antipsychotic (Investigational)	sertindole

*Available in Canada Only

BRAND NAME	GENERIC NAME

Serutan
Classification:
Laxative, bulk-producing

psyllium

Shur-Seal Gel
Classification:
Spermicide

nonoxynol

Sibelium
Classification:
Calcium channel blocker (Orphan)

flunarizine

Silace
Classification:
Laxative, softener

docusate sodium

Silapap Children's
Classification:
Analgesic; antipyretic

acetaminophen

Silapap Infants
Classification:
Analgesic; antipyretic

acetaminophen

Silphen Cough
Classification:
Antihistamine

diphenhydramine HCl

Silphen DM
Classification:
Non-narcotic antitussive

dextromethorphan

Siltussin
Classification:
Expectorant

guaifenesin

Silvadene
Classification:
Antibacterial

silver sulfadiazine

Silver Nitrate 1%
Classification:
Ophthalmic antiseptic

silver nitrate, ophthalmic

Silver Nitrate
Classification:
Ophthalmic antiseptic

silver nitrate, topical

BRAND NAME	GENERIC NAME
Simron Classification: Iron preparation	ferrous gluconate
Sinarest 12-Hour Classification: Nasal decongestant	oxymetazoline HCl, nasal
Sinemet-10/100 Classification: Antiparkinson agent	levodopa/carbidopa
Sinemet-25/100 Classification: Antiparkinson agent	levodopa/carbidopa
Sinemet-25/250 Classification: Antiparkinson agent	levodopa/carbidopa
Sinemet-CR Classification: Antiparkinson agent	levodopa/carbidopa
Sinequan Classification: Antianxiety; antidepressant	doxepin HCl
Sinequan Concentrate Classification: Antianxiety; antidepressant	doxepin HCl
Sinex Classification: Nasal decongestant	phenylephrine HCl, nasal
Singulair Classification: Bronchodilator; leukotriene antagonist	montelukast sodium
Sinografin Classification: Radiopaque agent	diatrizoate meglumine 52.7% and iodipamide meglumine 26.8%
Sinumist-SR Classification: Expectorant	guaifenesin

*Available in Canada Only

BRAND NAME	GENERIC NAME
Sinustat Classification: Nasal decongestant	pseudoephedrine HCl
Sitzmarks Classification: Radiopaque agent	radiopaque polyvinyl chloride
Skelaxin Classification: Skeletal muscle relaxant, centrally acting	metaxalone
Skelid Classification: Bone resorption inhibitor	tiludronate
Sleep-Aid Classification: Antihistamine	doxylamine succinate
Sleep-Eze 3 Classification: Antihistamine	diphenhydramine HCl
Slim-Mint Classification: Local anesthetic	benzocaine
Slo-bid Gyrocaps Classification: Bronchodilator; xanthine	theophylline
Slo-Niacin Classification: Vitamin, water soluble	niacin (vitamin B_3, nicotinic acid)
Slo-Phyllin Gyrocaps Classification: Bronchodilator; xanthine	theophylline
Slow-Fe Classification: Iron preparation	ferrous sulfate
Slow-Mag Classification: Electrolyte replacement	magnesium chloride

*Available in Canada only

BRAND NAME	GENERIC NAME

Slow K
Classification:
Electrolyte replacement; potassium

potassium chloride

Snooze Fast
Classification:
Antihistamine

diphenhydramine HCl

Sodium Acetate
Classification:
Electrolyte replacement

sodium acetate

Sodium Ascorbate
Classification:
Vitamin, water soluble

sodium ascorbate

Sodium Bicarbonate
Classification:
System alkalinizer

sodium bicarbonate

Sodium Chloride
Classification:
Electrolyte replacement

sodium chloride

Sodium Dichloroacetate
Classification:
Antilactic acidosis agent (Orphan)

sodium dichloroacetate

Sodium Fluoride
Classification:
Electrolyte replacement; fluoride

sodium fluoride

Sodium Iodide
Classification:
Antiseptic

iodine products

Sodium Iodide I 123
Classification:
Thyroid function test

sodium iodide I 123

Sodium Iodide I 131
Classification:
Antithyroid agent

sodium iodide I 131

Sodium Lactate
Classification:
Electrolyte replacement

sodium lactate

BRAND NAME	GENERIC NAME
Sodium Nitroprusside Classification: Antihypertensive; vasodilator	nitroprusside sodium
Sodium Phosphate P32 Classification: Antineoplastic; radiopharmaceutical	sodium phosphate P32
Sodium Phosphates Classification: Laxative, saline	saline laxatives
Sodium Polystyrene Sulfonate Classification: Potassium-removing resin	sodium polystyrene sulfonate
Sodium Salicylate Classification: Salicylate analgesic	sodium salicylate
Sodium Sulamyd Classification: Antibiotic; sulfonamide	sulfacetamide sodium, ophthalmic
Sodium Sulfacetamide Classification: Antibiotic; sulfonamide	sulfacetamide sodium, ophthalmic
Sodium Thiosalicylate Classification: Salicylate analgesic	sodium thiosalicylate
Sodium Thiosulfate Classification: Cyanide antidote	sodium thiosulfate
Soft'n Soothe Classification: Local anesthetic	benzocaine, topical
Solaquin Classification: Depigmentation agent	hydroquinone
Solaquin Forte Classification: Depigmentation agent	hydroquinone

*Available in Canada only

BRAND NAME	GENERIC NAME
Solarcaine Classification: Local anesthetic	benzocaine, topical
Solazine* Classification: Antipsychotic	trifluoperazine HCl
Solfoton Classification: Sedative-hypnotic; barbiturate	phenobarbital/phenobarbital sodium
Solganal Classification: Gold compound	aurothioglucose
Solium* Classification: Antianxiety; benzodiazepine	chlordiazepoxide HCl
Solu-Cortef Classification: Glucocorticoid	hydrocortisone sodium succinate
Soluble Complement Receptor (recombinant) Type 1 Classification: Biologic response modifier (Orphan)	soluble complement receptor (recombinant) type 1
Solurex Classification: Glucocorticoid	dexamethasone sodium phosphate
Solurex LA Classification: Glucocorticoid	dexamethasone acetate
Soma Classification: Skeletal muscle relaxant, centrally acting	carisoprodol
Somatostatin Classification: Sclerosing agent (Orphan)	somatostatin
Sominex Caplets Classification: Antihistamine	diphenhydramine HCl

*Available in Canada Only

BRAND NAME	GENERIC NAME
Sominex 2 Classification: Antihistamine	diphenhydramine HCl
Somnol* Classification: Sedative-hypnotic; benzodiazepine	flurazepam
Sopamycetin* Classification: Antibacterial	chloramphenicol, otic
Sorbitol Classification: Genitourinary irrigant	sorbitol
Sorbitrate Classification: Antianginal	isosorbide dinitrate, oral
Sorbitrate Classification: Antianginal	isosorbide dinitrate sublingual and chewable
Sorbitrate SA Classification: Antianginal	isosorbide dinitrate, oral
Soriatane Classification: Antipsoriatic	acitretin
Sotradecol Classification: Sclerosing agent	sodium tetradecyl sulfate
Span-FF Classification: Iron preparation	ferrous fumarate
Spancap No. 1 Classification: CNS stimulant	dextroamphetamine sulfate
Sparine Classification: Antipsychotic	promazine HCl

BRAND NAME	GENERIC NAME

Spec-T Anesthetic
Classification:
Local anesthetic

benzocaine, oral

Spectazole
Classification:
Antifungal

econazole nitrate

Spectrobid
Classification:
Antibiotic; aminopenicillin

bacampicillin HCl

Spexil
Classification:
Antibiotic; aminocyclitol (Investigational)

trospectomycin

Spherulin
Classification:
In vivo diagnostic

coccidioidin

Spironolactone
Classification:
Potassium-sparing diuretic

spironolactone

SPL-Serologic Types I and II
Classification:
Vaccine

staphage lysate

Sporanox
Classification:
Antifungal; triazole

itraconazole

Sportscreme
Classification:
Analgesic

trolamine salicylate

Spray-U-Thin
Classification:
Alpha-adrenergic agonist

phenylpropanolamine HCl

SPS
Classification:
Potassium-removing resin

sodium polystyrene sulfonate

S-P-T
Classification:
Thyroid hormone

thyroid USP (desiccated)

BRAND NAME	GENERIC NAME
SSD Classification: Antibacterial	silver sulfadiazine
SSD AF Classification: Antibacterial	silver sulfadiazine
SSKI Classification: Expectorant	potassium iodide
ST1-RTA Immunotoxin (SR 44163) Classification: Immune serum (Orphan)	ST1-RTA immunotoxin (SR 44163)
St. Joseph Adult Chewable Aspirin Classification: Salicylate analgesic; antipyretic	aspirin
St. Joseph Cough Suppressant Classification: Non-narcotic antitussive	dextromethorphan
St. Joseph Measured Dose Classification: Nasal decongestant	phenylephrine HCl, nasal
Stadol Classification: Opioid agonist-antagonist analgesic	butorphanol tartrate
Stadol NS Classification: Opioid agonist-antagonist analgesic	butorphanol, nasal
Staphcillin Classification: Antibiotic; penicillinase-resistant penicillin	methicillin sodium
Staticin Classification: Antibiotic; macrolide	erythromycin, topical

BRAND NAME	GENERIC NAME
Stelazine Classification: Antipsychotic	trifluoperazine HCl
Stemgen Classification: Biologic response modifier (Investigational)	stem cell factor
Stemetil* Classification: Antipsychotic	prochlorperazine
Sterapred Classification: Glucocorticoid	prednisone
Sterapred DS Classification: Glucocorticoid	prednisone
Sterecyt Classification: Antineoplastic (Orphan)	prednimustine
Stilboestrol* Classification: Estrogen	diethylstilbestrol
Stilphostrol Classification: Estrogen	diethylstilbestrol
Stimate Classification: Posterior pituitary hormone	desmopressin acetate
Stimulon Classification: Vaccine (Investigational)	stimulon
Stop Classification: Electrolyte replacement; fluoride	sodium fluoride
Streptase Classification: Antithrombotic	streptokinase

*Available in Canada Only

BRAND NAME	GENERIC NAME
Streptococcus Immune Globulin, group B Classification: Immune serum (Orphan)	streptococcus immune globulin, group B
Stress-Pam* Classification: Antianxiety; benzodiazepine	diazepam
Stromectol Classification: Anthelmintic	ivermectin
Strong Iodine Solution (Lugol's Solution) Classification: Iodine product	iodine product
Strong Iodine Tincture Classification: Iodine product	iodine products
Stye Classification: Ophthalmic lubricant	ocular lubricants
SU-101 Classification: Antineoplastic (Orphan)	SU-101
Sublimaze Classification: Opioid analgesic	fentanyl citrate
Succinate Classification: Glucocorticoid	methylprednisolone sodium succinate
Succinylcholine Chloride Min-i-Mix Classification: Depolarizing neuromuscular blocker	succinylcholine chloride
Sucralfate Classification: Protectant	sucralfate

BRAND NAME	GENERIC NAME
Sucrets 4-Hour Cough Classification: Non-narcotic antitussive	dextromethorphan
Sucrets Cough Control Classification: Non-narcotic antitussive	dextromethorphan
Sudafed Classification: Nasal decongestant	pseudoephedrine HCl
Sudafed 12 Hour Classification: Nasal decongestant	pseudoephedrine HCl
Sufenta Classification: Opioid analgesic	sufentanil citrate
Sufentanil Citrate Classification: Opioid analgesic	sufentanil citrate
Sular Classification: Calcium channel blocker	nisoldipine
Sulcrate* Classification: Protectant	sucralfate
Sulf-10 Classification: Antibiotic; sulfonamide	sulfacetamide sodium, ophthalmic
Sulfadiazine Classification: Antibiotic; sulfonamide	sulfadiazine
Sulfacetamide Sodium 10% Classification: Antibiotic; sulfonamide	sulfacetamide sodium, ophthalmic
Sulfacetamide Sodium 30% Classification: Antibiotic; sulfonamide	sulfacetamide sodium, ophthalmic

*Available in Canada Only

BRAND NAME	GENERIC NAME
Sulfalax Calcium Classification: Laxative, softener	docusate calcium
Sulfamethoxazole Classification: Antibiotic; sulfonamide	sulfamethoxazole
Sulfamylon Classification: Antibacterial; sulfonamide	mafenide acetate
Sulfamylon Solution Classification: Antibacterial (Orphan)	mafenide acetate
Sulfasalazine Classification: Anti-inflammatory; sulfonamide	sulfasalazine
Sulfatrim Classification: Antibiotic; sulfonamide	trimethoprim and sulfamethoxazole (TMP-SMZ)
Sulfinpyrazone Classification: Uricosuric	sulfinpyrazone
Sulindac Classification: Nonsteroidal anti-inflammatory	sulindac
Sulmasque Classification: Anti-acne product	sulfur
Sulpho-Lac Classification: Anti-acne product	sulfur
Sultrin Triple Sulfa Classification: Antibiotic; sulfonamide	triple sulfa
Sumycin 500 Classification: Antibiotic; tetracycline	tetracycline HCl

*Available in Canada only

BRAND NAME	GENERIC NAME

Sumycin Syrup
Classification:
Antibiotic; tetracycline

tetracycline HCl

Supasa*
Classification:
Antipyretic

aspirin

Superdophilus
Classification:
Antidiarrheal

lactobacillus

Superoxide Dismutase (human)
Classification:
Antioxidant (Orphan)

superoxide dismutase (human)

**Superoxide Dismutase
(recombinant human)**
Classification:
Antioxidant (Orphan)

superoxide dismutase (recombinant human)

Supeudol*
Classification:
Opioid analgesic

oxycodone HCl

Supprelin
Classification:
Gonadotropin-releasing hormone

histrelin acetate

Suppress
Classification:
Non-narcotic antitussive

dextromethorphan

Suprane
Classification:
General anesthetic

desflurane

Suprax
Classification:
Antibiotic; cephalosporin

cefixime

Surfak
Classification:
Laxative, softener

docusate calcium

Surgicel
Classification:
Hemostatic

oxidized cellulose

*Available in Canada Only

BRAND NAME	GENERIC NAME
Surital Classification: General anesthetic; barbiturate	thiamylal sodium
Surmontil Classification: Antidepressant	trimipramine maleate
Survanta Classification: Lung surfactant	beractant
Sus-Phrine Classification: Adrenergic agonist	epinephrine
Sustaire Classification: Bronchodilator; xanthine	theophylline
Sustiva Classification: Antiviral (Investigational)	efavirenz
Sux-Cert* Classification: Depolarizing neuromuscular blocker	succinylcholine chloride
Syllact Classification: Laxative, bulk-producing	psyllium
Symmetrel Classification: Antiviral; antiparkinson	amantadine HCl
Synacort Classification: Glucocorticoid	hydrocortisone, topical
Synalar-HP Classification: Glucocorticoid	fluocinolone acetonide
Synarel Classification: Gonadotropin-releasing hormone	nafarelin acetate

*Available in Canada only

BRAND NAME	GENERIC NAME

Synemol
Classification:
Glucocorticoid

fluocinolone acetonide

Synercid
Classification:
Antibiotic (Investigational)

quinupristin-dalfopristin

Synkavite*
Classification:
Vitamin K

menadione/menadiol sodium diphosphate (vitamin K_4)

Synovir
Classification:
Immunosuppressive agent (Orphan)

thalidomide

Synsorb Rx
Classification:
Anti-infective (Orphan)

synsorb Rx

Synthroid
Classification:
Thyroid hormone

levothyroxine sodium (T_4; L-Thyroxine sodium)

Syntocinon
Classification:
Oxytocic

oxytocin, parenteral

Syntocinon
Classification:
Oxytocic

oxytocin, synthetic, nasal

Synvisc
Classification:
Viscoelastic

hylan G-F 20

Syprine
Classification:
Chelating agent

trientine HCl

T

T-Gen
Classification:
Antiemetic; anticholinergic

trimethobenzamide HCl

BRAND NAME	GENERIC NAME
T-Phyl Classification: Bronchodilator; xanthine	theophylline
T-Stat Classification: Antibiotic; macrolide	erythromycin, topical
T/Scalp Classification: Glucocorticoid	hydrocortisone, topical
T4, Endonuclease V, liposome encapsulated Classification: Enzyme (Orphan)	T4 endonuclease V, liposome encapsulated
T4, Soluble Human, recombinant Classification: Antiviral (Investigational)	T4, soluble human, recombinant
TA-HPV Classification: Antineoplastic (Orphan)	recombinant vaccinia (human papillomavirus)
Tac-3 Classification: Glucocorticoid	triamcinolone acetonide
Tac-40 Classification: Glucocorticoid	triamcinolone acetonide
Tace Classification: Estrogen	chlorotrianisene
Tagamet Classification: Histamine H_2 receptor antagonist	cimetidine
Tagamet HB Classification: Histamine H_2 receptor antagonist	cimetidine

BRAND NAME	GENERIC NAME

Talwin
Classification:
Opioid agonist-antagonist analgesic

pentazocine

Tambocor
Classification:
Antiarrhythmic

flecainide acetate

Tamofen*
Classification:
Antineoplastic; hormone

tamoxifen citrate

Tamone*
Classification:
Antineoplastic; hormone

tamoxifen citrate

Tamoxifen
Classification:
Antineoplastic; hormone

tamoxifen citrate

TAO
Classification:
Antibiotic; macrolide

troleandomycin

Tapanol Extra Strength
Classification:
Analgesic; antipyretic

acetaminophen

Tapanol Regular Strength
Classification:
Analgesic; antipyretic

acetaminophen

Tapazole
Classification:
Antithyroid

methimazole

Tarabine PFS
Classification:
Antineoplastic; antimetabolite

cytarabine (Ara-C; cytosine arabinoside)

Targocid
Classification:
Antibiotic; glycopeptide (Investigational)

teicoplanin

Tarka
Classification:
Antihypertensive; angiotensin converting
enzyme inhibitor

trandolapril

BRAND NAME	GENERIC NAME
Tasmar Classification: Antiparkinson agent	tolcapone
TAT Antagonist Classification: Antiviral (Investigational)	TAT antagonist
Tavist Classification: Antihistamine	clemastine fumarate
Taxol Classification: Antineoplastic, miscellaneous	paclitaxel
Taxotere Classification: Antineoplastic, miscellaneous	docetaxel
Tazicef Classification: Antibiotic; cephalosporin	ceftazidime
Tazidime Classification: Antibiotic; cephalosporin	ceftazidime
Tazorac Classification: Anti-acne	tazarotene
Teargard Classifications: Ophthalmic lubricants	artificial tears solution
Teargen Classification: Ophthalmic lubricants	artificial tears solution
Tearisol Classification: Ophthalmic lubricants	artificial tears solution
Tears Naturale Classification: Ophthalmic lubricants	artificial tears solution

*Available in Canada only

BRAND NAME	GENERIC NAME
Tears Naturale Free Classification: Ophthalmic lubricants	artificial tears solution
Tears Naturale II Classification: Ophthalmic lubricants	artificial tears solution
Tears Plus Classification: Ophthalmic lubricants	artificial tears solution
Tears Renewed Classification: Ophthalmic lubricants	artificial tears solution
Tebamide Classification: Antiemetic; anticholinergic	trimethobenzamide HCl
Tebrazid* Classification: Antitubercular	pyrazinamide
Teejel* Classification: Salicylate analgesic	choline salicylate
Tega-Cort Classification: Glucocorticoid	hydrocortisone, topical
Tega-Cort Forte Classification: Glucocorticoid	hydrocortisone, topical
Tegison Classification: Antipsoriatic	etretinate
Tegopen Classification: Antibiotic; penicillinase-resistant penicillin	cloxacillin sodium
Tegretol Classification: Anticonvulsant	carbamazepine

*Available in Canada Only

BRAND NAME	GENERIC NAME

Tegretol-XR
Classification:
Anticonvulsant

carbamazepine, extended release

Tegrin Medicated
Classification:
Keratolytic

coal tar

Teladar
Classification:
Glucocorticoid

betamethasone dipropionate

Telepaque
Classification:
Radiopaque agent

iopanoic acid

Teline
Classification:
Antibiotic; tetracycline

tetracycline HCl

Teline-500
Classification:
Antibiotic; tetracycline

tetracycline HCl

Temazepam
Classification:
Sedative-hypnotic; benzodiazepine

temazepam

Temovate
Classification:
Glucocorticoid

clobetasol propionate

Temovate Emollient
Classification:
Glucocorticoid

clobetasol propionate

Tempra
Classification:
Analgesic; antipyretic

acetaminophen

Tempra 2 Syrup
Classification:
Analgesic; antipyretic

acetaminophen

Tempra 3
Classification:
Analgesic; antipyretic

acetaminophen

BRAND NAME	GENERIC NAME

Tempra Children's Syrup
Classification:
Analgesic; antipyretic

acetaminophen

Tempral
Classification:
Analgesic; antipyretic

acetaminophen

Ten-K
Classification:
Electrolyte replacement; potassium

potassium chloride

Tenex
Classification:
Antihypertensive, centrally acting

guanfacine HCl

Tenormin
Classification:
Antihypertensive; beta-adrenergic blocker

atenolol

Tensilon
Classification:
Anticholinesterase

edrophonium chloride

Tenuate
Classification:
CNS stimulant; anorexiant

diethylpropion HCl

Tenuate Dospan
Classification:
CNS stimulant; anorexiant

diethylpropion HCl

Terazol 3
Classification:
Antifungal

terconazole

Terazol 7
Classification:
Antifungal

terconazole

Terfenadine
Classification:
Antihistamine

terfenadine

Terfluzine
Classification:
Antipsychotic

trifluoperazine HCl

BRAND NAME	GENERIC NAME
Terpine Hydrate Classification: Expectorant	terpin hydrate
Terramycin Classification: Antibiotic; tetracycline	oxytetracycline HCl
Tesamone Classification: Androgen	testosterone aqueous suspension
Teslascan Classification: In vivo diagnostic	mangafodipir
Teslac Classification: Antineoplastic; hormone	testolactone
Tessalon Perles Classification: Non-narcotic antitussive	benzonatate
Testoderm Classification: Androgen	testosterone transdermal
Testoderm TTS Classification: Androgen	testosterone transdermal
Testopel Classification: Androgen	testosterone pellet
Testosterone Aqueous Classification: Androgen	testosterone aqueous suspension
Testosterone Cypionate Classification: Androgen	testosterone cypionate (in oil)
Testosterone Enanthate Classification: Androgen	testosterone enanthate (in oil)

*Available in Canada only

BRAND NAME	GENERIC NAME
Testosterone Propionate Classification: Androgen	testosterone propionate (in oil)
Testred Classification: Androgen	methyltestosterone
Tetanus Toxoid Adsorbed Classification: Toxoid	tetanus toxoid adsorbed
Tetanus Toxoid Plain Classification: Toxoid	tetanus toxoid
Tetracaine HCl Classification: Local anesthetic	tetracaine HCl, ophthalmic
Tetracap Classification: Antibiotic, tetracycline	tetracycline HCl
Tetracycline HCl Classification: Antibiotic; tetracycline	tetracycline HCl
Tetracycline HCl Syrup Classification: Antibiotic; tetracycline	tetracycline HCl
Tetrahydrozoline HCl Classification: Ophthalmic vasoconstrictor	tetrahydrozoline HCl, ophthalmic
Tetralean* Classification: Antibiotic; tetracycline	tetracycline HCl
Tetramune Classification: Toxoid	diphtheria and tetanus toxoids and whole-cell pertussis and haemophilus influenzae type b conjugate vaccines (DtwP-HIB)

BRAND NAME	GENERIC NAME

Teveten
Classification:
Antihypertensive; angiotensin II
antagonist

eprosartan

Texacort
Classification:
Glucocorticoid

hydrocortisone, topical

Thalitone
Classification:
Thiazide-like diuretic

chlorthalidone

Tham
Classification:
Systemic alkalinizer

tromethamine

Theo-24
Classification:
Bronchodilator; xanthine

theophylline

Theo-Dur
Classification:
Bronchodilator; xanthine

theophylline

Theo-Sav
Classification:
Bronchodilator; xanthine

theophylline

Theo-X
Classification:
Bronchodilator; xanthine

theophylline

Theobid Duracaps
Classification:
Bronchodilator; xanthine

theophylline

Theochron
Classification:
Bronchodilator; xanthine

theophylline

Theoclear-80
Classification:
Bronchodilator; xanthine

theophylline

Theoclear LA
Classification:
Bronchodilator; xanthine

theophylline

*Available in Canada only

BRAND NAME	GENERIC NAME

Theolair-SR
Classification:
Bronchodilator; xanthine

theophylline

Theophylline
Classification:
Bronchodilator; xanthine

theophylline

Theophylline Extended Release
Classification:
Bronchodilator; xanthine

theophylline

Theophylline Oral
Classification:
Bronchodilator; xanthine

theophylline

Theophylline SR
Classification:
Bronchodilator; xanthine

theophylline

Theophylline and 5% Dextrose
Classification:
Bronchodilator; xanthine

theophylline

Theospan-SR
Classification:
Bronchodilator; xanthine

theophylline

Theostat 80
Classification:
Bronchodilator; xanthine

theophylline

Theovent
Classification:
Bronchodilator; xanthine

theophylline

TheraCys
Classification:
Antineoplastic, miscellaneous

BCG, intravesical

Thera-Flur
Classification:
Electrolyte replacement; fluoride

sodium fluoride

Thera-Flur-N
Classification:
Electrolyte replacement; fluoride

sodium fluoride

BRAND NAME	GENERIC NAME
Theramycin Z Classification: Antibiotic; macrolide	erythromycin, topical
Theraplex T Classification: Keratolytic	coal tar
Theraplex Z Classification: Antiseborrheic	pyrithione zinc
Thiamilate Classification: Vitamin, water soluble	thiamine HCl (vitamin B_1)
Thiamine HCl Classification: Vitamin, water soluble	thiamine HCl (vitamin B_1)
Thimerosal Classification: Antiseptic	thimerosal
Thioguanine Classification: Antineoplastic; antimetabolite	thioguanine (TG; 6-thioguanine)
Thiola Classification: Anticystinuria agent (Orphan)	tiopronin
Thiopental Sodium Classification: General anesthetic; barbiturate	thiopental sodium
Thioplex Classification: Antineoplastic; alkylating agent	thiotepa (triethylenethiophos-phoramid; TSPA; TESPA)
Thioridazine HCl Classification: Antipsychotic	thioridazine HCl
Thiosulfil Forte Classification: Antibiotic; sulfonamide	sulfamethizole

BRAND NAME	GENERIC NAME

Thiothixene
Classification:
Antipsychotic

thiothixene

Thorazine
Classification:
Antipsychotic

chlorpromazine HCl

Thorazine Spansules
Classification:
Antipsychotic

chlorpromazine HCl

Threonine
Classification:
Amino acid

threonine

Threostat
Classification:
Amino acid (Orphan)

L-threonine

Thrombate III
Classification:
Antithrombin

antithrombin III, human

Thrombinar
Classification:
Hemostatic

thrombin, topical

Thrombin-JMI
Classification:
Hemostatic

thrombin, topical

Thrombogen
Classification:
Hemostatic

thrombin, topical

Thrombostat
Classification:
Hemostatic

thrombin, topical

Thymic Humoral Factor
Classification:
Biologic response modifier
(Investigational)

thymic humoral factor

Thymosin Alpha-1
Classification:
Biologic response modifier (Orphan)

thymosin alpha-1

*Available in Canada Only

BRAND NAME	GENERIC NAME

Thymostimuline (TP-1)
Classification:
Biologic response modifier
(Investigational)

thymostimuline (TP-1)

Thypinone
Classification:
Thyroid function test

protirelin

Thyrar
Classification:
Thyroid hormone

thyroid USP (desiccated)

Thyrel-TRH
Classification:
Thyroid function test

protirelin

Thyrogen
Classification:
In vivo diagnostic (Orphan)

thyroid stimulating hormone, human
(TSH)

Thyroid USP
Classification:
Thyroid hormone

thyroid USP (desiccated)

Thyrolar
Classification:
Thyroid hormone

liotrix

Thytropar
Classification:
Thyroid function test

thyrotropin (thyroid stimulating
hormone, or TSH)

Tiamate
Classification:
Calcium channel blocker

diltiazem HCl

Tiazac
Classification:
Calcium channel blocker

diltiazem HCl

Ticar
Classification:
Antibiotic; extended spectrum penicillin

ticarcillin disodium

Ticaripen*
Classification:
Antibiotic; extended spectrum penicillin

ticarcillin disodium

BRAND NAME	GENERIC NAME

TICE BCG
Classification:
Antineoplastic, miscellaneous

BCG, intravesical

TICE BCG
Classification:
Vaccine

BCG vaccine, percutaneous

Ticlid
Classification:
Antiplatelet

ticlopidine HCl

Ticon
Classification:
Antiemetic; anticholinergic

trimethobenzamide HCl

Tigan
Classification:
Antiemetic; anticholinergic

trimethobenzamide HCl

Tilade
Classification:
Antiasthmatic

nedocromil sodium

Timentin
Classification:
Antibiotic; extended spectrum penicillin

ticarcillin and clavulanate potassium

Timolol Maleate
Classification:
Antihypertensive; beta-adrenergic blocker

timolol maleate

Timodol Maleate Ophthalmic
Classification:
Beta-adrenergic blocker

timolol maleate, ophthalmic

Timoptic
Classification:
Beta-adrenergic blocker

timolol maleate, ophthalmic

Timoptic-XE
Classification:
Beta-adrenergic blocker

timolol maleate, ophthalmic

Timunox
Classification:
Biologic response modifier
(Investigational)

thymopentin

*Available in Canada Only

BRAND NAME	GENERIC NAME
Timunox Thymopentin Classification: Biologic response modifier	timunox thymopentin
Tinactin Classification: Antifungal	tolnaftate
TinBen Classification: Protectant	benzoin
TinCoBen Classification: Protectant	benzoin
Tine Test PPD Classification: In vivo diagnostic	tuberculin PPD multiple puncture device
Ting Classification: Antifungal	tolnaftate
Tirend Classification: Analeptic	caffeine
Tirilazed Mesylate Classification: Antiviral (Investigational)	tirilazed mesylate
TOBI Classification: Aminoglycoside	tobramycin, inhalation
Tobramycin Ophthalmic Classification: Aminoglycoside	tobramycin, ophthalmic
Tobramycin Sulfate Classification: Aminoglycoside	tobramycin sulfate
Tobrex Classification: Aminoglycoside	tobramycin, ophthalmic

BRAND NAME	GENERIC NAME
Tocopherol Classification: Vitamin, fat soluble	vitamin E
Tofranil Classification: Antidepressant	imipramine HCl
Tofranil-PM Classification: Antidepressant	imipramine pamoate
Tolazamide Classification: Antidiabetic; sulfonylurea	tolazamide
Tolbutamide Classification: Antidiabetic; sulfonylurea	tolbutamide
Tolbutone* Classification: Antidiabetic; sulfonylurea	tolbutamide
Tolectin 200 Classification: Nonsteroidal anti-inflammatory	tolmetin sodium
Tolectin 600 Classification: Nonsteroidal anti-inflammatory	tolmetin sodium
Tolectin DS Classification: Nonsteroidal anti-inflammatory	tolmetin sodium
Tolinase Classification: Antidiabetic	tolazamide
Tolmetin Sodium Classification: Nonsteroidal anti-inflammatory	tolmetin sodium
Tolnaftate Classification: Antifungal	tolnaftate

*Available in Canada Only

BRAND NAME	GENERIC NAME

Tomocat
Classification:
Radiopaque agent

barium sulfate

Tonocard
Classification:
Antiarrhythmic

tocainide HCl

Tonopaque
Classification:
Radiopaque agent

barium sulfate

Toothache Gel
Classification:
Local anesthetic

benzocaine, oral

Topamax
Classification:
Anticonvulsant

topiramate

Topicort
Classification:
Glucocorticoid

desoximetasone

Topicort LP
Classification:
Glucocorticoid

desoximetasone

Topicycline
Classification:
Antibiotic; tetracycline

tetracycline HCl, topical

Toposar
Classification:
Antineoplastic; mitotic inhibitor

etoposide (VP-16-123)

Toprol XL
Classification:
Antihypertensive; beta-adrenergic blocker

metoprolol

Toradol
Classification:
Nonsteroidal anti-inflammatory

ketorolac

Torecan
Classification:
Antiemetic

thiethylperazine maleate

*Available in Canada only

BRAND NAME	GENERIC NAME
Tornalate Classification: Bronchodilator; beta-adrenergic agonist	bitolterol mesylate
Totacillin Classification: Antibiotic; aminopenicillin	ampicillin, oral
Totacillin-N Classification: Antibiotic; aminopenicillin	ampicillin sodium parenteral
Touro Ex Classification: Expectorant	guaifenesin
Toxoids, adsorbed (for pediatric use) Classification: Toxoid	diphtheria and tetanus toxoids, combined (Td)
Tracrium Classification: Nondepolarizing neuromuscular blocker	atracurium besylate
Trancopal Caplets Classification: Antianxiety	chlormezanone
Trandate Classification: Antihypertensive	labetalol
Trans-Ver-Sal Adult Patch Classification: Keratolytic	salicylic acid, topical
Trans-Ver-Sal PediaPatch Classification: Keratolytic	salicylic acid, topical
Trans-Ver-Sal Plantar Patch Classification: Keratolytic	salicylic acid, topical
Transderm-Nitro Classification: Antianginal	nitroglycerin, transdermal systems

*Available in Canada Only

BRAND NAME	GENERIC NAME
Transderm-Scōp Classification: Anticholinergic	scopolamine, transdermal
Tranxene-SD Classification: Antianxiety; benzodiazepine	clorazepate dipotassium
Tranxene-SD Half Strength Classification: Antianxiety; benzodiazepine	clorazepate dipotassium
Trasylol Classification: Hemostatic	aprotinin
Travamine* Classification: Antiemetic; anticholinergic	dimenhydrinate
Travasol Classification: Nitrogen product	amino acid solution
Trazodone HCl Classification: Antidepressant, tetracyclic	trazodone HCl
Trecator-SC Classification: Antitubercular	ethionamide
Trental Classification: Hemorrheologic agent	pentoxifylline
Tresortil* Classification: Skeletal muscle relaxant, centrally acting	methocarbamol
Trexan Classification: Narcotic antagonist	naltrexone HCl
Trexan (Orphan) Classification: Narcotic antagonist	naltrexone HCl

*Available in Canada only

BRAND NAME	GENERIC NAME
Tri-Buffered Bufferin Classification: Salicylate analgesic; antipyretic	aspirin
Tri-Chlor Classification: Cauterizing agent	trichloroacetic acid
Tri-Immunol Classification: Toxoid	diphtheria and tetanus toxoids and pertussis vaccine adsorbed (DPT)
Tri-K Classification: Electrolyte replacement; potassium	potassium bicarbonate/acetate/citrate
Tri-Kort Classification: Glucocorticoid	triamcinolone acetonide
Triacana Classification: Antineoplastic agent (Orphan)	tiratricol
Triacet Classification: Glucocorticoid	triamcinolone acetonide, topical
Triadapin* Classification: Antianxiety; antidepressant	doxepin HCl
Triam-A Classification: Glucocorticoid	triamcinolone acetonide
Triam Forte Classification: Glucocorticoid	triamcinolone diacetate
Triamcinolone Classification: Glucocorticoid	triamcinolone diacetate
Triamcinolone Acetonide Classification: Glucocorticoid	triamcinolone acetonide

BRAND NAME	GENERIC NAME
Triamcinolone Acetonide Classification: Glucocorticoid	triamcinolone acetonide, topical
Triaminic AM Decongestant Formula Classification: Nasal decongestant	pseudoephedrine HCl
Triamonide 40 Classification: Glucocorticoid	triamcinolone diacetate
Triaz Classification: Anti-acne product	benzoyl peroxide
Triazolam Classification: Sedative-hypnotic; benzodiazepine	triazolam
Triban Classification: Antiemetic; anticholinergic	trimethobenzamide HCl
Trichlorex Classification: Thiazide diuretic	trichlormethiazide
Trichlormethiazide Classification: Thiazide diuretic	trichlormethiazide
Trichosanthin Classification: Antiviral (Investigational)	trichosanthin
Tricor Classification: Antilipemic	fenofibrate
Triderm Classification: Glucocorticoid	triamcinolone acetonide, topical
Tridesilon Classification: Glucocorticoid	desonide

*Available in Canada only

BRAND NAME	GENERIC NAME

Tridil
Classification:
Antianginal

nitroglycerin, intravenous

Tridione
Classification:
Anticonvulsant; oxazolidinedione

trimethadione

Trifluoperazine HCl
Classification:
Antipsychotic

trifluoperazine HCl

Triflurin
Classification:
Antipsychotic

trifluoperazine HCl

Trihexy-2
Classification:
Anticholinergic

trihexyphenidyl HCl

Trihexy-5
Classification:
Anticholinergic

trihexyphenidyl HCl

Trihexyphenidyl HCl
Classification:
Anticholinergic

trihexyphenidyl HCl

Trikacide*
Classification:
Antibacterial; amebicide

metronidazole

Trilafon
Classification:
Antipsychotic

perphenazine

Trileptal
Classification:
Anticonvulsant (Investigational)

oxcarbazeprine

Trilisate
Classification:
Salicylate analgesic

choline magnesium trisalicylate

Trilog
Classification:
Glucocorticoid

triamcinolone acetonide

BRAND NAME	GENERIC NAME
Trilone Classification: Glucocorticoid	triamcinolone diacetate
Trimazide Classification: Antiemetic; anticholinergic	trimethobenzamide HCl
Trimethobenzamide Classification: Antiemetic; anticholinergic	trimethobenzamide HCl
Trimethobenzamide HCl Classification: Antiemetic; anticholinergic	trimethobenzamide HCl
Trimethoprim (TMP) Classification: Antibiotic; folic acid antagonist	trimethoprim
Trimox 125 Classification: Antibiotic; aminopenicillin	amoxicillin trihydrate
Trimox 250 Classification: Antibiotic; aminopenicillin	amoxicillin trihydrate
Trimox 500 Classification: Antibiotic; aminopenicillin	amoxicillin trihydrate
Trimpex Classification: Antibiotic; folic acid antagonist	trimethoprim
Triostat Classification: Thyroid hormone	liothyronine sodium (T_3)
Tripedia Classification: Toxoid	diphtheria and tetanus toxoids and acellular pertussis vaccine (DTaP)
Tripelennamine HCl Classification: Antihistamine	tripelennamine HCl

*Available in Canada only

BRAND NAME	GENERIC NAME

Triple Sulfa
Classification:
Antibiotic; sulfonamide

triple sulfa

Triptone Caplets
Classification:
Antiemetic; anticholinergic

dimenhydrinate

Trisoject
Classification:
Glucocorticoid

triamcinolone diacetate

Trisoralen
Classification:
Psoralen

trioxsalen, oral

Tritec
Classification:
H. pylori agent

ranitidine bismuth citrate

Trobicin
Classification:
Antibiotic; aminocyclitol

spectinomycin HCl

Trocaine
Classification:
Local anesthetic

benzocaine, oral

Tronolane
Classification:
Local anesthetic

pramoxine HCl, topical

Tronothane HCl
Classification:
Local anesthetic

pramoxine HCl, topical

TrophAmine
Classification:
Nitrogen product

amino acid solution

Tropicacyl
Classification:
Mydriatic

tropicamide, ophthalmic

Tropicamide
Classification:
Mydriatic

tropicamide, ophthalmic

BRAND NAME	GENERIC NAME
Trovan Classification: Antibiotic; fluroquinolone	trovafloxacin
Trovan I.V. Classification: Antibiotic; fluoroquinolone	alatrofloxacin mesylate
Truphylline Classification: Bronchodilator; xanthine	aminophylline (theophylline ethylenediamine)
Trusopt Classification: Carbonic anhydrase inhibitor	dorzolamide HCl
Trysul Classification: Antibiotic; sulfonamide	triple sulfa
Tubarine* Classification: Nondepolarizing neuromuscular blocker	tubocurarine chloride
Tuberculin, Old, Tine Test Classification: In vivo diagnostic	tuberculin (Old) multiple puncture devices
Tubersol Classification: In vivo diagnostic	tuberculin purified protein derivative (mantoux, PPD)
Tubocurarine Classification: Nondepolarizing neuromuscular blocker	tubocurarine chloride
Tucks Classification: Astringent	hamamelis water (witch hazel)
Tumor Necrosing Factor-binding Protein I and II Classification: Biologic response modifier (Orphan)	tumor necrosing factor-binding protein I and II

BRAND NAME	GENERIC NAME
Tumor Necrosis Factor Classification: Biologic response modifier (Investigational)	tumor necrosis factor
Tums Classification: Antacid; calcium supplement	calcium carbonate
Tums 500 Classification: Antacid; calcium supplement	calcium carbonate
Tums E-X Extra Strength Classification: Antacid; calcium supplement	calcium carbonate
Tusibron Classification: Expectorant	guaifenesin
Tusstat Classification: Antihistamine	diphenhydramine HCl
TVC-2 Dandruff Shampoo Classification: Antiseborrheic	pyrithione zinc
Twice-A-Day Nasal Classification: Nasal decongestant	oxymetazoline HCl, nasal
Twilite Classification: Antihistamine	diphenhydramine HCl
Twin-K Classification: Electrolyte replacement; potassium	potassium bicarbonate/acetate/citrate
Tylenol Classification: Analgesic; antipyretic	acetaminophen
Tylenol Caplets Classification: Analgesic; antipyretic	acetaminophen

*Available in Canada Only

BRAND NAME	GENERIC NAME
Tylenol Chewable Classification: Analgesic; antipyretic	acetaminophen
Tylenol Children's Suspension* Classification: Analgesic; antipyretic	acetaminophen
Tylenol Extended Relief Classification: Analgesic; antipyretic	acetaminophen
Tylenol Extra Strength Classification: Analgesic; antipyretic	acetaminophen
Tylenol Infant's Drops Classification: Analgesic; antipyretic	acetaminophen
Tylenol Infant's Suspension* Classification: Analgesic; antipyretic	acetaminophen
Tyloxapol Classification: Mucolytic (Orphan)	tyloxapol
Typhim Vi Classification: Vaccine	typhoid vaccine
Typhoid Vaccine (AKD) Classification: Vaccine	typhoid vaccine
Typhoid Vaccine (H-P) Classification: Vaccine	typhoid vaccine
Tyzine Classification: Nasal decongestant	tetrahydrozoline HCl, nasal
Tyzine Pediatric Drops Classification: Nasal decongestant	tetrahydrozoline HCl, nasal

*Available in Canada only

BRAND NAME	GENERIC NAME

U

U-Cort
Classification:
Glucocorticoid

hydrocortisone acetate

Uendex
Classification:
Mucolytic (Orphan)

dextran sulfate inhalation

Ultane
Classification:
General anesthetic

sevoflurane

Ultiva
Classification:
Opioid analgesic

remifentanil HCl

Ultra Mide 25
Classification:
Emollient

urea (carbamide), topical

Ultra Tears
Classification:
Ophthalmic lubricant

artificial tears solution

Ultralente*
Classification:
Antidiabetic

insulin, zinc suspension extended
(ultralente)

Ultram
Classification:
Analgesic

tramadol HCl

Ultramicrosize Griseofulvin
Classification:
Antifungal

griseofulvin ultramicrosized

Ultrase MT 12
Classification:
Digestive enzyme

pancrelipase

Ultrase MT 20
Classification:
Digestive enzyme

pancrelipase

*Available in Canada Only

BRAND NAME	GENERIC NAME

Ultravate
Classification:
Glucocorticoid

halobetasol propionate

Ultravist
Classification:
Radiopaque agent

iopromide

Unasyn
Classification:
Antibiotic; aminopenicillin

ampicillin sodium and sulbactam sodium

Uni-Ace
Classification:
Analgesic; antipyretic

acetaminophen

Uni-Bent Cough
Classification:
Antihistamine

diphenhydramine HCl

Uni-Dur
Classification:
Bronchodilator; xanthine

theophylline

Uni-tussin
Classification:
Expectorant

guaifenesin

Unipen
Classification:
Antibiotic; penicillinase-resistant
penicillin

nafcillin sodium

Uniphyl
Classification:
Bronchodilator; xanthine

theophylline

Unisom Nighttime
Classification:
Antihistamine

doxylamine succinate

Unitrol
Classification:
Alpha-adrenergic agonist

phenylpropanolamine HCl

Uracid
Classification:
Amino acid

methionine

BRAND NAME	GENERIC NAME
Ureacin-10 Classification: Emollient	urea (carbamide), topical
Ureacin-20 Classification: Emollient	urea (carbamide), topical
Ureacin-40 Classification: Emollient	urea (carbamide), topical
Ureaphil Classification: Emollient	urea
Urecholine Classification: Cholinergic stimulant	bethanechol chloride
Urex Classification: Urinary anti-infective	methenamine hippurate
Uridine 5'-triphosphate Classification: Mucolytic (Orphan)	uridine 5'-triphosphate
Urispas Classification: Urinary antispasmodic	flavoxate HCl
Uritol* Classification: Loop diuretic	furosemide
Uro-KP Neutral Classification: Electrolyte replacement	phosphorous (replacement products)
Uro-Mag Classification: Electrolyte replacement	magnesium oxide
Urobak Classification: Antibiotic; sulfonamide	sulfamethoxazole

BRAND NAME	GENERIC NAME
Urocit-K Classification: Urinary alkalinizer	potassium citrate
Urodine Classification: Urinary analgesic	phenazopyridine HCl
Urogastrone Classification: Ophthalmic (Orphan)	urogastrone
Urolene Blue Classification: Urinary anti-infective	methylene blue
Urovist Cysto Classification: Radiopaque agent	diatrizoate meglumine 30%
Urovist Meglumine DIU/CT Classification: Radiopaque agent	diatrizoate meglumine 30%
Urovist Sodium 300 Classification: Radiopaque agent	diatrizoate sodium 50%
Urozide* Classification: Thiazide diuretic	hydrochlorothiazide
URSO Classification: Antilithic	ursodiol
Ursofalk Classification: Antilithic (Orphan)	ursodeoxycholic acid

V

V-Cillin K Classification: Antibiotic; penicillin	penicillin V potassium

BRAND NAME	GENERIC NAME
V-Lax Classification: Laxative, bulk-producing	psyllium
V.V.S. Classification: Antibiotic; sulfonamide	triple sulfa
Vagistat-1 Classification: Antifungal	tioconazole
Valergen 20 Classification: Estrogen	estradiol valerate
Valergen 40 Classification: Estrogen	estradiol valerate
Valisone Classification: Glucocorticoid	betamethasone valerate
Valisone Reduced Strength Classification: Glucocorticoid	betamethasone valerate
Valium Classification: Antianxiety; benzodiazepine	diazepam
Valium Roche Oral* Classification: Antianxiety; benzodiazepine	diazepam
Valproic Acid Classification: Anticonvulsant	valproic acid
Valtrex Classification: Antiviral	valacyclovir HCl
Vancenase AQ Nasal Classification: Glucocorticoid	beclomethasone dipropionate, nasal

BRAND NAME	GENERIC NAME
Vancenase Pockethaler Classification: Glucocorticoid	beclomethasone dipropionate, nasal
Vanceril Classification: Glucocorticoid	beclomethasone dipropionate
Vanceril Double Strength Classification: Glucocorticoid	beclomethasone dipropionate
Vancocin Classification: Antibiotic; tricyclic glycopeptide	vancomycin HCl
Vancoled Classification: Antibiotic; tricyclic glycopeptide	vancomycin HCl
Vancomycin HCl Classification: Antibiotic; tricyclic glycopeptide	vancomycin HCl
Vanoxide Classification: Anti-acne product	benzoyl peroxide
Vansil Classification: Anthelmintic	oxamniquine
Vantin Classification: Antibiotic; cephalosporin	cefpodoxime proxetil
Vaponefrin Classification: Adrenergic agonist	epinephrine
Vaqta Classification: Vaccine	hepatitis A vaccine, inactivated
Varicella-Zoster Immune Globulin (Human) Classification: Immune serum	varicella-zoster immune globulin (human) (VZIG)

BRAND NAME	GENERIC NAME
Varivax Classification: Vaccine	varicella virus vaccine
Vascor Classification: Calcium channel blocker	bepridil HCl
Vascoray Classification: Radiopaque agent	iothalamate meglumine 52% and iothalamate sodium 26%
Vasoclear Classification: Ophthalmic vasoconstrictor	naphazoline HCl, ophthalmic
Vasocon Regular Classification: Ophthalmic vasoconstrictor	naphazoline HCl, ophthalmic
Vasodilan Classification: Peripheral vasodilator	isoxsuprine HCl
Vasomax Classification: Vasodilator	phentolamine
Vasotec Classification: Antihypertensive; angiotensin converting enzyme inhibitor	enalapril maleate
Vasotec I.V. Classification: Antihypertensive; angiotensin converting enzyme inhibitor	enalaprilat
Vasoxyl Classification: Adrenergic agonist	methoxamine HCl
VaxSyn HIV-1 Classification: Vaccine (Investigational)	AIDS vaccine

*Available in Canada Only

BRAND NAME	GENERIC NAME

Vectrin
Classification:
Antibiotic; tetracycline

minocycline HCl

Veetids 125
Classification:
Antibiotic; penicillin

penicillin V potassium

Veetids 250
Classification:
Antibiotic; penicillin

penicillin V potassium

Veetids 500
Classification:
Antibiotic; penicillin

penicillin V potassium

Velban
Classification:
Antineoplastic; mitotic inhibitor

vinblastine sulfate (VLB)

Velbe*
Classification:
Antineoplastic; mitotic inhibitor

vinblastine sulfate (VLB)

Veldona
Classification:
Biologic response modifier
(Investigational)

veldona

Velosef
Classification:
Antibiotic; cephalosporin

cephradine

Velosulin
Classification:
Antidiabetic

insulin injection

Veltane
Classification:
Antihistamine

brompheniramine maleate

Venoglobulin-I
Classification:
Immune serum

immune globulin intravenous (IGIV)

Ventolin
Classification:
Bronchodilator; beta-adrenergic agonist

albuterol

*Available in Canada only

BRAND NAME	GENERIC NAME

Ventilin Nebules
Classification:
Bronchodilator; beta-adrenergic agonist

albuterol sulfate

Ventolin Rotacaps
Classification:
Bronchodilator; beta-adrenergic agonist

albuterol

Vepesid
Classification:
Antineoplastic; mitotic inhibitor

etoposide (VP-16-213)

Verapamil HCl
Classification:
Calcium channel blocker

verapamil HCl

Verazinc
Classification:
Electrolyte replacement; zinc

zinc sulfate

Verelan
Classification:
Calcium channel blocker

verapamil HCl

Vergon
Classification:
Antiemetic; anticholinergic

meclizine

Vermox
Classification:
Anthelmintics

mebendazole

Versed
Classification:
General anesthetic; benzodiazepine

midazolam HCl

Vesanoid
Classification:
Antineoplastic, miscellaneous

tretinoin

Vesprin
Classification:
Antipsychotic

triflupromazine HCl

Vexol
Classification:
Ophthalmic glucocorticoid

rimexolone

*Available in Canada Only

BRAND NAME	GENERIC NAME
Viagra Classification: Smooth muscle relaxant	sildenafil
Vianain Classification: Enzyme (Orphan)	ananain
Vibra-Tabs Classification: Antibiotic; tetracycline	doxycycline hyclate
Vibramycin Classification: Antibiotic; tetracycline	doxycycline hyclate
Vibramycin IV Classification: Antibiotic; tetracycline	doxycycline hyclate
Vicks Children's Chloraseptic Classification: Local anesthetic	benzocaine, oral
Vicks Dry Hacking Cough Classification: Non-narcotic antitussive	dextromethorphan
Vicks Inhaler Classification: Nasal decongestant	desoxyephedrine
Vicks Sinex 12-Hour Classification: Nasal decongestant	oxymetazoline HCl, nasal
Videx Classification: Antiviral; nucleoside	didanosine (ddI, dideoxyinosine)
Vimicon* Classification: Antihistamine	cyproheptadine HCl
VIMRxyn Classification: Antiviral (Investigational)	hypericin

*Available in Canada only

BRAND NAME	GENERIC NAME
Vinblastine Sulfate Classification: Antineoplastic; mitotic inhibitor	vinblastine sulfate (VLB)
Vincasar PFS Classification: Antineoplastic; mitotic inhibitor	vincristine sulfate (VCR; LCR)
Vincristine Sulfate Classification: Antineoplastic; mitotic inhibitor	vincristine sulfate (VCR; LCR)
Vioform Classification: Antifungal	clioquinol (iodochlorhydroxyquin)
Vioform Classification: Antifungal	iodochlorhydroxyquin
Viokase Powder Classification: Digestive enzyme	pancrelipase
Vira-A Ophthalmic Classification: Antiviral	vidarabine, ophthalmic
Viracept Classification: Antiviral; protease inhibitor	nelfinavir mesylate
Viramune Classification: Antiviral; non-nucleoside	nevirapine
Virazole Classification: Antiviral	ribavirin
Virilon Classification: Androgen	methyltestosterone
Viroptic Classification: Ophthalmic antiviral	trifluridine

*Available in Canada Only

BRAND NAME	GENERIC NAME
Visine L.R. Classification: Ophthalmic vasoconstrictor	oxymetazoline HCl, ophthalmic
Visken Classification: Antihypertensive; beta-adrenergic blocker	pindolol
Visipaque Classification: Radiopaque agent	iodixanol
Vistacon Classification: Antianxiety	hydroxyzine
Vistaril Classification: Antianxiety	hydroxyzine
Vistazine 50 Classification: Antianxiety	hydroxyzine
Vistide Classification: Antiviral; nucleoside	cidofovir
Vita-C Classification: Vitamin, water soluble	ascorbic acid (vitamin C)
Vita-Plus E Softgels Classification: Vitamin, fat soluble	vitamin E
Vitacarn Classification: Amino acid	levocarnitine
Vitamin A Classification: Vitamin, fat soluble	vitamin A
Vitamin B$_6$ Classification: Vitamin, water soluble	pyridoxine HCl (vitamin B$_6$)

*Available in Canada only

BRAND NAME	GENERIC NAME
Vitamin B₁₂ Classification: Vitamin, water soluble	cyanocobalamin (vitamin B₁₂)
Vitamin D₃ Classification: Vitamin, fat soluble	cholecalciferol
Vitamin E Classification: Vitamin, fat soluble	vitamin E
Vitinoin* Classification: Anti-acne product	tretinoin (vitamin A acid, retinoic acid)
Vitrasert Classification: Antiviral	ganciclovir sodium (DHPG)
Viva-Drops Classification: Ophthalmic lubricants	artificial tears solution
Vivactil Classification: Antidepressant, tricyclic	protriptyline HCl
Vivari Classification: Analeptic	caffeine
Vivelle Classification: Estrogen	estradiol transdermal system
Vivol* Classification: Antianxiety; benzodiazepine	diazepam
Vivotif Berna Vaccine Classification: Vaccine	typhoid vaccine
Volmax Classification: Bronchodilator; beta-adrenergic agonist	albuterol sulfate

BRAND NAME	GENERIC NAME
Voltaren-SR* Classification: Nonsteroidal anti-inflammatory	diclofenac sodium
Voltaren-XR Classification: Nonsteroidal anti-inflammatory	diclofenac sodium
Voltaren Classification: Nonsteroidal anti-inflammatory	diclofenac sodium
Voltaren Classification: Ophthalmic nonsteroidal anti- inflammatory	diclofenac sodium ophthalmic
Voltaren Rapide* Classification: Nonsteroidal anti-inflammatory	diclofenac sodium
Vontrol Classification: Antiemetic	diphenidol
Voxsuprine Classification: Peripheral vasodilator	isoxsuprine HCl
Vumon Classification: Antineoplastic; mitotic inhibitor	teniposide
VX478 Classification: Antiviral (Investigational)	VX478

W

Warfarin Sodium Classification: Anticoagulant	warfarin sodium
Warfilone Sodium* Classification: Anticoagulant	warfarin sodium

*Available in Canada only

BRAND NAME	GENERIC NAME
Warnerin* Classification: Anticoagulant	warfarin sodium
Wart-Off Classification: Keratolytic	salicylic acid, topical
Wart Remover Classification: Keratolytic	salicylic acid, topical
Wellbutrin Classification: Antidepressant	bupropione HCl
Wellbutrin SR Classification: Antidepressant	bupropion HCl
Wellcovorin Classification: Folic acid antagonist	leucovorin calcium (citrovorum factor; folinic acid)
Wellferon Classification: Biologic response modifier (Orphan)	interferon alfa-n1
Westcort Classification: Glucocorticoid	hydrocortisone valerate
WinRho SD Classification: Immune serum	Rho immune globulin IV (Human)
Winstrol Classification: Anabolic steroid	stanozolol
Witch Hazel Classification: Astringent	hamamelis water (witch hazel)
Wyamine Sulfate Classification: Adrenergic agonist	mephentermine sulfate

*Available in Canada Only

BRAND NAME	GENERIC NAME
Wycillin Classification: Antibiotic; penicillin	penicillin G procaine, aqueous (APPG)
Wydase Classification: Enzyme	hyaluronidase
Wymox Classification: Antibiotic; aminopenicillin	amoxicillin trihydrate
Wytensin Classification: Antihypertensive, centrally acting	guanabenz acetate

X

Xalatan Classification: Prostaglandin	latanoprost
Xanax Classification: Antianxiety; benzodiazepine	alprazolam
Xenical Classification: Antilipemic	orlistat
Xylo-Pfan Classification: In vivo diagnostic	D-Xylose
Xylocaine Classification: Local anesthetic	lidocaine HCl, local
Xylocaine Classification: Local anesthetic	lidocaine HCl, topical
Xylocaine HCl IV for Cardiac Arrhythmias Classification: Antiarrhythmic	lidocaine HCl IV

*Available in Canada only

BRAND NAME	GENERIC NAME

Xylocaine MPF
Classification:
Local anesthetic

lidocaine HCl, local

Xylocaine Viscous
Classification:
Local anesthetic

lidocaine HCl, topical

Y

YF-Vax
Classification:
Vaccine

yellow fever vaccine

Yocon
Classification:
Alpha-adrenergic blocker

yohimbine HCl

Yodoxin
Classification:
Amebicide

iodoquinol (diiodohydroxyquin)

Yohimbine HCl
Classification:
Alpha-adrenergic blocker

yohimbine HCl

Yohimex
Classification:
Alpha-adrenergic blocker

yohimbine HCl

Yutopar
Classification:
Uterine relaxant

ritodrine HCl

Z

Zagam
Classification:
Antibiotic; fluoroquinolone

sparfloxacin

Zanaflex
Classification:
Skeletal muscle relaxant

tizanidine HCl

*Available in Canada Only

BRAND NAME	GENERIC NAME

Zanosar
Classification:
Antineoplastic; alkylating agent

streptozocin

Zantac
Classification:
Histamine H_2 receptor antagonist

ranitidine

Zantac 75
Classification:
Histamine H_2 receptor antagonist

rantidine

Zantac EFFERdose
Classification:
Histamine H_2 receptor antagonist

rantidine

Zantac GELdose
Classification:
Histamine H_2 receptor antagonist

rantidine

Zantryl
Classification:
CNS stimulant; anorexiant

phentermine HCl

Zarontin
Classification:
Anticonvulsant; succinimides

ethosuximide

Zaroxolyn
Classification:
Thiazide-like diuretic

metolazone

Zeasorb-AF
Classification:
Antifungal

tolnaftate

Zebeta
Classification:
Antihypertensive; beta-adrenergic blocker

bisoprolol fumarate

Zefazone
Classification:
Antibiotic; cephalosporin

cefmetazole sodium

Zeldox
Classification:
Antipsychotic (Investigational)

ziprasidone

BRAND NAME	GENERIC NAME
Zemuron Classification: Nondepolarizing neuromuscular blocker	rocuronium bromide
Zenapax Classification: Immunosuppressive	daclizumab
Zephiran Classification: Germicidal	benzalkonium chloride
Zephiran Chloride* Classification: Germicidal	benzalkonium chloride
Zerit Classification: Antiviral; nucleoside	stavudine (d4T)
Zestril Classification: Antihypertensive; angiotensin converting enzyme inhibitor	lisinopril
Zetar Classification: Keratolytic	coal tar
Zetar Emulsion Classification: Keratolytic	coal tar
Zetran Classification: Antianxiety; benzodiazepine	diazepam
Zilactin Medicated Classification: Protectant	tannic acid
Zilactin-B Medicated Classification: Local anesthetic	benzocaine, oral
Zinacef Classification: Antibiotic; cephalosporin	cefuroxime sodium

*Available in Canada Only

BRAND NAME	GENERIC NAME
Zinc 15 Classification: Electrolyte replacement; zinc	zinc sulfate
Zinc-200 Classification: Electrolyte replacement; zinc	zinc sulfate
Zinc Gluconate Classification: Electrolyte replacement; zinc	zinc gluconate
Zinc Oxide Classification: Protectant	zinc oxide
Zinc Sulfate Classification: Electrolyte replacement; zinc	zinc sulfate
Zinca-Pak Classification: Electrolyte replacement; zinc	zinc sulfate
Zincate Classification: Electrolyte replacement; zinc	zinc sulfate
Zincon Classification: Antiseborrheic	pyrithione zinc
Zinecard Classification: Antineoplastic adjuvant; cardioprotective	dexrazoxane
Zintevir Classification: Antiviral (Investigational)	zintevir
Zithromax Classification: Antibiotic; macrolide	azithromycin
Zixoryn Classification: Anti-hyperbilirubinemia agent (Orphan)	flumecinol

BRAND NAME	GENERIC NAME
ZNP Bar Classification: Antiseborrheic	pyrithione zinc
Zocor Classification: Antilipemic	simvastatin
Zofran Classification: Antiemetic	ondansetron HCl
Zoladex Classification: Antineoplastic; hormone	goserelin acetate
Zolicef Classification: Antibiotic; cephalosporin	cefazolin sodium
Zoloft Classification: Antidepressant	sertraline HCl
Zomig Classification: Antimigraine	zolmitriptan
Zonalon Classification: Antihistamine	doxepin, topical
ZORprin Classification: Salicylate analgesic; antipyretic	aspirin
Zostrix Classification: Analgesic	capsaicin
Zostrix-HP Classification: Analgesic	capsaicin
Zosyn Classification: Antibiotic; extended spectrum penicillin	piperacillin sodium and tazobactam sodium

BRAND NAME	GENERIC NAME
Zovirax Classification: Antiviral	acyclovir
Zovirax Classification: Antiviral	acyclovir sodium
Zyban Classification: Smoking deterrent	bupropion HCl
Zyflo Classification: Bronchodilator; 5-lipoxygenase inhibitor	zileuton
Zyloprim Classification: Uricosuric	allopurinol
Zyloprim for Injection Classification: Uricosuric (Orphan)	allopurinol sodium
Zymase Classification: Digestive enzyme	pancrelipase
Zyprexa Classification: Antipsychotic	olanzapine
Zyrtec Classification: Antihistamine	cetirizine HCl

SKIDMORE-ROTH PUBLISHING, INC. ORDER FORM

Title	ISBN #	Price	Qty
NURSING CARE PLANS SERIES			
Critical Care	1-56930-035-6	$38.95	
Geriatric (2nd ed.)	1-56930-052-6	$38.95	
HIV/AIDS (2nd ed.)	1-56930-097-6	$38.95	
Oncology	1-56930-004-6	$38.95	
Pediatric (2nd ed.)	1-56930-057-7	$38.95	
SURVIVAL SERIES			
Geriatric Survival Handbook	1-56930-061-5	$29.95	
Nurse's Survival Handbook	1-56930-040-2	$39.95	
Obstetric Survival Handbook (2nd ed.)	1-56930-083-6	$35.95	
Pediatric Nurse's Survival Guide	1-56930-018-6	$29.95	
NURSING/OTHER			
AIDS/HIV Instant Instructor	1-56930-010-0	$9.95	
The Body in Brief (3rd ed.)	1-56930-055-0	$35.95	
Diagnostic and Lab Cards (3rd ed.)	1-56930-065-8	$29.95	
Drug Comparison Handbook (3rd ed.)	1-56930-075-5	$36.95	
Essential Laboratory Mathematics	1-56930-056-9	$29.95	
Geriatric Long-Term Procedures & Treatments (2nd ed.)	1-56930-045-3	$34.95	
Geriatric Nutrition and Diet (3rd ed.)	1-56930-096-8	$25.95	
Handbook of Long-Term Care (2nd ed.)	1-56930-058-5	$23.95	
Handbook for Nurse Assistants (2nd ed.)	1-56930-059-3	$23.95	
Hemodialysis Instant Instructor	1-56930-020-8	$9.95	
I.C.U. Quick Reference (2nd ed.)	1-56930-071-2	$35.95	
Infection Control	1-56930-051-8	$99.95	
Nursing Diagnosis Cards (2nd ed.)	1-56930-060-7	$29.95	
Nurse's Trivia Calendar	1-56930-098-4	$11.95	
OBRA Guidelines (3rd ed.)	1-56930-047-X	$149.95	
OSHA Handbook (2nd ed.)	1-56930-069-0	$119.95	
Oncology Instant Instructor	1-56930-023-2	$9.95	
Procedure Cards (3rd ed.)	1-56930-054-2	$24.95	
Pharmacy Tech	1-56930-005-4	$25.95	
Spanish for Medical Personnel	1-56930-001-1	$25.95	

Title	ISBN #	Price	Qty
OUTLINE SERIES			
Diabetes Outline	1-56930-031-3	$23.95	
Fundamentals of Nursing Outline	1-56930-029-1	$23.95	
Geriatric Outline	0-944132-90-1	$23.95	
Hemodynamic Monitoring Outline	1-56930-034-8	$23.95	
Critical & High Acuity Outline	1-56930-028-3	$23.95	
Medical-Surgical Nursing Outline (2nd ed.)	1-56930-068-2	$23.95	
Obstetric Nursing Outline (2nd ed.)	1-56930-070-4	$23.95	
Pediatric Nursing Outline (2nd ed.)	1-56930-067-4	$23.95	
NCLEX REVIEW SERIES			
PN/VN Review Cards (3rd ed.)	1-56930-093-3	$32.95	
RN Review Cards (3rd ed.)	1-56930-092-5	$32.95	
ALLIED HEALTH			
Paramedic Survival Handbook	1-56930-090-9	$29.95	
EMS Field Protocol Manual	1-56930-091-7	$14.95	

Order Total $_____

CO Sales Tax $_____

Name_____

Address_____

City_____ State_____ Zip_____

Phone   (_____)_____

❑ VISA   ❑ Master Card   ❑ American Express   ❑ Check/Money Order

Card #_____ Exp. Date_____

Signature (required)_____

Prices subject to change without notice. Shipping and handling will be added. Colorado residents add sales tax.
For faster service, call 1-800-825-3150, or fax your order to us at (303) 662-8079. Orders are accepted by mail.

MAIL ORDER TO:
SKIDMORE-ROTH PUBLISHING, INC.
400 Inverness Drive South, Suite 260
Englewood, Colorado 80112

Visit our website at: http://www.skidmore-roth.com